Urological Nu

Urological Nursing

EDITED BY

Clive Laker

RGN, RNT, DipN (Lond), DipNEd, BSc (Hons)
Lecturer,
Riverside College of Health Studies

Illustrations by

Sarah Ponder

SCUTARI PRESS • LONDON

© Scutari Press 1994

A division of Scutari Projects Ltd., the publishing
company of the Royal College of Nursing

First published 1994, reprinted 1995

British Library Cataloguing in Publication Data
  Laker, Clive
  Urological Nursing
  I. Title
  610.73

  ISBN 1-871364-84-1

Typeset and printed by Alden Press Limited,
Oxford and Northampton, Great Britain

Contents

THE ST. PETER'S GROUP OF HOSPITALS

The majority of the contributors to this textbook are currently employed within the St. Peter's Hospital, London.

St. Peter's is an amalgamation of four smaller hospitals, which were originally situated around the Covent Garden area of London.

The four hospitals offered a considerable range of urological and renal expertise, as well as an established research and teaching facility.

The original hospitals were closed, at the end of 1992, and relocated to Mortimer Street, WC2, where they now constitute the new St. Peter's Hospital (sited within the existing Middlesex Hospital building).

Contributors

Patricia Cattini, RGN, Clinical Nurse Specialist, Kingston Hospital, Surrey

Jane Champion, RGN, Ward Sister, St. Peter's Hospital, London

Daphne Colpman, RGN, Ward Sister, St. Peter's Hospital, London

Kevin Dennison, RGN, Charge Nurse, St. Peter's Hospital, London

Jean Douglas, RGN, DipN (Lond), SCM, In-service Facilitator, St. Peter's Hospital, London

Susan Fell, RGN, Formerly Ward Sister, St. Peter's Hospital, London

Sharon Fillingham, RGN, Clinical Nurse Specialist, Stoma Care, St. Peter's Hospital, London

Helen Forristal, RGN, Ward Sister, St. Peter's Hospital, London

Sue Keeble, RGN, RSCN, Senior Ward Sister (Paediatrics), St. Peter's Hospital, London

Clive Laker, RGN, RNT, DipN (Lond), DipNEd, BSc (Hons) Lecturer, Riverside College of Health Studies, London

Rachel Busuttil Leaver, RGN, Clinical Nurse Specialist (Urinary Diversion), St. Peter's Hospital, London

Rachel M Lockett, RGN, DipN (Lond), Formerly Clinical Nurse Specialist, (Stone Management), St. Peter's Hospital, London

Alison Lungley, RGN, RSCN, Ward Sister (Paediatrics), St. Peter's Hospital, London

Margaret Macaulay, RGN, DN, Continence Adviser, Wandsworth Community Health Unit, London

Jane Maxfield, RGN, St. Peter's Hospital, London

Sharon E Rainsbury, RGN, Formerly Ward Sister, St. Peter's Hospital, London

Kate Welford, RGN, Clinical Nurse Specialist, Urodynamics, St. Peter's Hospital, London

Preface

This book addresses the many recent innovations and treatments within urological nursing in relation to their required nursing management.

During the last ten years, the practice of urology has undergone major change. Percutaneous surgery, the use of extracorporeal lithotripsy and, more recently, lasertripsy, innovations within catheter and stent design and management, new treatments for the management of prostatic obstruction and the use of continent urinary diversions are all examples of changes which have exerted a direct influence upon the nursing care and management of urological patients.

In addition, Chapter 13 addresses the issue of nursing care within paediatric urology and Chapter 12 describes the controversial area of gender reassignment surgery, with its potential ethical dilemmas.

None of the contributors have been constrained by a particular framework of presentation; neither a universal nursing model nor a 'standard' chapter layout has been adopted. It is hoped that such an approach will make the text more approachable, providing the reader with a nursing resource which is both readable and user-friendly.

Our aim is to provide a book which will appeal to pre-registration students and those involved in post-registration studies within the sphere of urology.

Clive Laker

1

Anatomy and Physiology of the

Urinary System

THE KIDNEY

The kidney is one of the most vital homeostatic organs we possess, although it occupies only 1 per cent of the total body mass. Without a functional kidney it would be impossible to maintain a constant internal ionic environment within which the cells and tissue systems of the body can function. It is the kidney, for example, that is responsible for removing a number of key waste products of normal cellular metabolism (e.g. ammonia), which, if allowed to accumulate, would rapidly disrupt 'normal' homeostasis. The kidney also exerts direct control over the plasma concentration of ions such as sodium and potassium, both of which are necessary for nerve and muscle function, but can rapidly create life-threatening disturbance if the normal physiological level is significantly altered. Thus potassium, for example, readily becomes cardiotoxic in either excess or deficiency, leading to significant dysrhythmias. It is therefore the aim of this chapter to illustrate how the kidney, in cooperation with an intact, functional urinary tract, contributes to overall homeostasis. Before considering its structure, the seven major homeostatic functions of the kidney are described. These are summarised in Figure 1.1.

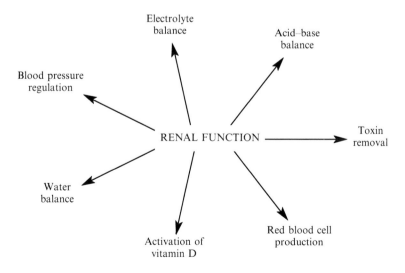

Fig 1.1 Summary of renal function

Macroscopically, the kidneys are reddish-brown organs which are loosely bean-shaped, and posterior to the parietal peritoneum, within the retroperitoneal space. The kidneys are surprisingly high up within the abdominal cavity and, relative to the spinal vertebrae, occupy a position between T12 (last thoracic) and L4, though the right kidney is slightly lower. The kidneys are also partially protected by the 11th and 12th rib pairs, the latter of which may need to be partly excised when the kidney is approached surgically. Other key anatomical relationships are shown in Figure 1.2.

In terms of size, the kidney measures only 10–12 cm in length, 5–7 cm in width and between 2 and 5 cm in thickness, which is very small when compared with, say, the spleen or liver. On the concave surface of the kidney, a notch-shaped region is very evident, through which the blood supply, lymphatic vessels and nerves both enter and exit, and from which the ureter drains urine (the processed waste product).

Because the kidney is so vascular, it clearly has the capacity to bleed very heavily if traumatised. The kidney also has a rich lymphatic supply, through which urine can reach the systemic circulation, if normal urinary drainage is in some way prevented (e.g. by obstruction). This mechanism acts as a safety valve, which helps to decompress the kidney, at least initially. However, such a route for drainage also means that microbes may also gain access to the circulation if obstruction is also present with infection, which is often the case. Fortunately, however, the kidney is normally well protected, being surrounded by three separate tissue layers.

The first of these tissue layers is the renal capsule, which is a smooth, fibrous membrane which can be stripped off to reveal the friable renal substance beneath. The capsule is continuous with the outer layer of the ureter, at the renal hilum, and provides a barrier to infection as well as to direct trauma. The second protective layer, outside the capsule, is the perinephric fat (or adipose capsule) which, apart from its protective function, helps to hold the kidney in place within the abdominal cavity. The outermost protective layer is the renal fascia, consisting of a thin layer of fibrous connective tissue, which anchors the kidney to its surrounding structures and

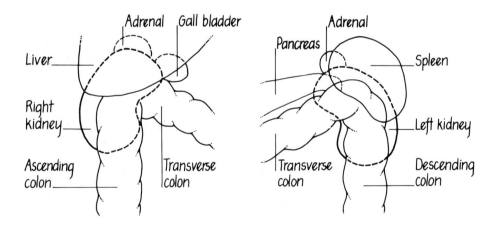

Fig 1.2   Key anatomical relationships of the kidney

to the posterior abdominal wall. As a result of these three layers, the kidney is normally well protected against direct trauma.

However, a crush injury to the abdomen, or a penetrating injury, e.g. a stab wound, or a severe blow to the posterior abdominal wall may directly damage the renal substance or renal blood vessels, thus creating a potential for extensive haemorrhage.

While considering the macroscopic kidney structure, it is interesting to note that, embryologically, the kidneys begin their development very much lower down in the abdomen, and actually migrate upwards to their normal anatomical position during intrauterine development. As a consequence, a number of developmental abnormalities are seen within the urinary system, which result from disorders/ disruption to this process of upward migration. For example, a 'horseshoe' kidney (a defect where the paired kidneys fail to separate and remain joined in the midline) relates to a failure of the early embryonic renal tissue to separate into two distinct renal organs. Likewise, duplication of the renal substance on one side may result either in 'double kidneys', or a duplex collecting system (e.g. duplex ureter). Also, the kidney may deviate from its normal migratory path, and thus come to occupy an ectopic position (e.g. pelvic, inguinal or lumbar).

The anatomical position of the normal kidney also poses some difficulty for open forms of surgery. Not only is the patient at risk of haemorrhage, but the typical surgical approach is a loin incision, just beneath the level of the 12th rib. Clearly this means that the incision is close to both diaphragm and pleura, and also directly involves the powerful muscles which normally drive respiration. Thus, post-operatively, patients can experience severe pain and discomfort, especially on breathing, and may also sustain a pneumothorax during surgery, particularly if the kidney is very fibrosed and difficult to mobilise. A longitudinal coronal section through the kidney, such that the organ is laid open into two halves, reveals several key macroscopic structures (see Figure 1.3).

The first point to note is that the kidney divides into an outer, darker area, the cortex, and an inner, lighter coloured area, the medulla. As will be seen, the primary functional units of the kidney (the nephrons) extend throughout both these distinct regions.

Within the inner medulla, between 10 and 18 striated, triangular structures are evident. Because of their shape, these are known as the renal pyramids, and their striated (or striped) appearance results from the presence of straight renal tubules (from the nephrons) and coexistent blood vessels. The pyramids are important structures, which direct the processed glomerular filtrate (urine) down into the initial part of the urine collecting system. It can be seen from Figure 1.3 that the cortex of the kidney extends from its outer boundary, down to the bases of the renal pyramids, as renal columns. Further, the cortex subdivides into an outer zone and an inner juxtamedullary zone. This is an important anatomical distinction, as those nephrons particularly responsible for water balance extend deeply into the juxtamedullary zone, whereas other nephrons do not. The renal cortex, in association with the pyramids, constitute the renal parenchyma, which in an average adult kidney, consists of approximately one million functional units, the nephrons.

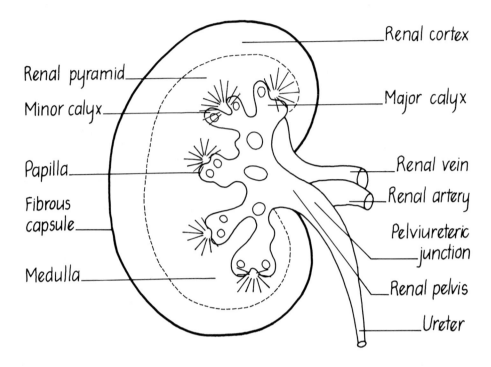

Renal cortex

Renal pyramid

Minor calyx

Major calyx

Papilla

Renal vein

Renal artery

Fibrous
capsule

Pelviureteric
junction

Medulla

Renal pelvis

Ureter

Fig 1.3   Macroscopic kidney structure

It is these vital structures (which have a limited ability to regenerate if damaged) that allow the kidney to exert its control over electrolyte absorption, water balance and selective reabsorption and secretion. They are, therefore, vital for the effective functioning of the kidney.

As the filtrate flows out of the pyramids, it enters a specialised collecting duct system, which then channels the urine into the renal pelvis, and from there down into the ureteric lumen. These protrusions of the pelvis, extending outward like fingers on a hand, and terminating at the base of the renal pyramids, are known as calyces (Greek *calyx*: wine goblet) and are divided into major and minor calyces, depending upon their size. Literally, the calyces collect the urine as it drips out of the individual pyramids.

The calyces are constructed of smooth muscle tissue, lined with a transitional cell epithelium, this being the histological nature of the epithelium which extends into the renal pelvis, and also lines both ureter and bladder. The highly homogeneous nature of the transitional cell epithelial lining of the calyces and urinary tract is one of the reasons why urological carcinoma can spread so rapidly, and underpins the rationale behind removing the ureter, as well as the kidney, in cases of renal carcinoma.

Contractions of the smooth muscle fibres, within the walls of the calyces and pelvis, propel urine down into the ureter. The rate of these contractions is controlled by intrinsic pacemaker cells, situated within the walls of the calyces. (These are not neuronally innervated, as the mechanism remains intact within transplanted kidneys.) These cells are able to monitor urine flow (via distension) and thus increase the role of peristaltic contraction when the urinary flow is high.

THE NEPHRON

As stated earlier, the functional unit of the mammalian kidney is the nephron (see Figure 1.4). Each nephron consists of two principal structures, first a 'tuft' of capillaries (approximately six to eight capillary loops in total) and then a renal tubule, approximately 6 cm long, and lined throughout by a modified columnar epithelium.

The 'tuft' of capillaries is collectively known as the glomerulus, and is very closely associated with the first portion of the tubule, the glomerular (or Bowman's) capsule. Anatomically, a good analogy of the close approximation between these two structures is that of a 'clenched fist' (the glomerulus) pushed into a water-filled balloon (the glomerular capsule) such that the balloon then completely engulfs the fist by a process of invagination.

This entire structure is approximately 150 nm in diameter, yet the entire glomerular capillary surface area is vast, enclosing approximately $1500 \, cm^2 / 100 \, g$

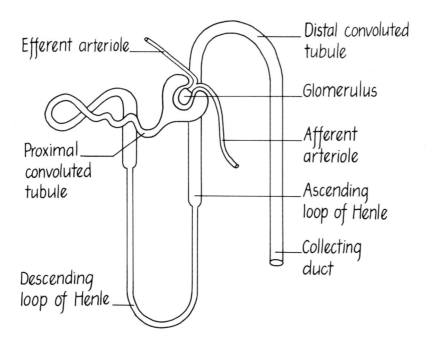

Fig 1.4   Diagrammatic representation of the nephron

tissue. It would seem that these capillaries are far more (approximately 100 times more) permeable to water and solutes than extra-renal capillaries, and contain pores (fenestrations) of 16–20 nm in diameter. This capillary endothelium then sits upon a basement membrane, on the other side of which rests the epithelial lining of the glomerular capsule. This arrangement is illustrated in Fig 1.5.

As can be seen, the capillary endothelium is a single layer, with large open pores. In contrast, the 'podocytes' of the glomerular epithelium all possess foot-like structures called 'pedicles', which cover the basement membrane, except for the pores. These cells are elongated and divide towards their base, thus forming the foot-like structures.

These foot-like processes contain numerous contractile filaments, which are thought to regulate the passage of substances through the basement membrane and filtration slits. These three layers therefore collectively constitute a selective barrier to filtration, in such a way as to inhibit progressively larger molecules. Thus the capillary endothelium allows the passage of large proteins, but not cells.

The basement membrane inhibits most large proteins, but not those of intermediate and smaller size, and the capsular epithelium prevents the passage of smaller proteins, and allows only electrolytes, water, urea, glucose, polypeptides and amino acids to pass through.

Filtration is therefore achieved within this first portion of the nephron. The other key functional areas of the nephron can be conveniently divided into the following five stages:

1. *Filtration*
2. *Mass salvage of essential substances*
3. *Water balance*, and the ability to create a medullary interstitium of high osmotic potential

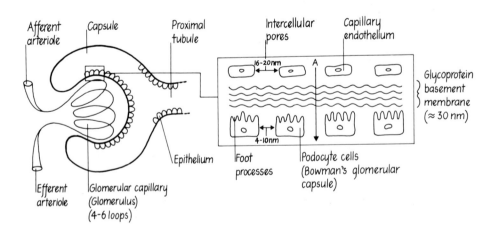

Fig 1.5   Fine structure of the glomerulus and Bowmans capsule (simplified). Arrow 'A' indicates direction of movement of filtrate

4. *Fine control of water, sodium and hydrogen* — also some selective secretion of specific substances

5. *Facultative water reabsorption*, under hormonal control (via the influence of anti-diuretic hormone)

Figure 1.6 illustrates the different types of cell found within the nephron.

When one considers the structure of the nephron, it becomes evident how the kidney is able to perform several of its specific homeostatic functions. For example, removal of nitrogenous wastes (e.g. urea, creatinine), regulation of acid–base balance and key electrolyte concentrations, and the maintenance of water balance all rely upon the ability of the nephron to filter the incoming plasma, selectively reabsorb and secrete specific compounds, and create an environment high in osmotic potential which facilitates water reabsorption.

In man, 15 per cent of the nephrons (the so-called juxtamedullary nephrons) have much longer loops of Henle, which pass deeply into the medulla. In addition, these nephrons possess a larger glomerulus and the efferent arteriole forms not only a peritubular network of capillaries but also a series of vascular loops known collectively as the vasa-recta.

The vasa-recta descend into the medulla and form a collective network of capillaries that surround the collecting ducts and ascending limbs of the loops of

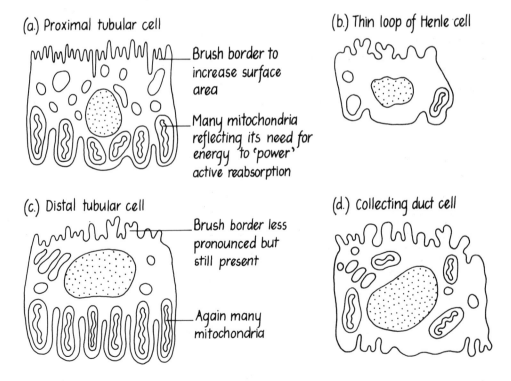

Fig 1.6   Histological appearance of cells within different functional areas of the nephron

Henle. Blood then returns to the cortex via ascending vasa-recta. Although less than 0.7 per cent of total renal blood flow enters the vasa-recta, they provide essential nutrients to the renal medulla and are also crucial for controlling the concentration of the urine produced (Stanton and Koeppen, 1990). The remaining 85 per cent of nephrons (the cortical nephrons) have far shorter loops of Henle, which barely reach the medulla, if at all.

These short-loop nephrons make no significant contribution to the maintenance of a high osmotic potential within the medullary interstitium. However, as the collecting ducts of all nephrons (both cortical and juxtamedullary) pass through the medulla, the long-loop nephrons produce a gradient of concentration that occurs in all nephrons. Thus as plasma flows through the glomerulus, an ultrafiltrate is produced, which progressively passes through the remaining nephron structure, finally reaching the collecting duct.

During this passage, essential substances such as water, glucose, amino acids, bicarbonate etc., are reabsorbed. However, waste products, secreted metabolites and surplus water and electrolytes (i.e. urine) pass into the collecting duct, prior to passage into the calyces and renal pelvis, and are then transported to the bladder. The process of selective reabsorption occurs by the action of both active and passive processes. Active reabsorption (transport) is invariably linked to specific, membrane-bound enzyme systems, which have a fixed capacity to reabsorb (i.e. if the tubular concentration of the specific substance is greater than the number of enzyme-binding sites available, then not all the filtered substance will be reabsorbed, and 'overspill' into the urine will occur; this process is responsible for glycosuria, for example). It is incredible to realise that the nephrons of an average adult kidney produce 180 litres of glomerular filtrate per day, yet only 1.5 litres of urine are actually lost, underlining the ability of the kidney not only to reabsorb water and electrolytes, but also to concentrate metabolic toxins into a small volume of fluid, for subsequent excretion. This ability to concentrate is one of the first functions of the kidney that is compromised in renal failure.

The major force to fluid movement out of the glomerular capillaries is clearly hydrostatic pressure, which underpins the kidneys' very high demand for blood. The following equation summarises the pressure relationships:

$$NEFP = GCP - COP + BCP$$

where NEFP is net effective filtration pressure; GCP is glomerular capillary pressure; COP is colloid osmotic pressure; and BCP is Bowman's capillary pressure. Thus GCP pushes blood against the leaky walls of the vessels, resulting in the production of an ultrafiltrate. This filtration pressure results from the afferent glomerular arteriole being significantly larger than the associated efferent vessel. COP helps to retain substances within the vessels, and is created by large molecular weight proteins.

BCP is a pressure-related force which opposes filtration and underlies the intimate relationship between capsule and glomerulus. Because the movement of fluid from the capillaries occurs in only one direction (outward), the oncotic pressure along the length of an individual capillary will increase until it equals the effective filtration (hydrostatic pressure). Therefore plasma filtration is limited to approximately 20 per cent of the total plasma volume entering the glomerular capillaries per minute.

Unlike the capillaries within the systemic circulation, the hydrostatic pressure within the glomerular capillaries changes only very slightly along the length of the vessel, thus maintaining net filtration throughout the glomerulus. In health, the volume of plasma filtered through the glomeruli in one minute is known as the glomerular filtration rate (GFR), and normally approximates to 120 ml/min.

The GFR provides a reliable measure of renal function, as it approximates well to the kidney's overall ability to filter, and is directly influenced by various disease processes, or by a lack of renal perfusion (thus, for example, the GFR falls very sharply in low BP or shock, resulting in acute oliguria).

At birth the effective GFR is approximately 30 ml/min, and rises steadily with maturity, reaching the 'normal' of 125 ml/min[2] by age 7–10 weeks. Clearly, however, with a GFR initially so low, fluid overloading in neonates is a major potential problem, as the kidney simply does not possess the excretory capacity to deal with excess fluid within the vascular space.

In older age, the GFR declines, such that an average value for an 80-year-old person would be approximately 60–70 ml/min, an effective decrease of 50 per cent. However, this is still sufficient renal function to allow effective renal homeostatic control to be maintained. Chapter 2 describes how the glomerular filtration rate is obtained clinically. A summary of the major absorptive/excretory processes within the nephron, which allow the modification of the glomerular filtrate and the formation of urine, is shown in Figure 1.7.

Table 1.1 illustrates the main components of the glomerular filtrate and their individual handling by the kidney.

Table 1.1 Major urinary components and renal handling

Component	Amount passing through glomeruli per day	Amount filtered per day	Amount reabsorbed from the filtrate per day	Amount excreted in urine per day
Water (litres)	180	180	178.5	1.5
Protein(s) (g)	7000–9000	10–20	10–20	< 0.2
Sodium (g)	540	540	537	3
Chloride (g)	630	630	625	5
Potassium (g)	28	28	24	4
Creatinine (g)	1.5	1.5	0	1.6*
Urea (g)	53	53	28	25
Bicarbonate (g)	300	300	299.7	0.3
Glucose (g)	180	180	180	0

After Tortora and Anagnostakos, 1990

* This figure for creatinine is higher because some creatinine is secreted from the distal tubule.

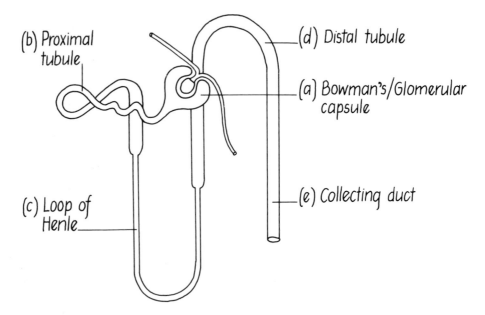

(a) Filtration of substances of atomic mass less than
    approx 70,000 (seventy thousand atomic mass units)
(b) Mass salvage of essential substances
(c) Maintenance of high osmotic potential within the medulla
(d) Fine control of reabsorption, plus selective secretion
(e) Water balance/reabsorption. Disposal of processed filtrate

Fig 1.7   Major absorptive/excretory processes within the nephron

Due to the high perfusion requirement of the adult kidney, the kidney possesses an intrinsic ability to autoregulate (i.e. to maintain its own blood flow) over a range of systemic arterial pressures. As volume decreases, the homeostatic response attempts to maintain sufficient blood flow to retain renal viability, and also to reduce filtration capacity in the short term (as the GFR falls) until normal levels of perfusion are restored.

This pressure range is approximately 80–180 mmHg, which allows the kidney to cope with a wide fluctuation in perfusion input from the aorta. Further, the glomerular filtration rate remains constant over this range, primarily due to the ability of the kidney to alter its vascular tone within the efferent and afferent glomerular arterioles.

These arterioles are smooth muscle structures, innervated with sympathetic nerve fibres, which primarily cause vasoconstriction. Thus, if afferent constriction occurs, the GFR will decrease as blood flow decreases. If the efferent vessels constrict, then GFR will increase, as effective filtration pressure will be increased. This mechanism, however, is not solely innervated neuronally, as transplanted kidneys still display an ability to autoregulate; it is therefore likely also to be under hormonal control, via adrenergic receptors on the smooth muscle cells of the arterioles. Sympathetic nervous system activity, via the influence of adrenaline, decreases the renal blood flow (via vasoconstriction) and thus the GFR. Blood is then transferred to the vital organs and results in small volumes of concentrated urine (oliguria) in conditions of low blood volume, for example, in patients suffering hypovolaemia.

Normal postural adjustments also require the sympathetic nervous system to adjust the level of arterial blood pressure, by constriction of vessels within the skin and viscera (and also the kidney). However, in these circumstances the GFR remains stable, as autoregulation occurs via the afferent or efferent arterioles, thus maintaining perfusion and therefore function.

A further potent homeostatic mechanism which aims to conserve blood flow to the kidney is that of the renin–angiotensin system, which also directly influences systemic blood pressure. The renin–angiotensin system is illustrated in Figure 1.8.

Angiotensinogen is an α_2 globulin, produced by the liver, with a molecular weight of 60,000 amu. It provides the substrate for renin (which therefore acts as an enzyme) to cleave the angiotensinogen molecule, as shown in Figure 1.9. Renin itself is produced by the polar cuff cells of the afferent arterioles, as shown in Figure 1.10.

As can be seen the afferent arteriole and distal tubule are in very close proximity. Within the wall of the distal tubule there are a number of specialised cells, known

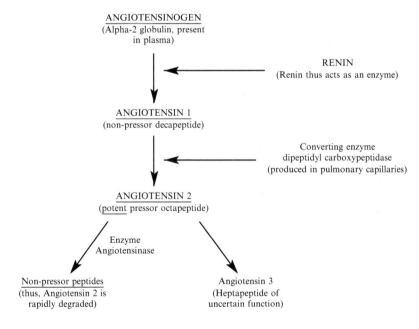

Fig 1.8 The renin–angiotensin system

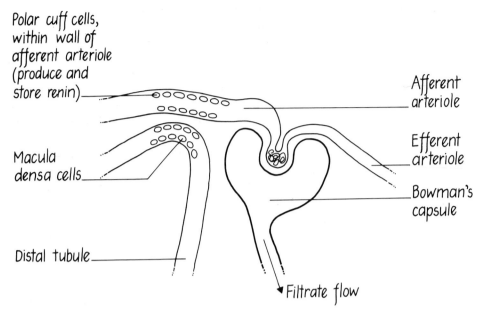

Fig 1.9   Renin and its site of production

collectively as the macula densa. These macula densa cells are primarily sodium sensitive. However, as a result of this close anatomical arrangement between the juxtaglomerular apparatus and the macula densa, renin release can be stimulated in response to three separate stimuli. These are:

1. *Low blood pressure*   Within the walls of the afferent arterioles there are pressure sensors (baroreceptors) which respond when the arteriole is stretched or contracted. Thus dilation of the arterioles (or increased blood flow) stretches the afferent arteriolar wall, causing a decrease in renin secretion. In conditions of low blood flow, stretch is obviously reduced and renin production therefore increases, in an attempt to compensate.

2. *Sodium signal*   Renal secretion would also seem to be controlled by the amount of sodium chloride within the glomerular filtrate, passing through the macula densa cells of the distal tubule. In circumstances of haemorrhage or low blood volume, the urine becomes more concentrated, and this stimulates the macula densa cells, which then transfer information to the polar cuff cells, thus initiating renin release. The sodium 'signal' therefore allows the kidney to respond to changes in sodium concentration as well as to blood volume, thus reflecting a tubular mechanism of regulation, rather than a vascular one.

3. *Adrenergic system*   This stimulus occurs via the sympathetic nervous system, being activated during situations of sympathetic nervous system activity (e.g. stressors such as haemorrhage or hypotension). Thus it constitutes a neuronal signal which causes renin release. In addition, the presence of adrenaline and noradrenaline also leads to renin release. From Figure 1.8 it can be seen that angiotensin II is a potent pressor substance, increasing the total peripheral resistance, and thus blood pressure. Its second major function, however, is its direct influence upon the adrenal cortex (zona glomerulosa), initiating the release of aldosterone (a hormone), a process which takes 45–60 minutes. Aldosterone is then renally active, causing an increase in tubular sodium reabsorption, which in turn increases the rate of passive water reabsorption. Thus, water is absorbed from the tubules with sodium, and the net effect is one of increasing the effective plasma volume (rather than plasma sodium in isolation).

Aldosterone is thought to exert its effect by inducing the formation of specific sodium carrier proteins within the epithelial cells of the renal tubules (Guyton, 1991).

Another hormone which exerts a crucial effect upon the renal tubules is the anti-diuretic hormone (ADH). ADH increases water reabsorption in the terminal portion of the distal tubule and within the individual collecting ducts. It would appear to exert this effect by initiating the formation of specific channels, which are highly permeable to water, within the distal tubule and collecting duct cells (Guyton, 1991). Water will therefore move from the tubule, due to the high osmotic potential of the renal interstitium, and is taken up by the vasa recta. From these vessels it then passes to the systemic circulation. In the absence of ADH, virtually no water is absorbed at all from the distal tubule and collecting duct cells, and huge amounts of very dilute urine are produced (an effect aptly demonstrated in cases of diabetes insipidus).

The renin–angiotensin system would be unable to exert its mechanism of increasing systemic volume, via the effect of aldosterone, without the influence of the neurosecretion ADH, produced from the posterior pituitary. As plasma sodium concentration increases, this is sensed within the hypothalamus (as well as in peripheral chemoreceptors) and ADH is released. ADH targets the cells of the collecting duct and changes their permeability to water, so increasing the intracellular pore size and facilitating increased water reabsorption (due to the high osmotic potential of the renal interstitium). The water reabsorbed then passes, via the vasa-recta, to the systemic circulation.

As previously stated, the kidney also plays a vital role in the maintenance of acid–base balance. This is achieved by:

1. The active reabsorption of virtually all filtered bicarbonate
2. The regeneration of new bicarbonate, to replace that used up in plasma buffering
3. The formation of titratable acid salts which can then be excreted in the urine

This process of urinary acidification provides the only means of removing non-volatile acid from the circulation. Thus, metabolic acidosis is a key problem in patients with renal failure. The urinary pH is normally between 4 and 8, which reflects the urinary route for acid excretion. Some bacteria (e.g. *Proteus* sp.) have the capacity to split the urea within urine (via the enzyme urease), so releasing ammonia and making the urine more alkaline. The alkalinity then causes the precipitation of key ionic species such as calcium and phosphate and may then lead to the formation of infection stones, if prolonged (e.g. stag-horn calculus).

Two remaining areas of renal function which do not directly relate to tubular absorption/secretion processes are the production of erythropoietin, and the activation of vitamin D. Erythropoietin is a hormone which forms the primary stimulus to bone marrow tissue, resulting in the production of new red blood cells (RBC). Such erythropoietic activity is stimulated by relative hypoxia, which then causes the release of renal erythropoietic factor from the kidney and liver (though the kidney produces by far the greater percentage, probably over 80 per cent). Once in the plasma, renal erythropoietic factor acts as a specific plasma protein, and is converted to the hormone erythropoietin, which then stimulates RBC production. Without this mechanism, chronic refractory anaemia results.

A most significant recent advance for patients suffering from chronic renal failure, who experience such anaemia, has been the successful production of human erythropoietin using recombinant DNA technology. This is given intravenously at the end of haemodialysis (or subcutaneously three times per week) and has resulted in the restoration of essentially normal haemoglobin levels in these patients, which gives a dramatic increase in quality of life. It is not known, at present, exactly where in the kidney erythropoietin is produced, though several sites are currently implicated. These include the mesangial cells of the glomerulus, which extend into the tuft of glomerular capillaries, and the renal tubular epithelial cells (Guyton, 1991).

In conditions of low oxygen tension, erythropoietin production begins within minutes/hours and reaches maximum production within 24 hours. If there is no renal function at all, anaemia is inevitable, as the 10–20 per cent of erythropoietin formed in other tissues is only adequate to sustain between 30 and 50 per cent of required RBC production (Guyton, 1991).

The kidney is also responsible for the activation of vitamin D. The term vitamin D refers to a group of compounds which are synthesised within the skin, from a precursor molecule already present. This process of synthesis is reliant upon the presence of ultra-violet radiation, from direct sunlight. The precursor substance is called 7-dehydrocholesterol, and sunlight converts this to cholecalciferol (vitamin D_3). The liver then converts vitamin D_3 to 25-hydroxycholecalciferol (i.e. adds an hydroxyl group). It is this substance that the kidney then further changes to 1,25-dihydroxycholecalciferol (or calcitriol), which is the most active form of vitamin D and acts as a hormone, stimulating calcium and phosphate absorption from the gut. This conversion process occurs within the proximal tubular cells of the nephrons.

Calcitriol is up to 1000 times more active than any of its precursor substances and thus, in the absence of kidney function, vitamin D loses almost all of its ability to induce calcium absorption (Guyton, 1991).

THE URINARY TRACT

For effective renal function it is essential that an intact and functional urinary tract is present. It is all too evident that renal damage can readily occur if the urinary tract is compromised (thus, for example, obstruction of the lower tract can induce significant urinary reflux and intra-renal pressure, leading to nephron damage).

Once urine is formed, and has been 'channelled' from the pyramids, via the calyces, to the renal pelvis, it is then pushed down the ureters which run outside the peritoneal cavity for most of their length.

Figure 1.10 shows the major structures comprising the lower urinary tract. As can be seen, two ureters are usually present (one per kidney), each comprising a hollow muscular tube, which extends from the renal pelvis (the so-called pelvi-ureteric junction, or PUJ) down to the posterior surface of the bladder. The ureters enter at the bladder base, close to the superior lateral angle. The ureters pass through the

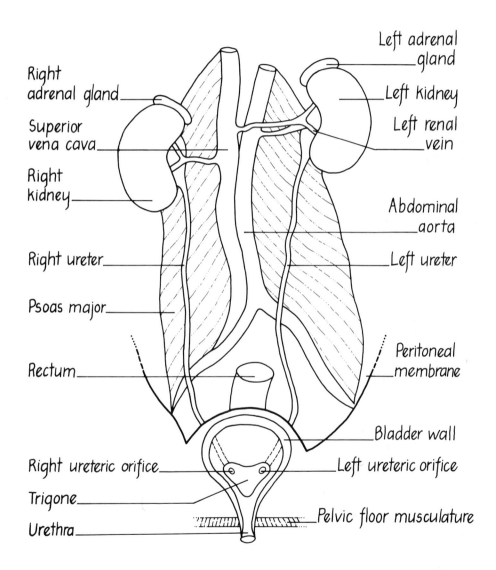

Fig 1.10 The lower urinary tract

bladder wall at an oblique angle, thus creating a functional valve, which acts to prevent retrograde reflux of urine by compressing the ureter when pressure within the bladder increases and the bladder wall therefore becomes stretched (for example, during the slow sustained pressure increase seen upon filling, or the sudden dramatic increase which occurs upon voiding).

However, this valve may be defective from birth, or destroyed by disease, leading to the possibility of recurrent urinary tract infection, reflux and renal damage, as already mentioned.

The wall of the ureter is constructed of three layers, as shown in Figure 1.11. The inner mucosa is a typical mucus-secreting transitional cell epithelium, congruent with the rest of the urinary tract. The mucus serves to both waterproof and protect the mucosal cells from urine, which is vastly different in its solute concentrations from that of the cells within the ureteric wall. The middle layer or muscularis comprises smooth muscle, laid down as a combination of inner longitudinal and outer circular fibres (the proximal one-third of the ureter also contains outer longitudinal muscle fibres), which actively propels urine down the ureter, in conjunction with hydrostatic pressure and gravity (thus allowing drainage of urine, whatever posture may be adopted). The outer layer of the ureter consists of fibrous tissue similar to that of the renal capsule, and extensions of the layer provide a means of anchoring the ureter within the retroperitoneal cavity.

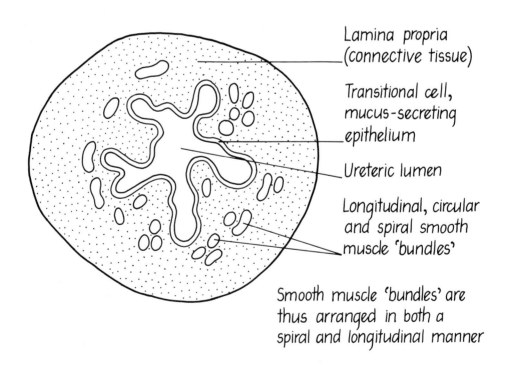

Fig 1.11   Ureter in cross-section

THE BLADDER

The bladder is a hollow muscular organ, which lies in the anterior half of the pelvic cavity. The bladder lies posterior to the symphysis pubis, lateral to the diverging walls of the bony pelvis.

In the female, the bladder is anterior to the rectum, and inferior to the peritoneal cavity. In both sexes, the rectum is separated from the bladder by the fascia of Denonvilliers, a combination of fused layers of peritoneum from the retrovesical pouch. This fascia is very important, as its tough, impenetrable nature produces a very effective barrier to rectal invasion from bladder or prostatic tumours. In addition, it also provides a useful plane of surgical cleavage between the bladder and rectum. The superior surface of the bladder is covered by the peritoneum, which is then reflected upward on to the anterior abdominal wall, and which peels upward and backward as the bladder rises out of the pelvic cavity on filling. Thus, it is possible to approach the anterior aspect of the bladder via the retropubic space, which effectively bypasses the peritoneal cavity. These anatomical relationships are summarised in Figure 1.12.

In the male, both the vas deferens and the seminal vesicles lie adjacent to the base of the bladder. Beneath the bladder, and attached to the bladder base, is the prostate gland, through which the urethra (the muscular tube carrying urine from the bladder base to the exterior) passes, prior to penetrating the pelvic floor muscles anteriorly (i.e. the levator ani and coccygeus muscles). The bladder draws its blood supply from branches of the internal iliac artery, principally the superior and inferior vesical arteries. The blood supply is extremely rich, which is clearly an important consideration in postoperative management, following surgery, or in cases of bladder trauma.

However, the profuse blood flow through the bladder tissue also allows it to be readily adapted for a variety of surgical procedures, as well as promoting healing following augmentation procedures. Venous drainage of the bladder (and prostate) is achieved via two principal routes. The first route utilises the internal iliac veins, and then the inferior vena cava. A second route, however, runs from the internal iliac veins to the veins of the innominate bones, femoral heads and lower vertebral bodies. Thus, it is very common to observe bony metastases within these sites, particularly the pelvis and upper femur, following primary malignancies within the bladder or prostate. The deep muscle layers of the bladder also contain a widespread lymphatic system which drains via the internal iliac and obturator groups of nodes, and also via the lymphatics of the bony pelvis and upper ends of the femur. The deep muscle layers therefore also provide a further route for metastatic spread. When empty, the bladder lumen is decreased, and the bladder wall appears thicker.

As the bladder fills it first becomes spherical, then 'pear shaped', as it rises up out of the pelvic cavity. The initial thickening when empty relates to the lining epithelium of the bladder, which contains several layers of transitional cells that can overlap and 'slip' over each other as the volume within the bladder increases. At the base of the bladder is a small triangular area known as the trigone. The trigone represents the

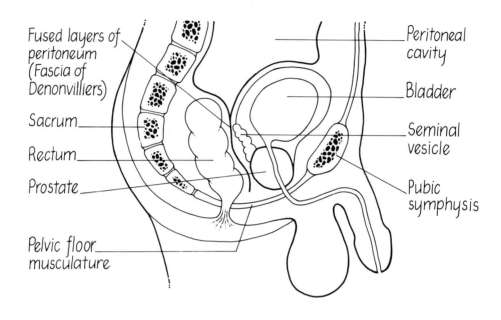

Fused layers of peritoneum (Fascia of Denonvilliers)

Sacrum

Rectum

Prostate

Pelvic floor musculature

Peritoneal cavity

Bladder

Seminal vesicle

Pubic symphysis

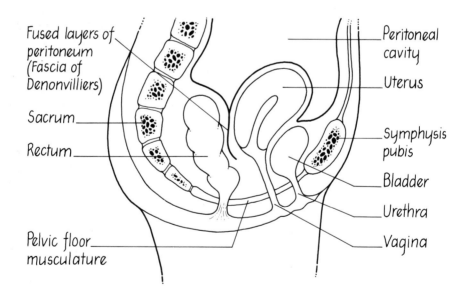

Fused layers of peritoneum (Fascia of Denonvilliers)

Sacrum

Rectum

Pelvic floor musculature

Peritoneal cavity

Uterus

Symphysis pubis

Bladder

Urethra

Vagina

Fig 1.12a and b   Anatomical relationships of the urinary bladder: (a) male; (b) female

area between the ureteric orifices and the internal urethral meatus, and undergoes little change in size during bladder filling. This makes it very sensitive to stretch and, because of its nerve supply, the whole trigonal area is easily irritated by foreign bodies such as urethral catheters, particularly if they are held in place by large volume balloons, such as those containing more than 30 or 50 ml of water.

The trigone is also probably responsible for causing bladder spasm in patients with indwelling urinary catheters, particularly if the balloon is sitting low down within the bladder. At this point the ureters run obliquely through the bladder muscle and mucosal layers for approximately 1.5–2 cm, prior to opening within the bladder at the left and right ureteric orifices. This oblique tunnel forms the antireflux valve, mentioned previously. The bladder is normally described as having four very distinct layers, though there is some argument over the exact nature of these (Bullock et al, 1991). Certainly there is little doubt that the inner layer is composed of a mucous secreting transitional cell epithelium. The transitional cells facilitate stretch, and rugae are also present within this layer. The second layer is normally called the submucosa and is constructed of connective tissue, which provides a bridge between the mucosa and the third, more muscular layer.

The exact nature of this third layer is probably the most debatable. The third layer contains the bladder muscle fibres (collectively known as the detrusor) and there is some controversy, at present, over the exact nature of this muscle. Certainly, the detrusor contains both longitudinal and circular fibres, though there is an opinion that the muscle consists of a network of smooth muscle 'bundles' distributed throughout the bladder wall, rather than in one discrete layer. The outermost layer, the serosa, is formed by peritoneum and so is not a distinct continuation of bladder tissue as such. Also, the serosa covers only the superior surface of the bladder.

The anatomical nature of the bladder neck (the so-called proximal or internal sphincter) is, at present, a further area of urological controversy. The sphincter also differs in its structure, between the sexes. In the male, a circular layer of smooth muscle is present, around the bladder neck, which then passes down into the prostatic capsule below, along with longitudinal muscle fibres. These muscle fibres are richly innervated with adrenergic, sympathetic nerves sensitive to noradrenaline, and are responsible for bladder neck contraction upon orgasm, thus preventing retrograde ejaculation of semen up into the bladder. The exact role of these muscle fibres in maintaining urinary continence is far less clear at this time, and it would seem likely that other mechanisms (e.g. circular, elastic muscle fibres) may be more important in keeping this area of the bladder neck closed.

In the female, there is no such circular muscle arrangement. Rather, the smooth muscle bundles/fibres run longitudinally (or obliquely) into the wall of the urethra and are innervated via cholinergic, rather than adrenergic, nerves. Interestingly, however, the bladder neck still remains closed at rest, probably due to the influence of circular elastic fibres and also the valve-like effect caused by the urethral mucosa, which is highly vascular. As stated earlier, the urine is expelled from the bladder via muscular contraction of the bladder wall, the urine then passing down the urethra. The urethra is also extremely important, because it contains the external sphincter, which is under voluntary control, and provides the mainstay of continence in both sexes.

Again, this is not an area without some degree of controversy, and authors such as Berne and Levy (1990) suggest that in the case of the female the external sphincter is actually poorly developed and therefore less important within the sphere of voluntary bladder control. The female urethra, however, does appear to fulfil the role of a urinary sphincter, particularly as it possesses mixed muscle fibres, i.e. smooth and striated muscle, within its wall (*see* Figure 1.14).

The male urethra divides conveniently into four distinct areas, as shown in Figure 1.13. These four distinct anatomical regions are:

1. *Prostatic urethra* (approximately 3–4 cm)
2. *Membranous urethra* (approximately 2 cm)
3. *Bulbar* (or spongy) *urethra* (approximately 1.5 cm)
4. *Penile urethra* (approximately 15 cm)

The male urethra is lined by transitional cell epithelium throughout most of its length except for a small region of squamous epithelium close to the external urethral meatus. The prostatic urethra is 3–4 cm in length, and receives ducts from the prostate on its posterior aspect (at the utriculus). This part of the urethra also contains a pyramid-shaped structure on its posterior wall, the verumontanum ('true mountain'), which is close to the prostate and above the level of the external

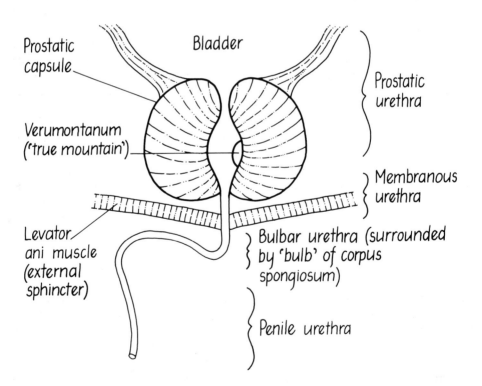

Fig 1.13   Anatomy of the male urethra

sphincter. The verumontanum is a crucial anatomical landmark for the surgeon, allowing prostatic resection to be carried out above the external sphincter mechanism, located within the membranous urethra, thus avoiding possible damage to the sphincter which could then subsequently render the patient incontinent. The ejaculatory ducts, which bring sperm from both vas deferens as well as secretions from the seminal vesicles, open on either side of the verumontanum. The urethra then pierces the pelvic floor musculature (the levator ani) as the membranous urethra, which extends from the prostatic apex to the bulb of the penis (a length of about 2 cm). The membranous urethra is relatively thin, and weaker than other urethral structures.

The penile or spongy urethra is surrounded by the corpus spongiosum (part of the erectile tissue within the penis), and receives many periurethral glands, whose ducts lie within the corpus spongiosum. The largest of these are a pair of four Cowper's glands, via the Cowper's ducts. The proximal part of the spongy urethra is surrounded by the bulbospongiosus muscle, and therefore is known as the bulbar urethra, or urethral bulb. It is a contraction of this muscle that assists in urethral emptying at the termination of voiding, and which also aids the expulsion of semen during orgasm and ejaculation. The spongy or penile urethra terminates at the fossa navicularis. As can be seen, the membranous urethra bridges the gap between the prostate, which is attached to the symphysis above, and the bulbar urethra below, which, due to its dense attachments to the corpora cavernosa on either side, is held firmly by the ischial tuberosities.

Thus any fracture which displaces the bones of the pelvis is likely to tear the membranous urethra. Fracture of the pubic and ischial rami on either side of the symphysis pubis causes the prostate to move posteriorly with the symphysis. As the bulbar urethra is firmly held by the corpora on either side, again, the membranous urethra may be stretched and consequently rupture.

In contrast to the length and complexity of the male urethra, the female urethra is only 4–5 cm in length, and lies directly posterior to the symphysis pubis and in front of the anterior vaginal wall (see Figure 1.12).

The female urethra passes through the pelvic floor musculature (levator ani) and its external meatus opens approximately 2–3 cm behind the clitoris (i.e. between the clitoris and the vaginal opening). As in the male, the female urethra is also lined by transitional cell epithelium for most of its length, and by squamous epithelium nearer to its external meatus. However, it occasionally can be lined totally by squamous epithelium, which continues up into the bladder neck. In addition, many mucus-secreting glands are also present. The muscular structure of the female urethra forms an intrinsic sphincter, which allows urethral closure to occur.

The sphincter is constructed of an inner longitudinal smooth muscle layer and an outer, circular, striated muscle layer. The action of the male external sphincter has been traditionally explained as arising from fibres of the levator ani muscle, which surrounds the membranous urethra. However, more recent anatomical studies have shown that these fibres do not constitute a 'complete' muscle ring, but rather only form an arrangement comparable to a 'urethral sling' (Bullock et al 1991). The main contribution to the external sphincter would seem to come from the urethral wall itself. At this point the urethral musculature contains an outer circular layer of

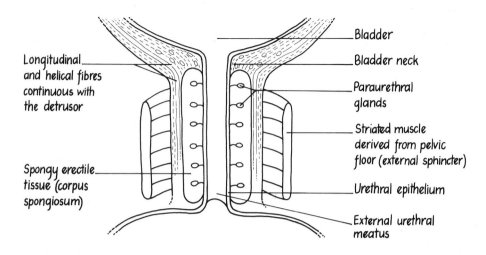

Fig 1.14   Structure of the female urethra

striated muscle fibres which are designed for prolonged contraction (so-called 'slow' twitch fibres). These fibres receive innervation via somatic (therefore voluntary) nerves from the level of sacral vertebrae 2 and 3 (S2 and S3). The periurethral sling of pelvic floor muscle fibres also plays a role in maintaining continence, by contracting for short periods. Its nature is one of 'fast' twitch fibres which seem to contract during sudden rises in intravesical pressure (caused by such events as coughing, laughing, running, etc.) and thus reinforce urethral closure and maintain continence.

The external or rhabdosphincter muscle (voluntary muscle) contains slow twitch fibres and is therefore capable of prolonged contraction. In the male there is no doubt that the external sphincter mechanism exerts a 'tighter' force of contraction (i.e. higher closure pressure) than the bladder neck itself, and is certainly a more powerful urinary sphincter. In the female, this rhabdosphincter extends throughout the length of the urethra, but is more pronounced in approximately the middle one-third. As in the male, a periurethral sling of first twitch fibres is also present. This muscle sling arises from levator ani fibres, and serves to raise urethral closure pressure during sudden episodes of high bladder pressure, such as coughing, etc. However, in females, the voluntary sphincter again plays the most profound role in protecting against urinary leakage.

Innervation of the Bladder

In terms of nerve supply, the bladder contains its own intrinsic system, yet it is also influenced by stimuli external to this system (i.e. from higher centres). Thus, for effective bladder function, autonomic plus somatic nerve fibres from the bladder and urethra pass to the spinal cord at the level of S2–S4, via the pelvic parasympathetic nerves. This area of the cord is known as the spinal micturition centre, acting as a 'switching centre' for both incoming sensory nerves and also providing the outflow route from the cord for parasympathetic motor nerves to the detrusor muscle (via autonomic fibres) and the sphincters (via somatic pudendal fibres).

From the spinal micturition centre, nerve fibres also ascend to the micturition centres with the pons and cerebral cortex, thus informing higher centres of bladder activity and also allowing inhibition of the micturition reflex, a voluntary response which is typically learnt at approximately age 3–4 years. Tragically, this very low position of the spinal micturition centre (lying at the border between the sacral and lumbar vertebrae) makes it very vulnerable to disruption via spinal injury, as any cord damage above this level is likely to cause loss of nervous innervation and therefore bladder dysfunction. Detrusor contraction occurs via impulses from parasympathetic, cholinergic nerves which pass to the detrusor along parasympathetic pelvic nerve fibres.

Sympathetic nerves also provide bladder innervation via the hypogastric nerves, and are mainly motor contractile fibres. The sphincter mechanism is innervated by both somatic voluntary nerves (from S2 to S3) and autonomic fibres, the autonomic innervation providing control for the smooth, slow twitch inner muscle layer of the urethra. The fast twitch, periurethral sling is innervated, as one would expect, by somatic voluntary nerves.

Figure 1.15 provides a diagrammatic overview of bladder innervation.

The bladder, acting as a most efficient storage reservoir for urine, has to be able to increase in size, yet not contract, so allowing urine to enter the bladder with little accompanying rise in intravesical pressure. As the bladder fills, the rugae flatten and the bladder volume is able to increase with very little change in the intravesical pressure.

Thus, the normal pressure rise on filling (e.g. from 10 ml up to say 400 ml) is only approximately 5–10 cm water, a fact which underlines the highly compliant nature of the bladder (Berne and Levy, 1990). Clearly, during filling, urinary leakage is prevented by contraction of the bladder neck and external sphincter. Voiding, however, is actually a most complex and superbly coordinated activity, involving relaxation of the external sphincter, relaxation of the bladder neck and contraction of the detrusor muscle, within the bladder wall.

This coordination of simultaneous relaxation and detrusor contraction is achieved via the so-called 'spino–pontine–spinal' reflex, which involves the higher micturition centre located within the pons. It is via the pontine centre that higher centre control (learned at about 4–5 years) can inhibit the normal reflex to void, thus bringing the reflex under voluntary control.

Such higher centre control is mediated via the cerebral cortex. During the period of bladder filling, stretch receptors within the detrusor muscle pass impulses to the spinal micturition centre, and then, via the spinal cord (via the lateral spinothalamic tracts), to the frontal cortex. These stretch receptor impulses 'create' the desire to void urine but are effectively suppressed by the higher centres (i.e. frontal cortex) until a convenient time for micturition is found. The cycle of voiding is initiated voluntarily, but relies also upon involuntary muscle activity, within the detrusor. First, relaxation of the urethral sphincter leads to a fall in pressure within the

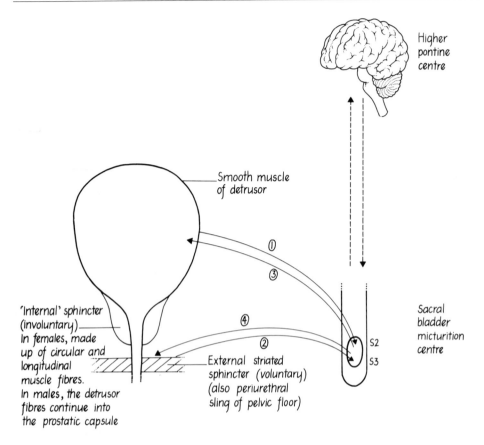

Higher
pontine
centre

Smooth muscle
of detrusor

'Internal' sphincter
(involuntary).
In females, made
up of circular and
longitudinal
muscle fibres.
In males, the detrusor
fibres continue into
the prostatic capsule

External striated
sphincter (voluntary)
(also periurethral
sling of pelvic floor)

Sacral
bladder
micturition
centre

S2
S3

Fig 1.15   Innervation of the bladder: 1, sensory input from detrusor stretch receptors; 2, sensory input from sphincter and pelvic floor; 3, motor output to detrusor (parasympathetic via pelvic nerves and sympathetic via hypogastric nerves); 4, motor output to sphincter and pelvic floor (via both somatic and autonomic nerves

urethral lumen. The pelvic floor muscles then also relax under conscious control, and the bladder neck opens (or 'funnels').

Simultaneous parasympathetic activity then leads to contraction of the detrusor muscle (within the bladder wall), which then actively expels the urine under pressure. As this occurs, the intravesical pressure rises markedly, achieving a typical value of 100 cm water. As the bladder empties and urine flow ceases the urethral sphincter closes under voluntary control. Any urine above the level of the external sphincter is 'milked back' into the bladder, as the proximal urethra also contracts prior to bladder neck closure. Once the emptying cycle is finished, higher centre inhibition again becomes active, so preparing the bladder for a new influx of urine, and a further filling cycle (Blandy, 1992).

Figure 1.16 illustrates the bladder cycle of filling and emptying.

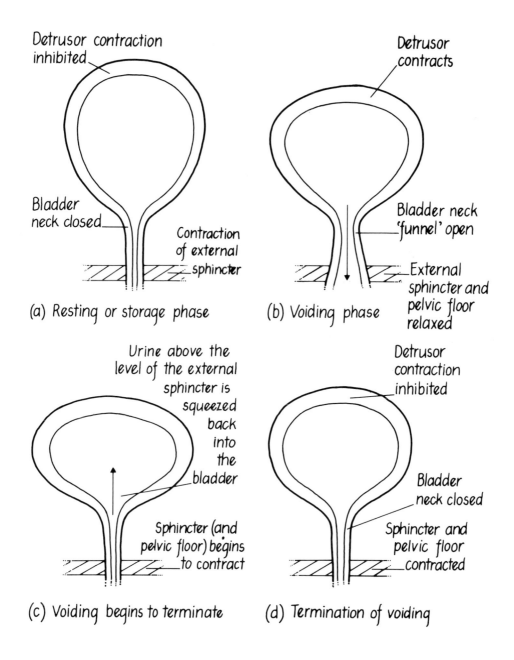

Detrusor contraction inhibited

Bladder neck closed

Contraction of external sphincter

(a) Resting or storage phase

Detrusor contracts

Bladder neck 'funnel' open

External sphincter and pelvic floor relaxed

(b) Voiding phase

Urine above the level of the external sphincter is squeezed back into the bladder

Sphincter (and pelvic floor) begins to contract

(c) Voiding begins to terminate

Detrusor contraction inhibited

Bladder neck closed

Sphincter and pelvic floor contracted

(d) Termination of voiding

Fig 1.16 Normal bladder cycle

THE PROSTATE

The prostate is probably the best known organ within the male urogenital system. Around 1 in 10 men over the age of 55 years will require surgery to relieve urinary obstruction caused by prostatic enlargement, and the gland therefore occupies a key position within the sphere of urological practice.

When one considers the anatomical nature and location of the prostate gland, it becomes evident why it is uniquely positioned to cause disruption to the normal passage of urine out of the bladder.

The prostate is situated around the bladder neck, and the portion of the urethra which emerges from the bladder at this point. It lies behind the symphysis pubis, to which it is attached by a tough layer of fascia (i.e. connective tissue). On either side, the pubis and ischial tuberosities curve around it. The size of the prostate shows considerable variability, increasing rapidly in size around the age of puberty. Its shape is often likened to a chestnut, which reflects its non-uniform nature. A normal gland is approximately 15 g in weight, and 3 cm in diameter, and this remains constant until approximately the age of 45–50 years, when the prostate may undergo enlargement of varying degrees.

One myth regarding such enlargement is that 'large' prostates invariably cause significant urinary obstruction, and smaller glands do not. This is not, in fact, the case, and small degrees of enlargement, which directly impinge within the urethral lumen, can be highly obstructive. The structure of the prostate gland and its key anatomical relationships are shown in Figure 1.17.

The prostate consists of a network of secretory tubules, surrounded by a capsule of smooth muscle. Each tubule is enclosed by contractile smooth muscle fibres and the whole gland is supported by connective tissue. These distinct ingredients tend to vary in their relative proportions, according to the age of the individual. In the case of the child, as one would expect, the glandular and muscular elements are far less developed, and they enlarge significantly at around the age of puberty. Further benign enlargement (to a greater or lesser degree) then occurs during 'middle age', which results in 'nodules' of prostatic hypertrophy.

The glandular ducts of the prostatic tissue empty into the prostatic urethra. As previously mentioned, lying on the posterior wall of the prostatic urethra is the distinct structure of the verumontanum. On either side of the verumontanum lie the two ejaculatory ducts, which deliver sperm from the vas deferens, which passes obliquely down through the posterior aspect of the prostate gland. The main area of glandular tissue is situated within the lateral and posterior portions of the prostate (the so-called 'outer' zone), whereas the mucosal glands, close to the urethra, lie in the middle of the gland (the so-called 'inner' zone). In the prostate of the young male, one does not see 'lobes', as such. However, what are known later in life as the 'middle' or 'lateral' lobes are really the result of regional hypertrophy within these specific regions of the prostate, an effect which is a result of the prostate having only a very limited space within which it can enlarge.

Benign prostatic hypertrophy is particularly common within the inner zone of the gland, which is then readily able to elongate and distort the prostatic urethra, and

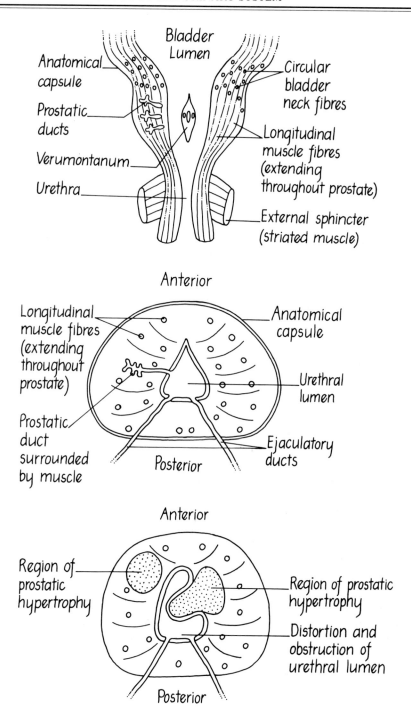

Fig 1.17 (a) and (b) Prostatic structure and key anatomical relationships. (c) Prostatic structure and mechanism of obstruction

thus impede the flow of urine. Unfortunately, fluid flow through a tube is proportional to the square of the radius, and therefore a small degree of enlargement can very seriously disrupt urinary flow.

The bulbo-urethral (or Cowper's glands) are approximately the size of a pea, lying between the prostate and penis, with ducts which open into the urethra. These glands produce a mucus-rich secretion, which serves as a urethral lubricant, prior to ejaculation.

In association with its rich network of smooth muscle fibres, the prostate serves an important contractile function during ejaculation and orgasm. It is vital that, upon orgasm, the bladder neck is simultaneously closed off, otherwise semen will reflux up into the bladder (so-called retrograde ejaculation), rather than be expelled down the urethra.

During ejaculation, the bladder neck and prostate therefore undergo muscular contraction, whereas the external sphincter relaxes, thus allowing semen to pass into the penile urethra. The prostatic gland produces a milky secretion, which makes up about 10–20 per cent of the total volume of the ejaculate. The fluid is watery in nature, slightly acidic and contains a variety of enzymes (e.g. acid phosphatase) and many other components (e.g. citrate, calcium, fibrinolysin). It is also responsible for giving semen its characteristic odour. At this time no *definitive* function has been proven for the prostatic secretion, though its ingredients have been variously suggested to stimulate sperm motility, cause coagulation of the secretion from the seminal vesicles, and also to help neutralise the natural acidity of the vagina (Blandy, 1992).

The prostate is dependent upon adequate amounts of circulating testicular hormones (i.e. androgens) for its secretory function, and both secretion and growth of the gland are intimately linked to changes in the plasma concentrations of these hormones. This fact is made use of in the treatment of prostatic carcinoma, where androgen antagonists are employed to block the effects of the testosterone, thereby reducing prostatic growth.

In the case of carcinoma, the process of enlargement commonly involves the outer or posterior portion of the gland, often felt (at least initially) as a hard nodule, on the surface of the gland, upon rectal examination.

Following prostatic surgery, not only is disruption caused to the anatomy of the bladder neck, but also prostatic tissue is removed during the process of resection. This results in a prostatic cavity of varying size (depending on the degree of resection) and an open (or partially open) bladder neck. As a result, semen will, to a greater or lesser degree, pass back up into the bladder on orgasm, and therefore a reduced amount of ejaculate, or no ejaculate, will be seen. The patient may then notice that their urine is cloudy when they next void, which is a result of semen being mixed with the urine. The patient will, however, remain continent, as the external striated sphincter, below the level of the prostate and verumontanum, is left intact.

Semen consists of a mixture of spermatozoa (male gametes) and secretions from both the prostate and other male accessory organs. Semen is also rich in the enzyme hyaluronidase, which breaks down mucopolysaccharides, thus helping the sperm pass through the cervical mucus. The bulk of the seminal fluid originates from the seminal vesicles and has a combined pH of about 7.2–7.4. This helps to neutralise the acidic vaginal pH, as the sperm become rapidly immobilised by an acid environment.

A diagram of the male genital system is shown in Figure 1.18. As can be seen the genital system in the male consists of the testes, their associated ducts, the accessory glands (e.g. prostate) and the penis. Each testis consists of a set of elongated tubules (seminiferous tubules), which contain a germinal epithelium responsible for producing the individual sperm cells, which are then released into the lumen of the tubule. These germinal tubules drain into the larger tubules (the rete testes) and then into the vasa efferentia (in some ways, analogous to the renal pelvis), which finally becomes the epididymis. The epididymis is essentially a long, highly convoluted tube, packed tightly within each testis and lined by a secretory columnar epithelium. If unwound, the epididymis would extend for approximately 6 metres, and is closely

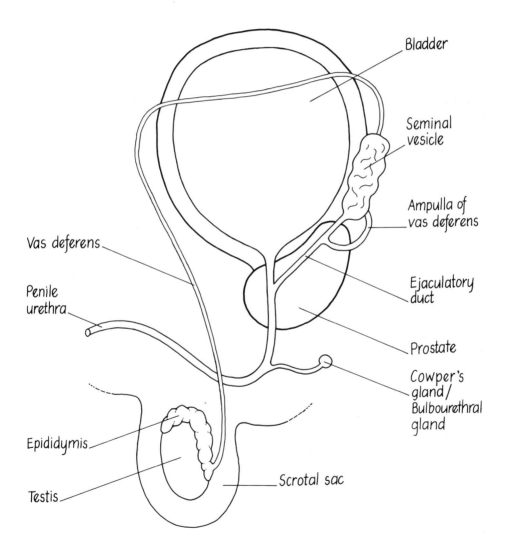

Fig 1.18 Male reproductive system

applied to the posterior aspect of the testis (e.g. it can be felt as a rough, string-like mass, by palpation of the posterior testicular surface).

The cilia attached to the luminal cells of the seminiferous tubules (sometimes called 'stereo cilia') beat continuously, in conjunction with regular smooth muscle contraction of the tubular wall, thus propelling the maturing spermatozoa towards the epididymis. The time taken to produce mature spermatozoa, including the journey from tubule to epididymis, is approximately 70 days, and it seems that the secretory epididymis produces a mixture of hormones, enzymes and nutrients that all play a role in sperm maturation. The sperm take approximately 2–4 weeks to traverse the epididymis and during this time they lose their remaining cytoplasm and acquire motility. The function of this epithelium is dependent upon adequate levels of circulating male androgen.

Classically, the epididymis is divided into three sections, head, body and tail, the tail region providing a storage space for sperm. Storage of sperm is necessary because, although production of mature sperm is a continuous process, ejaculation occurs only irregularly. Interestingly, if no ejaculation occurs (within 40–50 days), the sperm stored within the epididymis degenerate, via a process of liquefaction, and are removed by phagocytosis. The tail of the epididymis then drains into the vas (or ductus) deferens, a muscular tube that ends within the pelvic cavity, whereupon it joins with the duct of the seminal vesicle, so forming the ejaculatory duct.

Thus there are two ejaculatory ducts (right and left). The seminal vesicles are really just a diverticulum of the vas deferens, lined with columnar epithelium, and holding between 2 and 5 ml of fluid. The vesicles are secretory, producing fructose and also a range of other substances, which would seem to influence sperm production. Upon sexual excitation, the seminal vesicles swell to five or ten times their original size, producing most of the ejaculate volume, via a process of secretion.

The wall of the vas deferens contains three layers of smooth muscle, held together with connective tissue and innervated via the autonomic nerve supply. This then allows the vas deferens to contract rapidly during ejaculation, ensuring that the sperm pass on into the seminal vesicles, and then into the urethra.

THE TESTES

The two individual testes lie within the scrotal sac, with the smooth testes in front and the 'lumpy' epididymis behind, both being suspended from the external inguinal ring by the spermatic cord (nerves, arterial and venous supply, lymphatics and some muscle fibres), which acts much like an umbilical cord. The spermatic cord is able to shorten, due to muscle fibres within it, so moving the testes upward and thus closer to the body core. Such an arrangement occurs because the testes need to be at a temperature of 35°C (approximately 2°C below core) if sperm production is to occur. Thus, suspension of the testes within the scrotum allows such a temperature differential to be maintained.

Should the external temperature fall, the cremaster and dartos muscles will contract, bringing the testes closer to the body. This muscle contraction allows greater heat exchange and maintains the temperature required for spermatogenesis. Conversely, if the external temperature is high, the cremaster muscle relaxes and the testes sit lower down in the scrotal sac, away from the direct heating effect of the core body temperature.

Because the testicles are suspended, any twisting of the testes (and thus the spermatic cord) within the scrotum may rapidly impair the venous drainage and/or arterial blood supply, resulting in pain and possible ischaemia. This is known as testicular torsion, and constitutes a surgical emergency. Around each testis is a thin layer of tissue, the tunica vaginalis, which helps protect it from injury. This sheathes the testis during intrauterine life. The cavity between the testis and tunica vaginalis contains a small amount of lubricating fluid, which further helps protect the testis from sudden movement. However, this 'potential' cavity can expand and fill with fluid (much like the pleural cavity, in cases of pleural effusion) in which case a hydrocele results.

The testicle derives its rich arterial blood supply from the testicular artery, which leaves the aorta at the level of the renal arteries. This passes via the retropubic space into the groin, then along the inguinal canal and down the spermatic cord via the inguinal ring (a slit-like opening in the transverse abdominis muscle).

The venous drainage from the testicle is also very rich, again occurring through the spermatic cord, and from there to the left renal vein and vena cava. However, such drainage is facilitated by a complex network of veins, surrounding the testes and epididymis, the pampiniform plexus, which is thought to act as a heat exchanger, and keep the testes cool, thus allowing spermatogenesis.

As mentioned earlier, each individual testis consists of an elongated tubule, which is lined by a germinal epithelial layer. Within the basement membrane of this epithelium are found two distinct types of cells. The first are germinal cells (so-called spermatogonia) which continually differentiate into spermatocytes (primitive sperm) and the second 'Sertoli' (or mother) cells. Sertoli cells are polymorphic, and attached to the basement membrane of the tubule, but actually extend into the tubule lumen. They are sometimes called 'mother' cells because they seem to have a role in the nutrition and nourishment of the developing germ cells (they may also have a phagocytic function). Just internal to the basement membrane, the Sertoli cells are joined together by junctional points that effectively form a blood–testis barrier. This barrier is important, because the sperm and developing cells produce surface antigens that are recognised as foreign by the immune system. Thus, this barrier prevents the initiation of an immune response against such antigens by effectively isolating the cells from the bloodstream (Tortora and Anagnostakos, 1990).

The process of sperm maturation (via a process of differentiation, which involves two separate meiotic divisions) takes approximately 70 days to occur. However, mature spermatozoa are produced at an incredible rate, resulting in a sperm concentration of 60–100 million sperm per ml of semen, in healthy males.

Figures 1.19 and 1.20 show a cross-section of such a seminiferous tubule, alongside the microscopic structure of the testis.

A third type of cell, which indirectly facilitates the process of spermatogenesis, is the Leydig cell which is found within the connective tissue surrounding the testes. Leydig cells (sometimes called interstitial cells) are responsible for the storage and

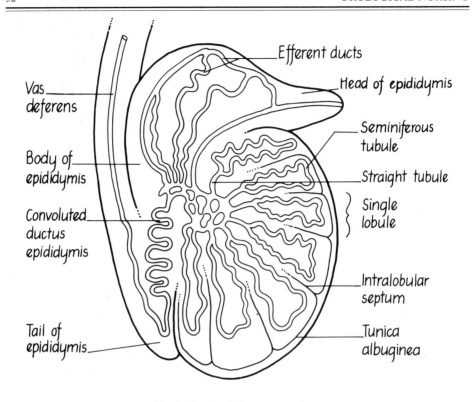

Vas deferens

Body of epididymis

Convoluted ductus epididymis

Tail of epididymis

Efferent ducts

Head of epididymis

Seminiferous tubule

Straight tubule

Single lobule

Intralobular septum

Tunica albuginea

Fig 1.19   Testis in cross-section

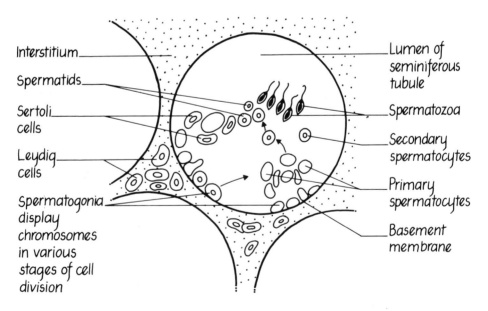

Interstitium

Spermatids

Sertoli cells

Leydig cells

Spermatogonia display chromosomes in various stages of cell division

Lumen of seminiferous tubule

Spermatozoa

Secondary spermatocytes

Primary spermatocytes

Basement membrane

Fig 1.20   Microscopic structure of the testis, showing cross-section of a seminiferous tubule

synthesis of testosterone. Thus, the Leydig cells actually control overall sperm production and testicular viability, as both of these processes are reliant upon a sufficient concentration of circulating androgen.

THE PENIS

The penis (male sexual organ) consists of three spongy sacs, two above and dorsal to the penile urethra (the corpora cavernosa) and one in the lower part of the penis, surrounding the urethra (the corpus spongiosum). The three corpora act as distensible storage reservoirs for blood, and are surrounded by a tough, rigid connective tissue layer, the Buck's fascia. The two reservoirs of the corpora cavernosa are able to intercommunicate, in terms of blood flow, but the corpus spongiosum is separate. The 'storage' property of the corpora allows them to fill with blood, so markedly increasing their rigidity (they are normally flaccid structures) and resulting in a state of erection, as shown in Figure 1.21.

As might be expected, relying upon such a mechanism for erection, the penis is highly vascular, and each corpus cavernosum possesses a large artery, running down the centre of its length. The corpus spongiosum also has two further arteries and the overall penile blood supply is further augmented by a variety of smaller arteries. The penis also possesses several veins, which provide an exit route for the blood.

The structure of the penis is shown in Figure 1.22. The head of the glans penis, upon which the urethra opens to the externa, is usually covered by a layer of loose fitting skin, the so-called prepuce or foreskin. This is often removed during the

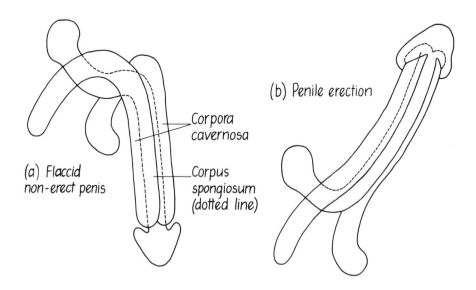

Fig 1.21 Penile structure and associated changes on erection

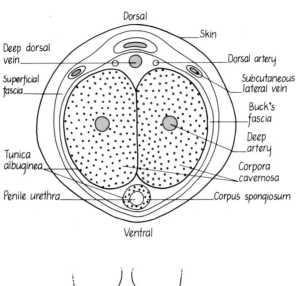

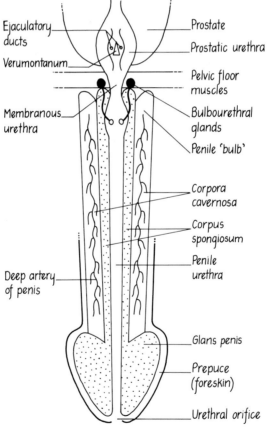

Fig 1.22 (a) Tranverse section through the penis. (b) Longitudinal section through the penis

procedure of circumcision. However, the foreskin is also extremely useful as a source of material for urethral reconstruction, should such a procedure be necessary (e.g. following possible urethral trauma). Normally, at rest, blood is shunted away from the penile veins, thus bypassing the corpora. However, during the process of erection, these shunts are closed, so channelling blood directly into the spongy reservoirs of each corpus. The shunts seem to be controlled by the parasympathetic nervous system, via neurones within the pelvic cavity. Thus, surgery low down within the pelvis, pelvic fracture or other lower abdominal trauma (or autonomic nervous lesions) may damage these nerves, and prevent adequate erection. Further, lesions to the actual vessels supplying the penile blood supply (e.g. as seen in diabetes or other vascular diseases) or a poor volume of blood supply will also adversely affect the ability of an individual to produce and sustain an adequate erection. In health, once erection is no longer desirable, the penis normally decompresses, by the shunts reopening, thus preventing further intake of arterial blood, and allowing the contents of the corpora to drain into the venous circulation.

As mentioned earlier, ejaculation is a further highly complex aspect of physiology. During sexual excitation, the seminal vesicles secrete a mucoid fluid, and significantly enlarge in size. As orgasm occurs, sperm stored within the vas deferens are expelled by muscular contraction (a process innervated via the α-adrenergic muscle fibres). Contraction of the seminal vesicles also occurs, so washing the spermatozoa outward with the rest of the ejaculate.

Clearly, therefore, ejaculation relies upon an intact bladder neck, which then prevents retrograde flow of semen.

References

Berne MR and Levy MN (1990) *Principles of Physiology*. St Louis: Wolfe.
Blandy JP (1992) *Lecture Notes on Urology*, 4th edn. Oxford: Blackwell Scientific Publications.
Bullock N, Sibley G and Whitaker R (1991) *Essential Urology*. Edinburgh: Churchill Livingstone.
Guyton AC (1991) *Textbook of Medical Physiology*, 8th edn. Philadelphia: WB Saunders.
Stanton BA and Koeppen BM (1990) *Elements of Renal Function*. In: Berne MR and Levy MN *Principles of Physiology*. St Louis: Wolfe.
Tortora GJ and Anagnostakos NP (1990) *Principles of Anatomy and Physiology*, 6th edn. New York: Harper and Row.

2

Urological Investigations

INTRODUCTION

The purpose of this chapter is to outline the common investigations which play an essential role in attempting to discover why a patient is presenting with a particular urological problem.

Technology has changed much over the previous decade, and there are now a variety of new investigative methods which can yield a great deal of information regarding the urinary tract and its function. However, there also still exist a number of other investigations which have been of benefit for many years, and which provide a valuable source of urological information (e.g. IVU intravenous urogram).

For each investigation considered, a description of the method and its underlying principle(s) is given, along with indications for use. Further information pertinent to specific patient preparation and patient teaching is given, followed by nursing care post-procedure and possible complications.

URINALYSIS

Urinalysis is a single, non-intrusive test, which can yield a great deal of information regarding renal and urinary function. Using chemically impregnated squares (e.g. Multistix), in combination with visual examination (and colour), a comprehensive urinary examination is possible.

Five factors are particularly useful, in relation to the urinary tract. These are as follows.

Urinary pH

Normal urinary pH should fall between the range 4–8 pH units, and this wide range underlines the role of the kidney in acid–base regulation (i.e. an acid or alkaline urine can be produced, according to bodily requirement). However, prolonged alkalinity of urine may well be an indication of urinary tract infection.

Certain organisms (bacteria) contain the enzyme urease, and are able to 'split' the urea molecules within urine, so releasing ammonium which causes the increased, alkaline pH. Such infection is commonly caused by *Proteus* sp., or other gram-negative bacilli.

Protein

The kidney normally excretes up to 200 mg of protein per day but this small amount remains undetected by routine urinalysis. However, significantly larger amounts than this will provide a positive urinary Multistix test result.

Such proteinuria may be an indication of urinary infection, or, more seriously, of a kidney which is 'leaking' protein, as a result of some form of underlying disease process (e.g. glomerulonephritis). In either case further investigation is likely to be required. Proteinuria can be a misleading finding in women, as the positive test result may arise from vaginal cells, shed into the urine, rather than from an infection.

Blood

The urinary Multistix test for blood is extremely sensitive, and may well prove positive in healthy individuals, due to the detection of very small numbers of red blood cells. This test has been responsible for a significant increase in patient referral for urological investigation as a result of routine urinalysis during medical examinations for insurance or pre-employment screening. In the vast majority of such cases, no underlying disease process is found.

Clearly, however, haematuria (blood in the urine) may be highly significant and may point to an underlying urinary tract infection (with an inflamed mucosal lining, which then loses red blood cells and leucocytes), stones within the kidney or urinary tract, a bleeding disorder or a more sinister condition such as urological cancer.

It is commonplace to find haematuria following instrumentation of the urinary tract or in patients with indwelling urethral or suprapubic catheters. Also, haematuria in females is often seen as a result of menstrual blood loss.

Leucocytes

The newer urinalysis reagent strips allow one to assay, at ward level, for leucocyte esterase, an enzyme found within white blood cells. A positive leucocyte assay is extremely reliable for the detection of white cells, which are usually present in the urine as a result of urinary tract infection (i.e. an increased leucocyte excretion correlates well with urinary tract infection, see for example Stevens, 1989 and Lowe, 1985).

However, a positive test for leucocytes does not necessarily imply a significant infection; rather, that a urinary pathogen is present (e.g. some patients may have organisms and white cells in their urine, but also may be asymptomatic and thus require no treatment).

Nitrites

Many organisms, especially gram-negative bacilli, are able to reduce nitrate to nitrite, as a result of a specific metabolic pathway within their cells. Thus, a positive nitrite assay, using Multistix, is indicative of a urinary infection but, again, does not necessarily indicate 'significance'.

In combination with a positive leucocyte assay, a positive nitrite result is extremely indicative of infection in the urine (Stevens, 1989, Lowe, 1985 and Hiscoke et al, 1990). Conversely, a negative nitrate and leucocyte result is approximately 97 per cent reliable in excluding the presence of urinary infection and thus provides a most useful way of screening urine at ward level for such infection (Stevens, 1989, Lowe, 1985). This provides an effective emergency diagnostic screen, or a routine screen for patients on admission.

URINARY MICROSCOPY

Microscopy of urine is an underused and inexpensive test, which involves simple urinary examination under a bright field or by use of phase contrast microscopy (to enhance the background and therefore make visualisation of bacteria easier). Centrifugation (as an attempt to concentrate the bacterial cells) is also used, but is both tedious to perform and inconvenient.

Bacteria can be seen in stained preparations of 90 per cent of specimens containing $> 10^5$ organisms (or colony-forming units per ml). An additional Gram stain also allows the morphology and staining reaction to be determined and therefore provides a useful guide to initial antimicrobial therapy, if required. Jenkins (cited in Stevens, 1989) carried out a review of urinary examination using this method, and concluded that stained, centrifuged urine provides the most sensitive screening test, and that unstained, uncentrifuged urine, which is most commonly used, is much less reliable.

Microscopic examination for pyuria (leucocytes in the urine) also provides an effective method for distinguishing between established urinary infection and simple contamination of the specimen. Greater than 10 leucocytes per ml of urine correlates well with established urinary tract infection.

Examination of the 'sediment', following centrifugation, may also show evidence of casts or crystals. The term 'casts' refers to the 'squeezed out' contents of the collecting tubules of individual nephrons, amd may be either *clear* or *granular* in nature.

Clear or hyaline casts are made of protein, whereas granular casts are formed either from red blood cells or leucocytes, or from a mixture of the two. Casts are commonly found in urine as a result of infection (e.g. pyelonephritis), or in renal diseases such as glomerulonephritis, or following either nephrotoxic or ischaemic lesions, which cause damage to the glomerular basement membrane, and thus allow 'leakage' of large cells, such as leucocytes, which is clearly abnormal. Crystals are commonly found in the urine of patients with renal stones, and are very characteristic of the type of material causing the stone. For example, calcium oxalate crystals are octahedral, cystine crystals hexagonal, and calcium ammonium phosphate stones (so called triple, or infection stones) square. Thus the shape of the crystal is very useful in terms of diagnosis.

In cases of infection with organisms such as *Schistosoma*, ova may be seen on microscopy, especially in an early morning specimen of urine.

Early Morning Urine (EMU)

EMU collection and examination is a further useful microscopic technique, especially when tuberculosis or cancer of the urinary tract is suspected. The principle here is that urine produced first thing in the morning is likely to be the most concentrated (due to increased ADH secretion at night, and the decreased fluid intake) and there is therefore a greater chance of finding either organisms or malignant cells.

Further, the urinary volume is generally smaller, and has been collected over a prolonged period (8–10 hours). The tubercule bacillus will not grow on ordinary culture media, but an EMU can be centrifuged and the sediment then stained using a Ziehl–Neelsen stain, which penetrates the lipid outer layer of the bacteria, which prevents the uptake of more common bacterial stains.

If cancer is suspected, the EMU should be voided into a fresh bottle containing 10 per cent formalin, which then 'fixes' any malignant cells, preventing their breakdown. The urine is then centrifuged and stained using a Pap stain, whereby malignant cells can be readily distinguished, if present.

URINARY CULTURE

Urinary culture is a very useful investigation, if infection is suspected, and involves plating out part of the specimen on to a nutrient medium, which is then incubated for 12–24 hours. A small paper inlay is often used, on top of the Petri dish of inoculated culture medium, which is impregnated with a range of antibiotics. Any organism present therefore grows over the surface of the culture plate, in direct contact with a range of antibiotic agents. This allows, when the plate is later examined, the sensitivity of any organism present to be determined, as far less growth (or no growth) will be seen in the areas of antibiotics to which the organism is sensitive. The colony can also be stained, and the causative pathogen then identified.

As urine is such an effective growth medium for microbes, urine specimens must be obtained with as few contaminents as possible (e.g. bacteria from the prepuce or vulva, or dust from the surrounding environment) and then kept at room temperature for as little time as possible, prior to plating out in the laboratory. At room temperature, any contaminent inoculated into the specimen at the time of collection will grow very rapidly and therefore invalidate the laboratory culture. Therefore, if a specimen cannot be sent to the laboratory at once, it should be refrigerated.

An estimation which can be performed within the laboratory is that of establishing the number of individual colonies from a given specimen which can then give a figure for the number of colony-forming units (CFU) per ml of urine. (Thus, a CFU can be either a single cell, or a group of identical cells.) It is normally taken that $> 10^5$ CFU/ml constitutes a significant urinary tract infection, which will then require medical treatment.

However, work by Stevens (1989) has shown that this figure is not completely reliable, although it has remained unchallenged for many years. The figure of 10^5 CFU/ml arose from work originally carried out by Kass (1957), who attempted to establish a diagnosis of urinary tract infection (UTI) by means of examining the number of bacteria found within early morning 'clean catch' specimens. However, Kass considered no other evidence of UTI at all, and thus, sadly, many urologists and nurses hold the 10^5 figure as sacrosanct, even though 'significant' symptomatic urinary tract infection may be associated with lower numbers of bacteria.

For example, Roberts (1986) found that 18 per cent of patients with UTI, in conjunction with bacteraemia, had counts of less than 10^5 CFU/ml, and similar results were reported by Strand et al (1985). Further, these patients had serious, life-threatening urinary infections, yet the 10^5 figure would deem such infections as insignificant, which is clearly ridiculous.

Catheterised patients may also have a lower number of organisms per ml of urine, yet still have symptomatic and often dangerous urinary infection (Kellogg et al, 1987).

Overall, the 10^5 figure is extremely useful, and used very widely, but it does need to be seen within the context of Kass' original study. It seems more valid therefore, to categorise a urinary infection as significant if it is causing adverse symptoms for the patient.

SPECIMENS FOR CULTURE

Urinary specimens for culture can be obtained in the following ways.

1. *Midstream urine specimen (MSU)* Here, the patient is asked to clean the prepuce or vulva area with a suitable topical agent (e.g. chlorhexidine or normal saline), and then void into a jug or other receptacle. The middle portion of the void is then collected into a sterile container, as this is less likely to be contaminated.

However, MSUs have a high rate of contamination, which would seem to indicate that many patients fail to understand what is required, or how to collect the specimen in the required manner. Also, a number of researchers have now cast considerable doubt upon the efficacy of pre-cleansing with such 'sterile' precautions prior to obtaining an MSU specimen (Morris et al 1979, Brown et al 1991, Immergut et al 1981).

2. *Catheter stream urine* Here, a sterile needle and syringe can be used to puncture the sample port in the catheter tubing (with or without a clamp) and between 1 and 2 ml of urine are then removed. This is placed within a sterile container, and sent to the laboratory for culture.

3. *Suprapubic aspiration* This is a quick and easy method to obtain a urine specimen for culture, but needs to be performed by a competent practitioner. A sterile needle is inserted through the anterior abdominal wall, into the bladder, and a specimen of urine then removed.

24-HOUR URINE SAVE

This is a simple yet important investigation, because it allows an assessment to be made of the 24-hour urinary excretion of a variety of key metabolites (e.g. Na^+, K^+, CA^{2+}, PO_4^{3-}, protein, creatinine, urinary catecholamines). The patient is first asked to void down the lavatory (generally, this is first thing in the morning, after waking) and this is taken as time zero. All subsequent voids are then collected, over the next 24-hour period.

The nature of the collecting vessel varies (e.g. plastic, glass) according to the specific assay being undertaken. Also, the vessel may or may not contain a variety of different preservatives.

URINARY CLEARANCE ESTIMATION

An important calculation that can be made from a 24-hour urine save is *renal clearance*. The concept of clearance is very widely utilised, as it provides a reliable estimation of overall renal function. The clearance value obtained is an expression of the theoretical volume of plasma that the kidney(s) are capable of clearing ('cleansing') of a designated substance, during one minute. Thus, the substance is present within blood, and filtered by the nephron as it passes through the renal vasculature.

Clearly, therefore, the degree of intact renal function will be reflected in how much substance is filtered, or, put another way, how many ml plasma/min are effectively *cleared* of the chosen urinary metabolite. The method relies on collecting all urine passed for a given 24-hour period and also taking a specimen of venous blood, during that period.

The urinary metabolite normally used for estimation of renal clearance is creatinine, a breakdown product of muscle metabolism (hence, this investigation is often called creatinine clearance). For clearance to be accurate, the substance passing through the kidney must pass unchanged (i.e. none must be reabsorbed into blood, via the tubules, nor any excreted from the tubules into the tubular fluid).

Creatinine, although widely used for renal clearance estimation, is not totally unchanged by the tubule. Some is actually excreted by the distal tubule, but as this is not a large amount, compared with overall creatinine excretion, it is insufficient to undermine the validity of the test. Conversely, because glucose is totally absorbed by the proximal tubule in healthy individuals, it cannot be used for calculating urinary clearance.

Urea is also not particularly effective, as its daily urinary excretion varies greatly, according to liver function, protein intake and nutritional status. It is more effective if the urea excretion over a prolonged period is estimated and compared with changes in glomerular filtration rate.

One of the most accurate substances for calculating renal clearance is the polyhydric alcohol inulin, which is freely filtered without any absorption or excretion. Thus a very close estimation of GFR is possible, but the disadvantage of inulin is its high cost, and it is for this reason that inulin is not widely used. The normal clearance figure for creatinine or inulin is dependent upon age, as renal function progressively deteriorates with advancing years, due to loss of nephrons, and/or disruption to the renal blood flow.

For a young, fit individual, a normal clearance figure is approximately 125 ml/min. Thus around 10 per cent of the effective plasma flow per minute, through the kidney, is actually 'cleared' of unwanted metabolites, such as creatinine. By the age of 70 years, the normal clearance figure has fallen to approximately 60–70 ml/min.

Clearance is calculated using the following formula:

$$\text{Clearance} = \frac{u \times v}{P}$$

where u is the urinary concentration of designated metabolite per 24 hours; v is the volume of urine passed during the 24-hour period; and P is the plasma concentration of designated metabolite. Renal clearance is therefore an inexpensive and very useful investigation, which causes minimal inconvenience to the patient, requiring only one blood specimen and the collection of urine for 24 hours.

BLOOD ASSAY

Blood assay is clearly a crucial part of the investigative process for the urological patient.

Table 2.1 illustrates some of the more important plasma constituents, relevant to urology, which can be directly estimated via venous blood sampling.

RADIOLOGICAL INVESTIGATIONS OF THE URINARY TRACT

Investigations which utilise imaging via X-ray, using either plain film or radio-opaque contrast dyes, form a large component of diagnostic assessment of the urinary tract. There are also now a number of newer, more advanced methods, which are described later in the chapter.

Plain Abdominal Film

This has limited use, as the normal plain film does not include the bladder. A kidney, ureter, bladder (KUB) film is of much greater value (see below).

Table 2.1   Possible diagnostic significance of plasma constituents

Plasma constituent	Possible diagnostic significance
Haemoglobin	Reduced in anaemia, severe haematuria, urological/renal cancer Glomerulonephritis
White blood cells	May be raised in cases of UTI, pyelonephritis, glomerulonephritis, tuberculosis, or cancer
Creatinine	May be raised in renal impairment or failure
Potassium (K^+)	Relates directly to level of renal function
Sodium (Na^+)	Relates to renal function. Raised levels may also be indicative of dehydration
Calcium (Ca^{2+})	High levels correlate closely to stone formation (either due to enzyme deficiency, or a high calcium diet)
Phosphate (PO_4^{3-})	Raised in patients with renal impairment or failure
Plasma proteins (e.g. albumin, globulin)	May be severely reduced in renal disease (e.g. glomerulonephritis) or in cases of malnutrition
Prostatic specific antigen	Significantly raised in cases of prostate carcinoma. Is a more reliable screen than acid phosphatase.
Tumour markers (e.g. human chorionic gonadotrophin, α-fetoprotein)	Allow determination of metastatic tumour spread, and provide a reliable means of assessing response to treatment

Kidney, Ureter, Bladder (KUB) Film

A KUB film is an X-ray of the kidneys, ureters, and bony pelvis, taken from both anterior and posterior aspects, without the use of contrast media. The patient is normally in the standing position, though, if only able to lay supine, then a single X-ray film of the anterior view is taken.

Indications

A KUB film is used to screen for renal calculi, in symptomatic patients, where a stone is suspected. However, not all stones are radio-opaque. KUB is also used prior to intravenous urogram (see below), or prior to endoscopic stone removal, as a final check on the presence and location of the stone.

Information

A KUB film can readily demonstrate both of the renal outlines (shadows), thus providing an estimation of the number, size and position of the kidneys. It is also possible to observe the psoas muscle shadows, bony pelvis and spinal column, and thus look for evidence of bony decalcification or damage, caused by metastatic spread from either bladder or prostatic carcinoma.

A KUB will also demonstrate radio-opaque calculi, such as calcium stones, but may not display radiolucent stones, or very small radio-opaque calculi.

Patient Preparation

Patient preparation is minimal, as the procedure is quick and painless. However, an explanation of the procedure is clearly necessary, particularly as a KUB film may also form part of a more complex investigation.

Intravenous Urogram (IVU)

An intravenous urogram is one of the 'mainstay' urological investigations, and is commonly performed on an out-patient basis. It is wrongly referred to as an IVP (intravenous pyelogram), as it visualises far more than just the renal pelvis, and also may then become confused with the completely separate pyelogram investigation.

The effectiveness of an IVU, within urological investigation, lies in the fact that it is able to image the entire urinary tract, including the urethra (although it is seldom used to do this, as an urethrogram provides a far superior method for looking at the urethra). An IVU consists of a series of X-ray films, which utilise a renally excreted contrast medium to enhance the morphology of the urinary tract, as the contrast passes from kidney to bladder. Thus, detailed information can be obtained regarding the kidneys (number, position, size), the ureters (e.g. number, possible obstruction or duplex systems, carcinoma or retroperitoneal fibrosis) and the bladder (e.g. size, capacity, space-occupying lesions).

The process of urinary transport from kidney to bladder is evaluated using a series of sequential films, at set intervals of time following the intravenous injection of the contrast medium. The contrast chosen is usually based upon the compound benzoic acid, and contains iodine atoms bonded to the ring structure of the benzoic acid molecule. Thus, the contrast contains virtually no 'free' iodine. The dosages administered vary, depending upon the individual patient (e.g. a patient with very poor renal function will require far more contrast, as the rate of renal excretion is so much lower).

Dosages are categorised as low, medium and high. A suitable adult dose is approximately 1 ml/kg body weight, of most commercially available preparations. In the case of children, an intravenous contrast medium of lower strength is used, as this exerts less influence upon both blood volume and red blood cells. The dose is given over 2–3 minutes, so that there is no sudden shift of fluid between body compartments. The contrast takes approximately 15–20 seconds to begin to reach the kidneys and the renal parenchyma.

Indicators

An IVU is performed on a wide variety of patients, particularly where an underlying structural abnormality is thought to be present within the urinary tract. IVU is thus a valuable investigation in cases of renal calculi, urinary calculi, recurrent urinary tract infection or pyelonephritis, haematuria, suspected space-occupying lesions within the kidney, suspected urinary malignancy, urinary obstruction (e.g. prostatic hypertrophy causing outflow obstruction) or in cases of congenital abnormality (e.g. ureteric reflux, where renal damage is suspected).

IVU, because it uses an intravenous, iodine band contrast reagent, is clearly contraindicated in patients who are allergic to iodine. IVU should also be performed with care in patients who have renal impairment of any sort, or who are suffering from either multiple myeloma or diabetes mellitus. In all these patient groups, excessive dehydration could result in further renal damage, and renal failure.

IVU consists of the following films.

1. *Pre-contrast KUB*   This acts as a control film, and will illustrate any opacities such as stones or other areas of tissue calcification.

2. *Immediate film (nephrogram)*   This is taken as an anterior–posterior view of the kidneys.

The film is taken 10–15 seconds after the injection of the intravenous contrast, the time delay reflecting the 'arm-to-kidney' transit time. The film aims to show the nephrogram, which consists of the renal parenchyma enhanced by contrast medium within the proximal tubules of the nephrons. The nephrogram film is dependent upon water absorption from the contrast.

The nephrogram displays the presence of more than one kidney, and particularly demonstrates the size and shape of the renal outlines, which allows assessment of any renal scarring. If excretion from either kidney is delayed, due to tubular obstruction (e.g. from stones or other ureteric obstruction), or if circulation through the renal substance is reduced, then a much denser nephrogram may be seen, which lasts for several hours.

If there are confusing overlying shadows on the film, caused by gas within the bowel, or if calculi or cancer is suspected, then tomograms may be taken, to enhance the view. Here, a series of films focus on a single plane of the kidney, effectively giving views of 'slices' through the kidney.

3. *5-minute film (pyelogram phase)*   This is taken as an anterior–posterior view of the renal areas.

This film allows one to estimate whether the excretion of contrast from both kidneys is symmetrical, and also allows the technique to be modified if there has been poor initial opacification of the kidneys (thus, further contrast can be given, at this point, to increase the quality of the image).

Often, once the 5-minute film has been taken, a compression band (essentially a wide belt) is applied around the patient's abdomen midway between the anterior iliac spines, i.e. over the point at which the ureters cross the pelvic brim (Doyle et al 1989). The aim of this procedure is to occlude the drainage of contrast temporarily, down the ureters, thus resulting in more effective distension of the renal pelvis and calyces by the contrast medium and therefore an enhanced image, which may reveal more detail. Compression is not used at this stage in cases of:

● Recent abdominal surgery
● Renal trauma
● A suspected abdominal mass (which could bleed)
● A 5-minute film already displaying evidence of calyceal distension

4. *15–20-minute film*   This is an anterior–posterior view of the renal areas.

This film further displays the renal calyces and pelvis, showing further enhancement of the image as more contrast has, by this stage, been filtered.

Compression is released if adequate films have been obtained, and the contrast allowed to proceed down the ureters into the bladder, without impairment.

5. *Release film (30 minutes)*   This is taken supine, as an anterior–posterior view of the abdomen.

This film allows visualisation of the whole urinary tract, including the ureters and bladder, and will readily display evidence of ureteric obstruction or trauma, or space-occupying lesions within the bladder. In patients where abdominal compression is not utilised, this view is normally taken between 15 and 20 minutes after injection of contrast.

The 30-minute film is also useful in patients with urinary stomas, as it allows visualisation of the residual volume within the stomal cavity, as well as the internal lumen of the cavity (although a stomogram is more effective at doing this).

6. *Post-micturition film*   This is taken supine and aimed at the bladder approximately 5 cm above the level of the symphysis pubis.

The patient is asked to empty his/her bladder and, as soon as possible after this, the post-micturition film is taken, which then provides an assessment of contrast retained within the bladder. This correlates very well with the patient's residual urine volume, following normal voiding, and also displays the size of the bladder. It is thus a valuable film if obstruction is suspected, where one may also see a large, floppy overextended bladder, particularly if the outflow obstruction is of a chronic nature.

Bladder pathology, such as a space-occupying lesion, may also be seen more clearly on this film.

A further film may be taken of the urethra during voiding (a so-called voiding urethrogram), although this is not commonly performed, as a urethrogram is so much more effective (i.e. much greater opacification is obtained when the contrast is instilled via a retrograde approach).

Delayed IVU films may be required in cases of obstructive uropathy, where excretion is very slow, or in cases of poor renal function. Also, prone abdominal films (with the patient lying on his/her front) may also provide enhanced visualisation of the ureters.

In patients with renal impairment, it must be ensured that the patient's fluid intake is not restricted, as this may further compromise already poor renal function. The maximum possible dose of contrast is used, to compensate for the poor function and lack of fluid restriction. Further tomograms are normally taken during the nephrogram phase, to eliminate bone and gas shadows, and a delayed nephrogram and pyelogram film is often taken, between 6 and 12 hours later.

Care must be taken in patients with diabetes, or multiple myeloma, where it is also crucial that the patient is not dehydrated, so protecting the kidney from further damage. Thus, it is crucial that fluids are taken normally, post-IVU, to decrease any likelihood of dehydration.

One misnomer regarding IVU is that a 'dense' image implies 'good' renal function. This may not, in fact, be the case, and may actually reflect very poor function, in a kidney which filters contrast slowly (due to poor tubular function) and is then unable to excrete it. Hence, the contrast builds up within the renal parenchyma, providing a dense X-ray image. The same mechanism also occurs in cases of obstruction.

Information

An IVU can yield a great deal of information about the urinary tract, including the number, size and position of kidneys and ureters, evidence of renal or ureteric stones, or other obstructive lesions, the size and shape of the bladder, evidence of bladder neoplasm and pre- and post-micturition volume. For this reason (i.e. the wealth of information generated) IVU is commonly performed on patients with urological symptoms.

Patient Preparation

Patients must be screened for potential allergy to iodine-based intravenous contrast media. Usually the patient is given nil by mouth (NBM) for 4–6 hours prior to the procedure, as this helps prevent nausea and also enhances the images obtained (due to slower excretion). In cases where dehydration could be a problem (see previous sections) the patient should still be kept NBM (to avoid nausea or vomiting during the procedure), but hydrated via a peripheral intravenous infusion. In such patients, enhanced doses of contrast will need to be given due to the slower rate of excretion. Clearly, diabetics could not be kept NBM without some form of intravenous glucose and insulin regimen, combined with suitable hydration.

The other main component of patient preparation consists of adequate bowel preparation, as the X-ray images have to pass through the colon, to visualise the kidneys. As the bowel should be as empty as possible, some form of bowel preparation is required. This will depend upon the patient's age and tolerance, although the better this aspect of care, the more effective will be the films obtained.

Common purgative agents used, to clear faecal mass out of the colon, include Picolax, Dulcolax or castor oil, and vary between individual units. Such agents are usually given 12–24 hours prior to the procedure. If the patient is severely constipated, he or she may require an enema, but this is not ideal as it causes a lot of residual air to be withheld, so obscuring the kidneys and ureters.

With older, more frail patients, a far more 'gentle' regimen is preferable, with an acknowledgement that the films obtained will be of poorer quality.

Patient Information

Patients will obviously require a full explanation of the procedure.

IVU is performed with the patient lying down, on his/her back, and the contrast given via a single needle, as a bolus (a small initial dose is given first to assess any hypersensitivity reaction).

Patients must be warned regarding initial nausea, or a feeling of 'flushing' or warmth (which proceeds up the arm to the whole body, but lasts only 20–30 seconds) or an unpleasant 'metallic' taste, as the contrast is being given, all of which can be quite anxiety provoking, if the patient is unprepared. Also, patients should be told that a tight compression belt may be used to enhance the quality of the images obtained, and that, as a series of films is to be taken, they are likely to be in the radiology department for some time. The radiation exposure during IVU is approximately three to four times that of a single chest radiograph.

The major complication of IVU relates to hypersensitivity reactions. These can be rapid (within seconds) and life threatening, as they may include glossopharyngeal and tracheal oedema, or widespread vasodilation and cardiac arrest. Over 20 per cent of patients experience some reaction to the dye, and the majority are trivial in nature (e.g. nausea, minor uriticaria). Severe reactions (e.g. circulatory collapse or bronchospasm) usually occur in the 5 minutes following injection and 90 per cent of such reactions occur within the first 15 minutes (Doyle et al 1989).

It is vital, therefore, that an IVU is only performed in a radiology suite where all resuscitation equipment (including equipment for intubation) and relevant drug therapy is available (e.g. adrenaline, antihistamines such as Piriton, hydrocortisone, plus oxygen).

Antegrade Urography

Antegrade urography may be utilised when other diagnostic methods (such as IVU, high-dosage IVU or tomograms) have failed to provide the information required concerning either a kidney or its ureter.

The pelvis of the kidney is located, commonly by use of ultrasound, and a fine bore needle then inserted through the skin and into the renal pelvis. A flexible, normally polythene cannula is then passed down the needle lumen into the pelvis, and the needle removed. This allows contrast to be injected directly into the renal pelvis via the cannula and a number of films are then taken, with the patient lying supine, prone or on his/her side.

Further, if previous intravenous urography has revealed what appears to be an obstructed ureter (i.e. a widened hydroureter) but there is uncertainty as to whether the ureter is actually obstructed, due to a secondary cause, or just swollen and oedematous, or has a functional obstruction (as in retroperitoneal fibrosis) where peristalsis is inhibited but the ureteric lumen is patent, then the indwelling cannula can be used to perform Whitaker's test.

Whitaker's test relies on the principle that, in an unobstructed ureter (or tube), fluid will flow *out* of the tube at the same rate as it flows into it. Thus, the patient is catheterised urethrally, and a nephrostomy cannula connected to an infusion pump which allows a *constant* flow of fluid into the renal pelvis. At the same time, the rate of fluid collection from the urinary catheter is measured.

If the two rates of flow are equal, then this indicates that no secondary cause of obstruction (e.g. a stone or cancer) is present, but that the patient has a swollen, dilated ureter or a functional obstruction (though this is much rarer).

The antegrade polythene cannula can also be left in place after the investigation if obstruction is diagnosed, or replaced with a wider-bore tube. Such an arrangement, which drains urine directly from the renal pelvis, is known as nephrostomy, and provides a simple and effective method of decompressing an obstructed kidney, which will sustain damage and loss of nephrons all the time that an outflow obstruction is present. Release of such obstruction is crucial, if renal function is to be preserved.

If cancer is suspected, antegrade cannulation of the pelvis should be carried out with care, as it is possible to cause spread of tumour cells, especially if significant haemorrhage is caused. However, fluid samples can be taken from the renal pelvis and sent for cytological examination, which is clearly useful.

Information

Antegrade urography can thus yield valuable information regarding renal size and also the integrity of the calyces, renal pelvis, pelviureteric junction and ureter. It can also demonstrate the presence of tumours (or other obstructive lesions) in any one of these locations and can be used to relieve outflow obstruction, via nephrostomy.

Patient Preparation/Information

The patient should be given nil by mouth for 3–4 hours prior to the procedure.

Antegrade urography is carried out in the radiology department, usually via ultrasound or X-ray image intensification (i.e. low-dose radiography). The patient is asked to lie on the opposite side to the kidney under investigation, and the skin is then prepared with iodine or another suitable reagent. The kidney is then visualised, and the point of entry marked on the skin. A small incision is then made, and the metal cannula inserted into the renal pelvis (using guidance via ultrasound or radiography). Therefore, patients require a full explanation of the procedure, and consent must also be obtained for nephrostomy insertion, if this is planned.

As an iodine-based contrast is used, the patient must have no sensitivity to iodine and, again, equipment for treating any hypersensitivity reaction must be present.

The affected side, over the kidney area, should be shaved if hair is present and some form of oral premedication can be given if the patient is particularly nervous.

The patient will return from the procedure with a cannula or nephrostomy tube sutured in place (with a suitable dressing) and connected to a drainage bag and tubing, if the kidney is found to be obstructed. Analgesia will usually be required after the procedure, and can be given as either an oral or intramuscular preparation.

Renal Arteriogram/Angiography

A renal arteriogram is a highly invasive investigation, involving direct cannulation of the renal artery and a high-speed series of X-ray films which allow detailed examination of the arterial supply of both kidneys.

Angiography is performed under local anaesthetic, but often with some sedation. The patient is taken to the radiology department, and a radio-opaque catheter is inserted into the femoral artery, after suitable skin preparation and the administration of a local anaesthetic. Once the artery has been cannulated, the catheter is threaded into the abdominal aorta and from there to the renal artery. The catheter, once in position, is connected to a 50 ml syringe, located within a powerful syringe driver, capable of emptying the syringe over a very short time (typically 2–5 seconds).

When ready, the machine is activated and simultaneously a series of films is automatically taken, at pre-set intervals, as the contrast is infused. (The technique uses a rapid serial film changer and is thus known as serial radiography.) The first films are taken over the initial 2–4 seconds following injection, and allow visualisation of the renal arteries (e.g. interlobar and arcuate arteries). A normal regimen is two per second for 2 seconds, and one per second for the next 5 seconds. A second series of films is then taken during the 5–10 second period and again at 15–20 seconds. These films provide visualisation of the renal substance. The venous phase follows, but is more limited in the amount of information that can be obtained.

Information

Renal angiography allows one to look for evidence of renal artery stenosis (in hypertensive patients) or tumour or to investigate the nature of a space-occupying lesion within the renal substance, as cancers will have their own 'corrupted' blood supply, which is very different from the normal architecture of the kidney. Angiography is also be undertaken prior to live donor-related transplanation, as it is crucial to know how many branches there are from the renal arteries to each kidney and where these branches are prior to attempting donor nephrectomy.

Some individuals possess a congenital abnormality which manifests as an increased number of arterial branches and therefore such a kidney would not be removed, because of the risk of severe haemorrhage.

Arteriography may also be undertaken following renal trauma if a laceration or contusion of the kidney is suspected.

Digital subtraction angiography is a refinement of the above technique, and utilises a computer to subtract images of surrounding tissues.

Patient Preparation/Teaching

Clearly, any allergy to iodine-bound contrast media is contraindicated. Because of the invasive nature of the investigation, the patient may be anxious and should be given a full explanation of the procedure. As the contrast is injected, patients often feel transient though significant discomfort (e.g. 'flushing' which spreads all over the body and/or acute nausea) and they should be prepared for this.

Patients are kept NBM for 4–6 hours, and given a suitable premedication as sedation. The groin is shaved in the radiology department and, following the procedure, it is essential to observe for haemorrhage from the cannulation site (which constitutes an arterial puncture, into a large and high-pressure vessel) and also for any allergic reactions (e.g. dyspnoea) from the contrast used. The patient will normally be kept on bed rest for 8–12 hours or longer if any oozing is seen from the puncture site.

Pedal pulses and nailbed flush are assessed every 30–60 minutes, at least for the first 12 hours, and a pressure dressing kept in situ (this is normally removed 48 hours later). It is normal for a large bruise to occur and a haematoma may also form, which should resolve spontaneously.

Renal Venogram

Taking a renal venogram is very similar to angiography in method, except that cannulation is carried out via the right femoral vein, and the catheter is then advanced to the opening of the left or right renal vein, as necessary. The image may be further enhanced by injecting adrenaline into the renal artery, thus delaying excretion of the contrast via the venous circulation, due to vasoconstriction within the kidney. Adrenaline is injected into the renal artery approximately 10 seconds after contrast is injected into the vein.

Venography is considered in cases of renal vascular hypertension, where blood may be sampled and assayed for plasma renin concentration. Venography may also be used in cases of renal vein thrombosis or where a renal mass or tumour is present. Here, injection of contrast into the vena cava may display loss of contour, caused by tumours spreading from the kidney into the renal vein and thus to the venae cavae.

Patient preparation and subsequent management are essentially the same as for angiography except that there is no need to assess pedal pulses following the procedure. However, both warmth and colour of the leg should be observed.

Retrograde Pyeloureterography

A retrograde pyelogram is a series of radiographs, taken either as distinct films or, more commonly, by the use of an image intensifier, with films taken of specific views. Retrograde pyelography thus provides detailed anatomical information regarding the ureter, any pelviureteric junction obstruction and the renal pelvis and calyces. The investigation is performed under general or epidural anaesthetic, with the patient in the lithotomy position. Patients are usually delivered to the radiography suite with the ureteric catheter in place.

Using a cystoscope, the surgeon identifies the ureteric orifice in question, and then proceeds in one of two ways.

The 'classic' approach is to insert a graduated ureteric catheter up the length of the ureter to the renal pelvis (in most adults this is a distance of 20–25 cm). Contrast can then be gently injected or else infused under gravity into the upper tract and X-ray films then taken of the renal pelvis and pelviureteric junction.

A more modern approach is the use of a bulb-ended catheter (e.g. a Prash bulb) which is used to seal the end of the ureter temporarily, prior to injection of contrast. This is particularly useful when ureteric catheterisation is not possible, and is less traumatic to the ureter, although pelvicalyceal filling may be incomplete, as filling occurs from the base of the ureter. The radiologist impacts the bulb against the ureteric orifice and 2–3 ml of contrast are slowly injected. As contrast runs up the ureter, image intensification may show the pelvis to be full of contrast or the presence of 'stones' or other space-occupying lesions.

Indications

Retrograde pyelography can be used in patients allergic to iodine-bound contrast media, or who have non-functioning kidneys which are incapable of concentrating and excreting contrast, and in whom no results are obtained with IVU. Patient preparation is minimal, and centres upon routine preoperative care. However, a full explanation of the procedure is clearly required, especially as the investigation is of an invasive nature.

Contraindications/Complications

Retrograde imaging must only be performed in patients who have a negative urinary screen prior to the procedure, as any significant urinary infection could easily be inoculated into the blood stream. Other possible complications include mucosal damage to the ureter and possible ureteric perforation (or perforation of the renal pelvis) by the catheter.

Occasionally, contrast may be absorbed and cause an allergic reaction, but the risk of such a reaction is far less than exists with excretion urography. Sterile pyelitis, caused by contrast stasis, and overdistension of the pelvis can also occur. Pyelonephritis as a result of instrumentation of the urinary tract is also possible and clearly more serious. Therefore, following the procedure the patient must be observed for loin pain, dysuria, fever or rigor, especially during the first 24–48 hours. Should such problems occur, aggressive treatment with urinary culture, intravenous antibiotics and fluids and appropriate analgesia is required.

Contrast extravasation is also possible, but temporary, as a water-based contrast is used, which is absorbed from the surrounding tissue space.

Cystogram

A cystogram is a complex investigation which involves radiographic examination of the bladder, using contrast media. It is normally performed as a single investigation (rather than as part of an IVU) when it is suspected that there may be a problem with urinary reflux into the ureters, from the bladder, upon voiding. Such reflux results from defective ureterovesical valves (which normally close upon voiding) and 'carries' urine which is commonly infected, upward to the renal pelvis and calyces, resulting in pyelonephritis and/or possible renal damage with scarring.

Usually a video film is taken, via image intensification, so that reflux from the bladder can actually be recorded as it occurs, thus avoiding the possibility of reflux being missed on a static film.

For a full description of the different types of cystogram, and typical patient profiles, please see Chapter 3.

Ascending Urethrogram

A urethrogram is a useful and commonly employed investigation which allows visualisation of the entire length of the male urethra. There are two methods to achieve this:

1. A *'viscous' contrast* is gently injected into the urethral meatus, via a syringe, and a penile clamp then applied to the glans. This provides an anatomical demonstration of the urethra and has the advantage of effecting greater urethral distension, thus enhancing the views obtained.

2. A *water-based contrast* is used, which is inserted into the urethra via a Foley catheter, positioned just inside the external penile meatus. The catheter balloon can be inflated with 1–2 ml of water after being inserted into the fossa navicularis. Use of a water-soluble contrast is good for demonstrating functional obstruction, but less urethral distension is obtained than with viscous contrast, and therefore the films obtained may not be as good.

Viscous contrast cannot be used with the catheter method because the pressure created within the urethra would dislodge the catheter.

A similar method can be used in women, if necessary, though it is far less common to visualise the female urethra.

The patient lies supine on the X-ray table, and three views are taken (supine, lateral and oblique), with the right leg abducted and the knee flexed. The same views are then taken for the left leg, with the left leg abducted and the knee flexed.

Chapman and Nakielny (1986) suggest that ascending urethrography should be followed by micturating cystourethrography or excretory micturating cystourethrography, to demonstrate the proximal urethra. Occasionally, it is only possible to see a urethral fistula or periurethral abscess on voiding examination, and reflux of contrast into dilated prostatic ducts is also better seen during micturition.

Information

The ascending urethrogram can yield valuable information regarding the anatomy of the urethra and will readily display abnormalities such as:

1. Urethral stricture
2. Urethral tear or false passage (e.g. following traumatic catheterisation)
3. Congenital abnormalities (e.g. urethral valves)
4. Periurethral or prostatic abscess
5. Fistulae or false passages

The urethrogram is contraindicated in urinary tract infection or following recent instrumentation.

Patient Preparation/Teaching

No specific preparation is required prior to urethrography but, clearly, adequate information should be given as the investigation may be uncomfortable, especially if a penile clamp is used. Also, it is potentially very embarrassing and the patient requires both support and a caring approach from staff.

Downagram

A downagram is a variation upon the ascending urethrogram, but is used following urethral surgery (e.g. for stricture repair) such as urethroplasty. A downagram is performed 10–14 days following surgery, to assess for urethral patency and thus healing, following the procedure. A water-based contrast is used, in case there is any leakage from the healing anastomosis.

Such patients usually have both a suprapubic and a urethral catheter in place and contrast is therefore inserted via the suprapubic catheter and allowed to drain out of the urethral stent catheter. The urethral stent is fenestrated and contrast therefore flows out of the holes, and around the catheter as well as down the catheter lumen. Thus the urethral outline can be visualised, and observation made of any extravasation of contrast into the soft tissues around the urethra. This would indicate that the anastomosis is not yet watertight, and therefore requires longer for healing.

An 'up and downagram' is a combination of both classic urethrogram (although without a clamp) and downagram. Clearly, any allergy to iodine-based contrast would be a contraindication but there is no specific patient preparation except adequate information and explanation.

Lymphangiogram

Lymphangiography is used much less frequently now, because of the availability of computer-assisted tomography, nuclear magnetic resonance scanning and ultrasound (see later sections for a description of these methods). Also, lymphangiography is very difficult to assess accurately (reliably) and the results obtained are often very poor.

For the technique, 2 ml of 1% lignocaine is mixed with 2 ml of 2.5% patent blue violet (a dye), and 0.5 ml of the mixture is then injected subcutaneously into each of the two medial web spaces of both feet. The feet are then exercised for 30–60 minutes until the lymphatics are visible on the dorsum of each foot.

Under local anaesthetic, a small incision is made over a lymphatic vessel, which is then cannulated and the needle secured with silk ties or suitable tape. The vessel is checked that it is not a vein, by aspiration, and the procedure then repeated for the other leg. An 'oily' contrast (10–20 ml in volume) is then inserted. Such 'oil'-based contrast media opacify both lymph nodes and vessels. The contrast fills up the lymphatics of the leg, lymph nodes in the groin and also the iliac and para-aortic nodes. Water-based contrast can also be used, but tends to opacify only the lymphatic vessels.

Indications

Lymphangiography is a lengthy investigation, used to look for abnormalities within lymph vessels caused by metastatic deposits or lymphoma (i.e. blockages) or filling defects in otherwise normal-looking lymph nodes. It was commonly used in cases of testicular cancer, for assessing tumour spread, although CT scanning and ultrasound are now far more effective and also have the advantage of being non-invasive.

Lymphangiography is not a good method for assessing spread of prostatic or bladder cancer and is also clearly unpleasant for the patient, particularly because it is time consuming and has a number of risks attached. Also the contrast ends up within the lung tissue, from where it is slowly absorbed; thus the technique is not advised if the patient has pre-existing respiratory disease.

Lymphangiography is also contraindicated in cases of active thrombophlebitis, localised sepsis or iodine sensitivity, and in patients who have had cytotoxic therapy. Small pulmonary emboli, caused by the oily contrast, produce fine 'pin-point' opacities on a 24-hour chest radiograph, but are normally asymptomatic. However, if a larger than normal volume of contrast reaches the pulmonary circulation, more significant pulmonary emboli may result.

If the patient is undergoing cytotoxic therapy, his/her lymph glands may be damaged and will therefore allow more contrast into the circulation. Systemic oil emboli are also possible, of which cerebral emboli are the most important. Also radiotherapy to the lung within 3 weeks of the procedure can disrupt the normal pulmonary architecture and therefore allow contrast into the systemic circulation.

Films are initially taken over the ankle (at 10 minutes), knees (15 minutes), thighs, AP pelvis and femora (30 minutes) and supine abdomen (at 40 minutes). Then a further supine abdominal film is taken every 15 minutes until the contrast reaches the level of the third lumbar vertebra (L3).

Two hours after injection, a PA chest film, supine abdominal film and AP of pelvis and upper femur are taken. These may be repeated for a 24-hour series, or as a delayed series up to 8 weeks later, to assess response to treatment.

Patient Preparation/Teaching

Adequate pre-procedure information and teaching are clearly important. If oedema of the ankles and/or legs is present, the limbs should be elevated for the preceding 24 hours, or a compression bandage applied, to help cannulation. Children may require a general anaesthetic, and the patient should empty his/her bladder prior to the start of the investigation.

The patient must also be told that his/her skin and urine may be blue for a few days following the test. After lymphangiography, the patient is kept in hospital overnight, and no general anaesthetic, radiotherapy or cytotoxic drugs should be given for at least 1 week. Sutures are removed 10 days later.

Patients should be observed for any allergic reaction or pulmonary problems and for any evidence of extravasation of contrast, infection or lymphangitis.

NON-INVASIVE INVESTIGATIONS OF THE URINARY TRACT

CT scanning and NMR provide two examples of much more recent investigative techniques which are non-invasive, yet provide a wealth of information regarding the structure of the kidney and lower urinary tract. The underlying principle of each method is completely different.

Computer-assisted Tomography (CT Scanning)

Computer-assisted tomography (CT scanning) has been used for approximately 10–15 years. It produces a much enhanced, high-resolution tomographic image, which provides films of 'slices' taken transversely at different levels through areas of the body (e.g. thorax, abdomen, head). For urological use, CT scanning is employed to provide computer-generated images of the abdomen, including the kidneys, ureters, bladder and renal blood vessels, and also the thorax, where metastatic spread of cancer to the lungs or para-aortic nodes may be present (e.g. in cases of testicular cancer, such as teratoma). CT scanning is also increasingly being utilised to search for enlarged lymph nodes, which again may be indicative of metastatic spread from a primary cancer. A CT scan provides an estimate of the densities of various tissues, which it calculates in Hounsfield units, named appropriately after the inventor of the machine. 'Normal' parenchymal tissues have a value of 80–100 units, bone + 1000 units, air –1000 units, fat –100 units and water zero.

Nuclear Magnetic Resonance (NMR) Imaging

NMR has many similarities in its methodology to CT scanning, but the image obtained is produced in a completely different way. Because the number of protons (positively charged particles, present in the nucleus of atoms) differs within living tissues of different types, each tissue creates a minute, but unique magnetic field, caused by the motion of the protons. Further, if exposed to a magnetic field of greater magnitude, then the protons within the cells align themselves along the direction (lines of force) of the stronger field at the lowest energy state possible (the 'ground' state). If the tissues under study are then exposed to a brief pulse of radio waves, due to the processes of interference and resonance a brief rise is seen in the energy state of the proton particles. When the radio waves are removed, this increase in energy from the ground state is lost, and the protons return to the ground state by the release of energy, in the form of electromagnetic radiation. It is this energy signal that NMR detects, and computer enhancement and processing allows images of the tissues under study to be produced.

Views can also be generated from sagittal, coronal and transaxial planes, which are more useful than transverse (sagittal) sections. NMR is not so effective, however, for detecting calculi or tissue calcification.

Indications

Generally, these are the same as for CT scanning (e.g. space-occupying lesions of the urinary tract or abdomen).

Contraindications

NMR is contraindicated in patients with pacemakers (because NMR may cause interference), or in patients with other metallic implants. Such implants should not be exposed to strong magnetic fields, especially if they are small (e.g. gut staples) because they may move during the procedure.

Patients who suffer from claustrophobia may also find the technique disturbing, as it generates the same 'closed in' feeling as does CT scanning.. This is because the person has to lie within a tube-like structure.

Patient Preparation/Teaching

As for CT, NMR requires careful preparation in terms of information and teaching, as the patient is required to lie still, within an enclosed space. The machine is again 'tube-like', and the patient lies supine on a table which then gradually advances into the detector. Patients with a history of claustrophobia, or who are confused, and young children may require sedation. Like CT, NMR is non-invasive and painless.

All metal objects such as rings, earrings, etc. must be removed prior to the procedure.

Ultrasound of the Urinary Tract

Ultrasound of the kidney and urinary tract is an investigation which has dramatically increased in diagnostic value over the past 10–15 years. It is entirely non-invasive, and a measure of its effectiveness and safety is indicated by the way in which it is used so widely in the monitoring of foetal growth and position during antenatal care. Ultrasonography uses a probe, which is placed upon the patient's skin, over the area to be imaged. The probe emits high-frequency sound waves (5–20 kHz) which enter the body and are reflected back off the organ being studied. The degree of reflection, as with any sound wave, is dependent upon the density of the surface acting as a reflector. Thus, dense structures such as bone reflect much more of the sound waves than would, say, a fluid-filled cyst or a hydronephrotic area of the kidney (or tumour mass).

The sound waves returning to the probe are detected, and fed to a computer, which analyses the difference between the sent and the returning signal and then constructs an image on a screen, which can be observed visually.

The equipment used is also able to take still photographs or moving film, as required. Since no radiation dose is involved, ultrasound offers many advantages. Multiple images can be obtained, from several angles, by moving the probe to different positions on the skin, over the area of interest. Further, the lack of radiation means that repeat studies are not dangerous, and can be carried out in any suitable room (i.e. an X-ray suite is not required).

Indications

Ultrasound is used in a variety of ways within urology. For example, suspected space-occupying lesions within the abdomen can be visualised and ultrasound study is very effective at distinguishing cystic structures from solid tumour. Also, ultrasound is used to locate urinary calculi, if a radio-translucent stone is suspected. This is particularly useful in patients with recurrent urinary tract infection, due to suspected stone disease, as there is no direct invasion of the urinary tract.

Ultrasound can also locate collections of fluid within the abdomen (e.g. subphrenic abscess, following nephrectomy) and will readily display liver metastases or invasion of cancer outside the bladder or kidney. (Ultrasound relies upon the differing densities between 'normal' and 'malignant' tissues.)

Ultrasound also plays an important role within radiology, where it is often used to pass guidewires etc., for example in nephrostomy.

A more recent urological application of ultrasound is in transrectal ultrasound, for the assessment of prostatic growth. Here, the patient is placed on his left side, with the legs drawn up toward the chest, and a rotating ultrasound probe, contained within a fluid-filled sac made of latex rubber (to prevent damage to the rectal mucosa) is placed within the rectum. The signals sent back allow a picture of the prostate to be obtained, any suspect areas to be assessed and exact sizes or volumes of tissue mass to be measured. Also, rectal ultrasound will display any invasion of tumour mass outside the prostatic capsule.

For routine renal ultrasound, images of the kidney, pelvis, ureters and bladder are obtained both supine and prone. A conducting jelly is placed on the skin, at the site of investigation, which prevents 'leakage' of sound waves (thus increasing picture quality) and both transverse and longitudinal images are obtained. The 'jelly' is removed with a tissue, once the investigation is completed. Ultrasound can thus image the renal substance and outline pyramids, calyces and pelvis as well as allow measurement of renal size. Also, any upper tract dilation or hydronephrosis can easily be seen, as these show up far darker due to absorption of the sound waves by the fluid. Stones within the urinary tract block transmission of sound waves almost completely.

Overall, ultrasonography of the urinary tract takes between 10 and 15 minutes to perform, with minimal patient discomfort. There are no contraindications, and bowel preparation is not required. Ultrasound can therefore be performed at short notice.

Patient Teaching

Explanation is clearly required and reassurance that ultrasound is simple, non-invasive and painless.

ISOTOPIC/RADIONUCLEOTIDE IMAGING OF THE KIDNEY
(RENAL SCANNING)

Isotopic/nuclear imaging of the kidney and urinary tract utilises a radioactive tracer molecule (e.g. ^{99}Tc) which is either bound to a substance freely filtered by the kidney (e.g. DTPA) or which is bound to a substance that binds directly to the tubular cells (i.e. is taken up and not filtered).

Thus, the first approach yields information regarding function of the kidney whereas the second is far more geared to providing information concerning the structure of the kidney. The radionucleotide (e.g. ^{99}Tc-EDTA) is injected intravenously, and its activity (or handling by the kidney) is then detected and measured by a computer-enhanced detection system, such as a gamma camera (sensitive to gamma radiation), which allows comparison between the kidneys to be made simultaneously.

A renal scan can thus provide very useful information regarding both structure and function of the kidney(s), as well as providing a quantitative comparison of renal function. Such functional information is given the generic term of renogram.

The approaches that may be used are shown in Table 2.2. The normal renogram, using a tracer substance, produces a graphical result, which can be divided into three phases. These are:

1. *Vascular phase*   This represents the uptake function of the kidney and will relate directly to renal blood flow: (0–2 minutes).

2. *Filtration phase*   This reflects the transport of the isotope from the nephron to the renal pelvis, and clearly will be prolonged if there is renal damage (e.g. acute tubular dysfunction from acute renal failure) or poor renal perfusion, when the renal blood flow is reduced: (2–6 minutes).

3. *Excretion phase*   This phase reflects the passage of the isotope from the renal pelvis down the ureter, and will clearly be lengthened by any pelviureteric junction or ureteric obstruction: (6–15 minutes). (Thus, the excretion phase will lengthen in hydronephrosis, caused by a ureteric stone, or in cases of a large, 'baggy' renal pelvis, or in cases of a tumour at the ureterovesical junction.)

Table 2.2   Methods of renal scanning

Name	Use
DTPA scan (renogram)	Differential renal function
	Suspected obstruction
	Assessment of single kidney function
DMSA scan	Differential function and detection of structural damage (e.g. cortical scarring)
Hippuran scan (renogram)	As for DTPA scan

Because some of the isotope is taken up by the soft tissues, it is normal to place an additional detector over an adjacent part of the loin, or arm, which measures the background uptake, and automatically subtracts this figure from the value obtained over the kidney.

^{99}Tc-DTPA (Technetium-99m Diethylenetriamine Penta-acetic Acid Scan)

^{99}Tc-DTPA is mainly excreted via glomerular filtration and can therefore be used to image kidneys, ureters and bladder. Its primary use is to assess any upper tract obstruction, although glomerular filtration rate and differential renal function may also be estimated.

Following an intravenous bolus injection, an initial film (similar to the nephrogram of an IVU) may be taken at 30 seconds, to provide an estimation of renal cortical blood flow. Subsequent pictures are then taken at 1, 5, 10, 15 and 20 minutes.

DTPA scanning provides more functional information than structural detail. Further, if pelviureteric junction (PUJ) or ureteric obstruction is suspected, radionucleotide washout can be imaged from each kidney, following the administration of an intravenous diuretic such as frusemide. If obstruction is present, a slower rate of removal or no removal of isotope will be seen. If a large, baggy, unobstructed pelvis is present, which is thought to be collecting urine and/or causing urinary tract infection, the use of intravenous diuretic will result in an increased excretion rate, and the baggy pelvis will be seen to empty.

^{99}Tc-DMSA (Technetium-99 Dimercaptosuccinic Acid Scan)

This mercurial compound is taken up and 'held' by the nephrons, where it binds to the basement membrane of proximal tubular cells.

It therefore allows evaluation of renal cortical structure. Following intravenous injection, it is usual to take a series of images, using a gamma camera, approximately 45–60 minutes later, and these will readily display any evidence of renal cysts, scarring or space-occupying lesions.

^{131}I-OIH (Iodine-131 Orthoiodohippurate)

This substance is excreted by both glomerular filtration and tubular excretion. It can yield the same information as DTPA, but emits far more gamma radiation (Brundage, 1992). Its use is therefore limited, but it may be of use where renal function is very poor and relatively little isotope is being filtered.

GFR via Isotopic Study

Radioactive tracer (isotope) can also be used to measure glomerular filtration rate, by accurately detecting and quantifying the clearance from blood or a designated tracer molecule. After the dosage is administered intravenously, serial measurements of vascular radioactivity are taken (over a 60-minute period) either by serial sampling or by the use of a counter placed over the forearm, which is less invasive. Isotopic GFR is especially useful in patients where a conventional 24-hour urine collection is hard to obtain, and has the advantage of being extremely accurate.

Bone Scan

A very useful, further application of radioisotope imaging is in screening for cancer of the prostate and bladder which may present with possible bony metastases. The specific investigation is called a bone scan, and normally uses ^{99}Tc-MDP (Tc-99 methylene diphosphonate).

This isotope is taken up by vascular areas of bone, and will readily detect bony metastases because the vascularity of such areas is increased, due to the higher metabolic rate. Metastatic deposits will therefore normally be observed before they are visible on conventional radiographs, by the use of isotopic imaging. Further, because of the low dosage of radiation, this investigation can be performed repeatedly over a prolonged period of time, to assess response to treatment.

Problematic, however, is that recent bony injury, or arthritic conditions or other degenerative changes, because they induce inflammation also increase vascularity within those bony areas affected, and thus will also display increased uptake of isotope. There is, therefore, a potential for false-positive results to be obtained, although, in the hands of a competent radiologist, this is unlikely, as such areas can be easily distinguished.

Further, these conditions also tend to occur within defined areas of the bony skeleton. Because spread of prostatic cancer is primarily to the bony pelvis, femurs and lower spine, a bone scan provides a very effective method for assessing tumour growth and patient response to treatment (Maisey et al, 1991). No specific patient preparation is required.

Contraindications of Imaging

Isotopic imaging is contraindicated during pregnancy, due to the emission of gamma radiation.

Patient Teaching/Nursing Care

Radioactive tracer substances are administered via intravenous injection, and therefore care of the site after the procedure is important, as irritation can result.

There is no other specific preparation, and no requirement for bowel preparation as gamma radiation will readily pass through the bowel, and any faecal material or gas. Also, the radiation dosage is significantly less than for an IVU, which is a great advantage of isotopic study, and the half-life of the tracer is only hours in length.

The patient's urine, following the procedure, should be disposed of in accordance with hospital policy. Clearly, because of the nature of the investigation, patients require careful explanation and information, particularly as the method will be more effective in a cooperative patient. Patients also need reassurance that the dose of radiation administered is very small.

DIRECT VISUALISATION METHODS

Direct visualisation of parts of the urinary tract rely upon the use of endoscopy, via a precision optical telescope containing an intrinsic light source (e.g. nephroscope, ureteroscope, cystoscope). Nephroscopy allows visualisation of the renal pelvis and calyces, via an antegrade approach, whereas ureteroscopy and cystoscopy both employ a urethral approach, ureteroscopy then proceeding further to cannulation of the ureteric orifice in question.

For nephroscopy, a percutaneous tract is first made, via radiography, with the patient under anaesthetic. The tract is made using an image intensifier and the use of contrast and either a rigid metal sheath inserted into the tract followed by a rigid endoscope ('rigid' endoscopy) or a smaller bore, flexible endoscope ('flexible' endoscopy). Either method allows biopsy specimens to be taken, and often is combined with endoscopic stone removal. Nephroscopy, although its principal use is for percutaneous nephrolithotomy, can also be of value in cases of recurrent urinary tract infection or congenital abnormality, where direct visualisation of the renal substance is therefore possible.

All endoscopic methods are contraindicated in patients with established urinary tract infection, as they could easily result in an inoculation of the causative organism into the blood stream. Urine must therefore be suitably screened, prior to investigation.

Nursing Care

Patients require work-up for either a general or spinal anaesthetic, plus a non-infected urine. Thus, any urinary infection must be treated, although with stone disease it may be impossible to eradicate all bacteria completely.

Following the procedure, patients require routine postoperative care, plus observation for haematuria (this is expected but should not be heavy or prolonged) and infection. Because of the possibility of mucosal damage and the spread of bacteria into the circulation, any evidence of fever or systemic infection must be aggressively treated.

Patients require adequate preoperative information, reassurance and preparation for the anaesthetic of choice. The nephroscopic 'tract' will close in 48–72 hours, unless a nephrostomy tube is left in position following the procedure.

Ureteroscopy is becoming more common, as it forms part of laser-assisted endoscopy for ureteric stones (lasertripsy). Here, a laser fibre (or extrahydraulic lithotripsy probe) is passed up the ureter, under direct visualisation, using a narrow bore fibreoptic telescope. The stone is visualised, and then broken up using either laser or sound waves.

Following the procedure, the ureteroscope allows examination of the whole length of the ureter, and therefore any obstruction or areas of oedema (which may be hard to distinguish from obstructive lesions on radiographs) can readily be seen. Ureteroscopy is thus very versatile, and allows video film or photographs to be taken.

Patient preparation is the same as for cystoscopy, and is performed under general or epidural anaesthetic, with the patient in the lithotomy position. Also, patients require information and reassurance, especially as they may have back pain on the side visualised after the procedure. Clearly, ureteroscopy is invasive and the urine must again be infection free.

After the procedure, the patient should be observed for evidence of infection, haematuria or excessive pain. Ureteroscopy is a new procedure, but becoming increasingly common, due to its use in the treatment of stones.

Cystoscopy

In many ways, cystoscopy is one of the best known of invasive urological investigations, allowing direct observation of both the urethra (especially in the male, where the urethra is a far more complex structure than in the female) and the interior of the bladder.

The cystoscope used can be either a rigid, metallic telescope or a flexible, polymer-based telescope, both using an intrinsic or fibreoptic light source. Cystoscopy is generally performed in theatre, under general anaesthetic, with the patient in the lithotomy position.

The technique utilises glycine irrigation fluid to maintain a clear visual field for the operator. However, in patients who have frequent cystoscopic examination (e.g. for follow-up after treatment of bladder cancer), many are now being successfully treated as out-patients, with a local anaesthetic, in a suitable clinic environment. This eliminates the need for hospital admission. In out-patients, cystoscopy is carried out via a flexible cystoscope, with the patient sitting in a specialised chair, after the use of a suitable intraurethral anaesthetic agent.

Clearly, the urine must have no infection.

Indications

Cystoscopy is one of the 'mainstay' urological investigations and, in cases of unexplained haematuria, allows visualisation of the bladder, ureteric orifices, trigone, sphincters and urethra.

Cystoscopy is also performed to investigate bladder dysfunction, obstruction (e.g. strictures or bladder neck obstruction) and for both the diagnosis and staging of bladder cancer, where it allows mucosal biopsy to be taken for histology as well as the depth of spread (and thus 'staging') assessed. Cystoscopy takes approximately 5–15 minutes.

Contraindications

These are very few, as even frail or cardiac/respiratory compromised patients can be cystoscoped with suitable precautions (e.g. by the use of flexible cystoscopy under local anaesthetic).

Patient Preparation/Teaching

Patients require preparation for general or epidural anaesthetic, and reassurance and information is important, especially if they have never experienced cystoscopy before. Often patients have some urethral discomfort postoperatively, and should be observed for significant haematuria and re-establishment of voiding.

Again the urine must be screened preoperatively, and any postoperative infection treated aggressively.

References

Brown J, Meikle J and Webb C (1991) Collecting mid-stream specimens of urine: the research base. *Nursing Times* **87** (13): 49–52.

Brundage D (1992) *Renal Disorders*. St Louis: Mosby.

Chapman S and Nakielny R (1986) *A Guide to Radiological Procedures*, 2nd edn. London: Baillière Tindall.

Doyle T, Hare W S C, Thomson K and Tress B (1989) *Procedures in Diagnostic Radiology*. Edinburgh: Churchill Livingstone.

Hiscoke C, Yoxall H, Greig D and Lightfoot N F (1990) Validation of a method for the rapid diagnosis of urinary tract infection suitable for use in general practice. *British Journal of General Practice* **40**: 403–405.

Immergut M A, Gilbert E G and Fresilli F J (1981) The myth of the clean catch urine specimen. *Urology* **17**: 339–340.

Kass E H (1957) Bacteriuria and the diagnosis of infections of the urinary tract. *Archives of Internal Medicine* **100**: 709–714. Cited in Stevens M (1989) Screening urines for bacteriuria. *Journal of Medical Laboratory Sciences* **46**: 194–206.

Kellogg J A, Manzella J P, Shaffer S N and Schwartz B B (1987) Clinical relevance of culture *versus* screens for the detection of microbial pathogens in urine specimens. *American Journal of Medicine* **83**: 739–745.

Lowe P A (1985) Chemical screening and prediction of bateriuria – a new approach. *Journal of Medical Laboratory Sciences* **42**: 28–33.

Maisey M N, Britton K E and Gilday D L (1991) *Clinical Nuclear Medicine*, 2nd edn. London: Chapman and Hall.

Morris R W, Watts M R and Reeves D S (1979) Perineal cleansing before midstream urine : a necessary ritual? *Lancet* **11**: 158–159.

Roberts F J (1986) Quantitative urine culture in patients with urinary tract infection and bacteremia. *American Journal of Clinical Pathology* **85**: 616–18.

Stevens M (1989). Screening urines for bateriuria. *Journal of Medical Laboratory Sciences* **46**: 194–206.

Strand C L, Bryant J K and Sutton K H (1985) Septicaemia secondary to urinary tract infection with colony counts less than 10^5 CFU/ml. *American Journal Clinical Pathology* **83**: 619–621.

3
Urodynamics

Urodynamics is the study of the neuromuscular function and dysfunction of the lower urinary tract. Urodynamic studies can be divided into three groups:

1. Urinary flow studies – uroflowmetry
2. Pressure studies of both bladder and urethra
3. Video studies – videocystourethrography

Not everyone with a urinary tract dysfunction requires a full urodynamic assessment with an evaluation of all phases of their bladder filling and voiding cycles. It is very important therefore to identify the appropriate tests for the various conditions. Techniques are largely invasive and care should be taken at all times to safeguard the patient's interests in the light of his/her condition and the information sought.

UROFLOWMETRY

Uroflowmetry measures the rate and volume at which urine is voided. It is measured as millilitres passed per second. Different types of equipment can be used to measure flow rates: dipstick, weight transducer and rotating disc. However, all involve the person either sitting on a commode seat or voiding directly into the funnel of the machine.

Dipstick Method

The dipstick is usually made of perspex with a metal plate on either side. As the level of urine in the jug rises, the electrical capacitance falls. This information is then fed into the computer which produces a tracing.

In order to obtain accurate results, the nurse needs to ensure the correct jug and dipstick combination is used. The bottom of the dipstick should be immersed in water prior to use (unless the metal plates touch the bottom of the jug) in order to ensure that all the urine voided is recorded. The rest of the dipstick should be dry and fitted in the jug vertically.

Weight Transducer Method

The collecting jug sits on a weight transducer. As the jug fills with urine, the weight increases and from this the flow rate can be calculated. Unlike in the dipstick method, the type of jug can differ as the machine is set to zero *after* the jug is placed on the transducer.

Rotating Disc Method

A disc at the bottom of the funnel spins continuously as urine is voided onto it. As this happens the motor demands more power in order to keep the disc rotating at a constant speed. The change in power required is then used to calculate the flow rate.

Here again, the collecting device is not important and the machine can therefore be directly plumbed into the sewerage system.

The equipment should be prepared before carrying out the investigation, ideally in a room set aside purely for flow rates with the equipment plumbed in and a lockable door to maintain privacy.

Patient Preparation

The investigation must be explained to the patient before he/she attends clinic so that he/she may arrive with a full bladder. The patient should be asked to void when comfortably full. Ideally the flow rate tests should be performed in a flow rate clinic where the patient produces a series of three consecutive flow rates over a morning, and is able to leave the clinic between tests.

A series of recordings gives a far more accurate picture than a one-off recording. However, if a one-off recording is made it is essential the patient is asked if the flow and volume were normal. If not it should be noted on the recording. Inhibition can greatly increase hesitancy and slow the flow, hence the importance of maintaining privacy at all times.

Following the final flow rate test the residual urine may be calculated – this is especially useful if the flow rate has been poor due to either obstruction or poor detrusor function. The residual can be done either by bladder ultrasound or by passing a urethral catheter.

Some typical flow rate profiles are shown in Figure 3.1.

CYSTOMETRY

For many years cystometry has been the main method of investigating bladder function. Simply put, when performing a cystometrogram (CMG) we are looking at the bladder pressure both when filling the bladder and whilst voiding. A straightforward non-video CMG is performed if it is felt that seeing the outline and neck of the bladder is not necessary to make an accurate diagnosis. It therefore follows that a video CMG is performed if it is necessary to see bladder outline and neck.

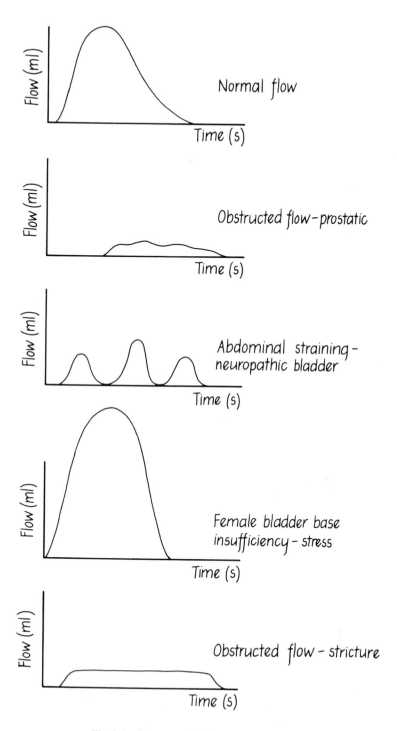

Fig 3.1 Some typical flow rate profiles

Non-Video CMG

Prior to the investigation a history of the patient's voiding problem is taken, which ensures an accurate current picture of the problem as the situation may have changed since the initial referral. However, the 'history' also enables the nurse or continence adviser to give advice on continence aids and other measures which might be required after the test. The nurse will also fully explain the test.

Investigation

The patient should arrive for the CMG with a full bladder, so that, once the procedure has been explained, the patient will be asked to void into the flow rate machine. This action indicates the patient's bladder capacity and uninhibited flow rate. After this the patient is urethrally catheterised with a Jacques (usually size 12 FG) catheter to allow filling and an intravesical pressure catheter (a polythene cannula, external diameter 1 mm). The patient has both catheters inserted at the same time using a sterile technique. Any residual urine is noted except in an atonic bladder which normally holds residual urine. (Having been completely emptied it may become very unstable on filling.)

The suprapubic route can also be used although this is rarely done unless there is a suprapubic catheter already in situ. Children, however, will often have suprapubic lines (filling and pressure) inserted under a general anaesthetic, usually at the same time as cystoscopy.

The pressure line is filled with water and connected to a pressure transducer, which is wired to a recorder. The filling catheter is connected to normal saline (room temperature) via an irrigation or intravenous giving set.

The bladder pressure line records the intravesical pressure, i.e. the detrusor pressure, together with the abdominal pressure caused by the position of the bladder in the body. In order to exclude a pressure rise due to an extravesical component, e.g. intra-abdominal pressure rise due to straining or coughing, a rectal plug is inserted. This records the intra-abdominal (rectal) pressure separately and then is electronically subtraced from the intravesical pressure, giving the intrinsic intravesical pressure or detrusor pressure.

The rectal pressure is recorded by using a 2-mm external diameter water-filled polythene cannula, protected by a finger cot against faecal contamination.

Both the bladder pressure line and the rectal line are flushed with water to allow recordings to be taken. Once the tubes are in and flushed, the patient is asked to cough; this will raise the abdominal pressure and therefore the total bladder pressure. However, the subtracted pressure (the detrusor pressure) should show no rise. The filling of the bladder can then commence whilst the patient is in the supine position.

A 'physiological' fill rate of 1 ml/min is impractical and would make routine cystometry impossible. A medium fill rate is therefore generally used (see Table 3.1).

In patients with a suspected neuropathic bladder, the filling rate is reduced to 10–20 ml/min as filling too quickly may give an abnormal rise in bladder pressure.

The fluid may be pumped into the bladder at a predetermined speed or else the bladder can be filled by gravity. The fluid bag or bottle will hang on a weight

Table 3.1   Accepted fill rates

Fill rates	ml/min
Slow	0–10
Medium	10–100
Fast	100+

transducer so that the volume of fluid entering the bladder can be measured. The patient is asked to inform the examiner when he/she gets the 'first sensation' or first desire to void, and the volume at this stage is noted. However, the filling continues until the patient has a strong desire to void. At this point women will be helped into a sitting position on the commode while men are helped to stand up. The pressure transducers stay level with the symphysis pubis to prevent an artificial pressure rise. Once in the new position the patient can often take more fluid. The examiner will try to fill to a volume at least equal to the first free void. When the patient has reached full capacity, the filling catheter is removed, leaving both the bladder and rectal pressure lines in place. The patient will then be asked to cough to recheck for subtraction and/or signs of leakage.

The examiner may try other methods to induce leakage such as asking the patient to jog on the spot or by running the taps. Once the examiner is satisfied that all is being recorded the patient is asked to void into the flow rate funnel. Halfway through voiding the patient may be asked to stop. After the stop test, the patient continues to void until completion. The volume voided should equal the filled volume. The pressure lines are then removed and the patient is given the opportunity to freshen up and change prior to seeing the doctor. At this point the doctor may be able to prescribe medication or explain possible surgery if required. The nurse/continence adviser will also be able to give advice.

Figure 3.2 illustrates a typical cystometrogram investigation.

Video CMG

This is essentially the same as a straight CMG except that a radio-opaque contrast is used as the filling medium. Radiographs are then taken intermittently throughout the procedure and shown on a TV monitor together with the pressure and flow recordings. This information is then stored on video tape. The additional video information means that the bladder and urethra can be observed during filling and voiding.

If outflow obstruction is suspected (although a straight CMG would indicate this) a video would indicate where the obstruction was (i.e. prostatic, bladder neck or urethral stricture). A video would also show evidence of bladder trabeculation, diverticulae and/or ureteric reflux, and this significantly enhances the diagnostic capability of the procedure. Some common profiles from CMG are illustrated in Figures 3.3–3.7.

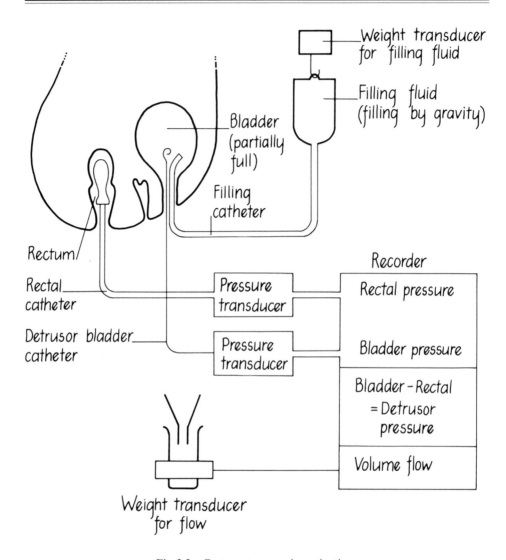

Fig 3.2   Cystometrogram investigation

Typical Figures for Normal CMG (Figure 3.3)

Filling

● First sensation about 250 ml
● Strong desire about 400 ml
● No rise in detrusor pressure. No urgency or leakage

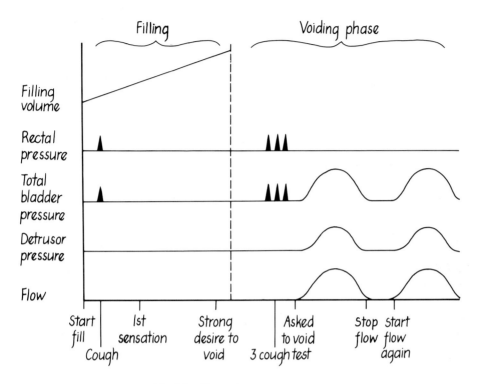

Fig 3.3 Normal cystometrogram

Voiding

- No leakage on pretest cough
- Voiding pressure 60 cmH$_2$O
- Able to stop and start
- Maximum flow rate 27 ml/s
- Volume voided 400 ml. No residual urine

Typical Figures for Stress Incontinence (Figure 3.4)

Filling

- First sensation about 250 ml
- Strong desire about 400 ml
- No rise in detrusor pressure
- No urgency or leakage

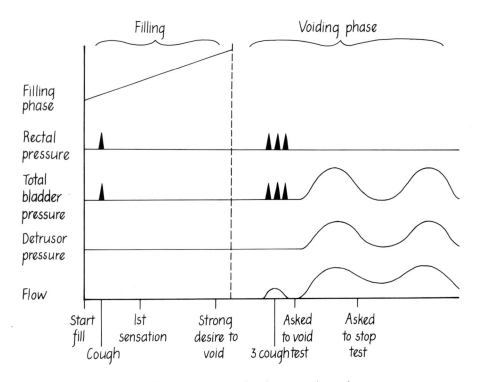

Fig 3.4 Cystometrogram showing stress incontinence

Voiding

● Leaks on three cough test
● Voiding pressure 60 cmH₂O
● Unable to stop test
● Maximum flow 35 ml/s
● Volume voided 400 ml, therefore no residual urine

Typical Figures for Atonic Bladder (Figure 3.5)

Filling

● No first sensation
● No desire (strong)
● No rise in detrusor pressure
● No urgency or leakage
● Filling stopped at 800 ml

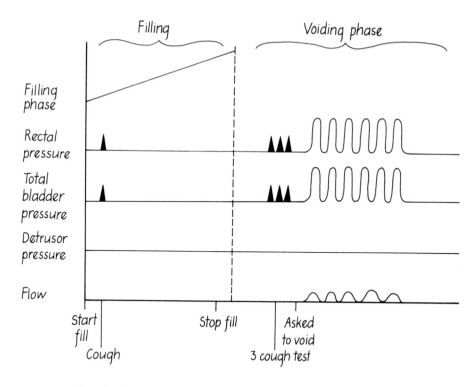

Fig 3.5 Cystometrogram showing bladder atonia (atonic bladder)

Voiding

● No leakage on coughing
● No detrusor pressure when asked to void although total pressure 100+ cmH$_2$O
● Void with abdominal straining
● Voided volume 150 ml, residual 650 ml at least (residual not drained at start)

Typical Figures for Bladder Instability (Figure 3.6)

Filling

● First sensation at about 50 ml
● Strong desire at about 125 ml
● Phasic rise in detrusor pressure unable to inhibit contraction and voids total amount prior to instruction to void
● Has marked urgency with leakage
● No residual

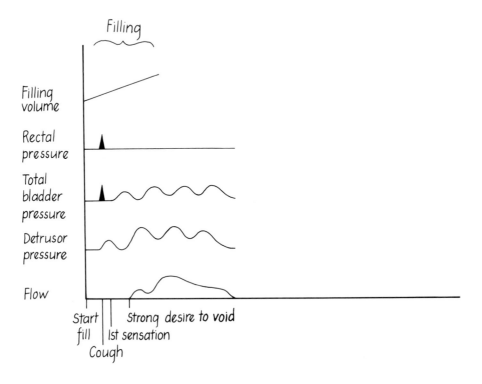

Fig 3.6 Cystometrogram showing bladder instability

Typical Figures for Outflow Obstruction (Figure 3.7)

Filling

- First sensation at about 250 ml
- Strong desire at about 400 ml
- No rise in detrusor pressure
- No urgency or leakage

Voiding

- No leakage on cough test
- Voiding pressure 80 cmH$_2$O
- Poor flow 7 ml/s
- Voided volume – 200 ml – may leave residual, may be able to void to completion over long period of time
- Has hesitancy

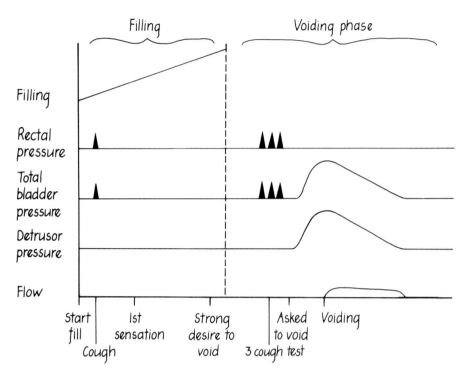

Fig 3.7 Cystometrogram showing bladder outflow obstruction

URETHRAL PRESSURE PROFILE (UPP)

UPP is the measurement of the intraurethral pressure from bladder neck to external meatus.

It involves passing a urethral pressure catheter into the bladder urethrally (rather than suprapubicly). The catheter is then mechanically withdrawn at a constant rate and the pressure along the urethra recorded. The test will normally be repeated three times for an accurate recording.

4
Urinary Drainage Systems

ESTABLISHING A URINARY DRAINAGE SYSTEM

It has been estimated that 12.6 per cent of patients admitted to hospital will be catheterised (Crow et al, 1986) and that 4 per cent of patients living in the community have a catheter (Roe, 1989a). These figures show that catheterisation, as a means of bladder drainage, is still a common procedure although the use of permanent indwelling catheters has declined in recent years. This is probably due to the complications they cause combined with advances in alternative forms of bladder drainage. Despite this, it has been found that nurses are very limited in their knowledge of the different equipment available and research-based practice (Crummey, 1989; McCullough, 1989). Therefore, the aim of this chapter is to provide nurses with the knowledge required to safely establish and manage a urinary drainage system.

A urinary drainage system (UDS) comprises a catheter, to ensure complete bladder drainage, to which is attached a collecting bag. The need for such a system may be temporary or permanent and the catheter is inserted into the bladder via the urethra or a suprapubic cystotomy and is referred to as 'indwelling'. Intermittent catheterisation does not require a drainage bag since the catheter is removed directly after drainage has ceased (see section on Clean Intermittent Self-Catheterisation, later in this chapter).

Indications for indwelling catheterisation are:

1. To ensure complete bladder emptying prior to surgery or an investigative procedure.
2. For the relief of acute and chronic urinary retention.
3. For post-surgical drainage when intermittent catheterisation is inappropriate or 'stenting' of the urethra is required.
4. To measure accurately urine output in the critically ill patient.
5. To manage intractable urinary incontinence when other methods of urine collection are inappropriate.

Catheterisation is contraindicated when there is a lack of cooperation from the patient which might result in deliberate removal.

Preparation for Establishing a UDS

The prospect of catheterisation is almost always alarming and frightening for the patient and it is important that it is handled sensitively. In hospital, most catheters are inserted on a temporary basis either immediately prior to or after surgery and it is important that the patient is prepared for this and is aware that it may be a temporary measure. If the catheter is inserted in a critical situation, when the patient may not be conscious, he/she should be told about the catheter as soon as possible.

In the community, most catheters are inserted for long-term drainage; thus it is even more important that the patient accepts this form of management. Thought should be given as to whether the patient can manage the equipment and who will change the catheter. This is not usually a problem with females but in many health authorities it is still not accepted practice that female nurses recatheterise males. It may be possible to teach the procedure to the patient, a friend or a relative unless there is easy access to a hospital.

Unless unplanned, the decision to catheterise should be a joint one between the medical and nursing practitioners and the patient. With all its attendant risks (see section on Management, later in this chapter), catheterisation is best avoided if at all possible and should never be considered for the convenience of the nurse. However, in the community, it may be the only acceptable way that a person can remain at home if cared for by relatives and thus, in some cases, it can be a very positive form of management.

Once the need for a catheter has been established, selection of the most suitable catheter and drainage bag can begin. The huge range of products available ensures that a catheter and drainage bag can be selected that fits in with the patient's life-style, level of activity and preferences.

Preparation for Insertion of a Urethral Catheter

Only once the correct equipment is available should the patient be catheterised. Unless in an emergency situation, the use of inappropriate catheters could be harmful and may cause unnecessary discomfort to the patient.

Catheterisation is an aseptic procedure and the local policies for aseptic technique and hand-washing should be followed. Catheterisation policies vary slightly in different health authorities but follow the same principles. A point to remember here is that the drainage bag should be sterile when connected to the catheter and, therefore, should be opened onto the sterile field with the other equipment.

Urinary Catheters

A catheter is a thin, hollow tube which may be passed intermittently into the bladder or held permanently in situ, originally by suturing to the skin. In 1935, Dr Foley invented the first retention catheter with two channels, one for drainage and the second as a means of inflating a balloon which is positioned around the proximal end of the catheter immediately below the drainage eyes. The balloon is inflated immediately after the catheter has been inserted into the bladder, allowing the catheter to be retained in the bladder, and can be deflated to facilitate removal.

Three-way catheters are available with a third channel to facilitate continuous bladder irrigation after urological surgery. The Nelaton catheter is made from PVC without a retention balloon and is used only for intermittent catheterisation and investigative procedures.

The most recent innovation in catheter design is the Conformocath (see Figure 4.1). This is a development of the Foley catheter which incorporates a collapsible urethral portion. This aims to reduce distortion of the female urethra which is a twisting, spiralling slit. Thus it is believed to increase patient comfort and reduce urethral trauma and related complications. At present the Conformocath is available only in female length and size 14 Charrière.

Selection of the Catheter

The huge range of products available ensures that a catheter and drainage bag can be selected that fits in with the patient's life-style, level of activity and preferences.

Restricted choice in hospitals is usually due to the limited range of products that the stores department is able to hold. If there are no suitable 'stock' items available, others can usually be obtained by special order. It is important to remember that the whole range of products will be available in the community on prescription and it is preferable that the patient goes home with the system he will continue to use.

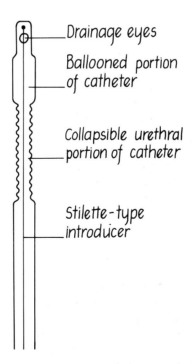

Fig 4.1 Conformocath

Material

The earliest catheters were fashioned from onion stalks, gold, silver and glass. The first Foley catheters were made from red rubber which caused severe urethral irritation, ultimately leading to stricture formation. This was superseded by latex which caused fewer problems but was still toxic.

Thus began the procedure of 'coating' catheters, first with silicone and silicone-elastomer and more recently Teflon and hydrogel. It is the surface material of the catheter which determines how long it can remain in the bladder and the catheter will thus be defined for short-term (0–14 days) or long-term (2–12 weeks) use. It should be remembered that the operating practitioner is responsible for the correct use of equipment and thus the manufacturers' recommendations should be followed when using catheters. Manufacturers are now bound to ensure that their products meet the specifications laid out in British Standard 1695.

Catheters for Short-term Use

Studies have shown that coating latex catheters with silicone reduces encrustation of the tip and lumen of the catheter which increases its life and also ensures a soft, pliable catheter which is comfortable for the patient (Blannin, 1982). Silicone-dipped catheters are for short-term use as delamination of the coating has been found to occur if they are left in for long periods.

Plastic (PVC) catheters have the advantage of a wider lumen relative to Charrière size as they are unabated. However, the plastic catheter is quite rigid and uncomfortable at room temperature and so can only be tolerated in the short-term. Also, as these are uncoated catheters, the part of the catheter to which the balloon is attached has a relatively greater Charrière size compared with the shaft. The balloon is incorporated into the Charrière size of coated catheters. Catheters of this type are more likely to be used after urological surgery when their rigidity helps to maintain the patency of the urethra and the wide lumen allows the passage of blood clots.

Catheters for Long-term Use

The all-silicone catheter, also uncoated, is better tolerated although still quite rigid, but the inert nature of the material means that it is more resistant to encrustation and thus is suitable for long-term use (Kennedy, 1983a). Silicone-elastomer catheters have silicone chemically bonded to the latex which prevents delamination of the coating.

Hydrogel-coated catheters, the most recent development, are biocompatible and when moistened by urethral secretions become slippery. Thus they are claimed to reduce encrustation and friction with the urothelium.

Colour

It is important to remember that the different colours of catheters denote the manufacturer rather than the material from which they are made. However, with the advent of 1992, manufacturers have had to conform with European standards that require all catheters to be the pale brown colour of the Teflon-coated catheter.

Catheter Size

Catheters are measured in the Charrière scale (CH) or French gauge (FG), one unit of which equals 0.3 mm. Thus a size 12CH catheter actually measures 4 mm in diameter. Sizes range from 8 and 10CH, for paediatric use, to 30CH. Although the diameter of the lumen varies between coated and uncoated catheters it does not increase significantly in relation to the Charrière size of the catheter. Therefore, inserting a larger Charrière catheter does not ensure a wide drainage channel.

The urethral mucosa contains elastic tissue which will close around the catheter. Larger catheters have been found to be associated with more catheter-related problems (see section on Management, later in this chapter) and the rule is to select the smallest size catheter that will provide drainage (Kennedy et al, 1983). Under normal circumstances, a size 12CH or 14CH is suitable for a woman and 12–16CH for a man. Sizes above this should be reserved for use after specific urological procedures.

Catheters have traditionally been manufactured in a single length, 40–43 cm, to accommodate the male urethra. However, female-length catheters are now widely available and are approximately 23–26 cm long. This reduces the external length of catheter which could be tugged or pulled. However, the longer catheter often remains preferable, particularly in obese women, because it allows easier access to the junction between the catheter and the drainage bag.

Balloon Size

The retention balloon should be inflated only after the catheter is in the bladder. Sterile water must always be used for this as diffusion of some of the contents of the balloon into the bladder is likely. Balloons come in three sizes: 3–5 ml for paediatric use; 5–10 ml for standard use; 30 ml for use after some urological procedures. The larger balloon size is used to provide traction haemostasis on a bleeding prostatic bed after transurethral resection of the prostate.

The valve at the end of the inflation channel has a Luer lock for connection to a water-filled syringe to inflate the balloon and deflate it prior to removal of the catheter. Some coated catheters are now available with prefilled balloons.

This ensures that the correct amount of sterile water is inserted, reduces the amount of equipment required for the procedure and means that there are no 'sharps' to deal with afterwards.

Tip Design

The standard tip is rounded with two staggered drainage eyes. However, there are a number of variations with specific uses (Figure 4.2).

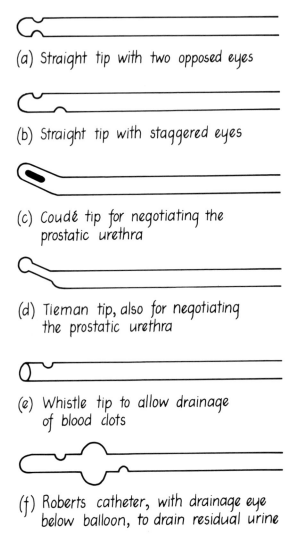

(a) Straight tip with two opposed eyes

(b) Straight tip with staggered eyes

(c) Coudé tip for negotiating the prostatic urethra

(d) Tieman tip, also for negotiating the prostatic urethra

(e) Whistle tip to allow drainage of blood clots

(f) Roberts catheter, with drainage eye below balloon, to drain residual urine

Fig 4.2 Tip designs

Packaging and Markings

Each catheter is double-wrapped and sterile. Information written on both the outer packet and the catheter includes the size of the catheter, a code number and the names of the manufacturer and the product. The outer packet also has printed on it the sterilisation and expiry dates. Out-of-date catheters should be discarded. The person performing the catheterisation is responsible for ensuring that the equipment used is in a satisfactory state. The code number is important so that faulty equipment can easily be traced by the manufacturers.

Cost

The cost of the catheter should not be the primary factor in the selection process. However, all else being equal, the nurse should be aware of the different costs and select accordingly. The price of catheters ranges from the fairly inexpensive Nelaton catheter to the more costly catheters with special features. Individual health authorities will make their own contractual arrangements with specific companies which will reduce the cost per item.

Storage

Catheters should be stored flat in the boxes in which they are dispatched and should not be tied in 'bunches' with elastic bands which might damage the wrapping or the catheters and compromise sterility. Catheters should not be exposed to direct heat or sunlight and should be kept in a dry, cool environment.

Catheter Supports

Many of the problems discussed later in this chapter are related to urethral trauma and can be minimized if the catheter is well supported. There are now available a number of catheter supports. Unfortunately, these are not yet available on prescription but can be obtained by special order. They aim to provide a firm, secure support for the catheter, allowing freedom of movement while ensuring that the catheter cannot be tugged.

Drainage Bags

Indwelling catheterisation requires a urine collection bag to allow periodic emptying. Originally catheters drained into open glass jars which stood on the floor. These days, drainage bags are made from moulded plastic and are designed to be either worn on the body or free-standing. There are design elements common to all drainage bags. Each bag has an inlet tube, the proximal end of which is connected to the catheter, a collecting chamber and a drainage tap.

If the drainage bag is to be connected directly to an indwelling catheter it must be sterile whichever design is used. Non-sterile, free-standing bags are available for connection to a body-worn bag in a 'link' system (see later) and non-sterile body-worn bags are available for use with urinary drainage sheaths.

Body-worn or leg bags should be used whenever possible. They are either attached to the leg or suspended from the waist thereby allowing maximum freedom of movement and can be concealed beneath clothing. This is an essential prerequisite in the community but is important during any period of rehabilitation.

Free-standing bags have much larger volumes and thus are used for overnight drainage or the bed-bound patient. Modified free-standing bags are available which have an inner measuring chamber which allows accurate measurement of urine in the critically ill patient.

All drainage bags are available on prescription in the community but availability in hospitals is subject to local purchasing agreements. However, as for catheters, the patients' needs must determine provision and it may be necessary to look further than this for the most appropriate appliance. Since there are many different types of bag available (Association of Continence Advisors, 1988) and no single bag will suit all users, it is recommended that patients and their carers should be given an opportunity to try different systems to determine which best suits their needs (Roe et al, 1988).

Selection of the Body-worn Bag

Principles for the selection of the drainage bag are similar to those for the catheter and there are a number of variables in the basic design to consider.

Length of the Inlet Tube

The inlet tube ranges from about 4 cm to 40 cm so that the bag can be attached to either the thigh or calf and concealed under various garments whilst still remaining accessible for emptying. The length of the inlet tube can be adjusted on some body-worn bags to suit individual needs by adding pieces of extension tubing or by cutting the existing tubing and reapplying the connecting piece.

Capacity

Leg-bags come in various sizes according to their capacity: 350 ml, 500 ml and 750 ml. Which size is most suitable depends on how frequently the bag is to be emptied and, in practice, the 500 ml bag is most popular.

Outlet Tap

There are various tap designs. It is important that the patient can manage the tap, particularly where manual dexterity is compromised. Most taps can be manipulated using just one hand.

Collecting Chamber

Originally all leg bags were designed with a single chamber which, as the bag begins to fill, results in 'sloshing' of urine which is embarrassing and uncomfortable, and causes a 'ballooning' of the bottom of the bag which makes it more obvious. A technique to reduce this effect is to break down the surface area of the urine by introducing bonded vertical lines. More recently a bag has been developed which uses the bonding process with pleated chambers so that, even when full, the bag lies relatively flat against the leg.

'Link' System Connector

All leg bags should have a facility for connection to an overnight drainage bag. This is usually a piece of tubing which is attached to and extends beyond the drainage tap.

This extension is usually bonded onto the outlet tap to minimise the risk of disconnection.

Sampling Port

All drainage bags have a facility for the aspiration of sterile urine for analysis. This is usually an area of inlet tube covered by a sleeve of resealable rubber through which a needle can be injected. However, many needle-stick injuries have occurred when the needle has been pushed out through the back of the tubing. This resulted in the development of a rigid plastic backing to the aspiration area. A sampling port has recently been developed that accepts a Luer-lock syringe, thus dispensing with the need for a needle for this procedure and significantly reducing the risk of injury.

Backing Material

Drainage bags are made from soft plastic and this may be uncomfortable when worn next to the skin. Some bags have a woven 'coverstock' on their posterior surface although this may suffer during bathing. One manufacturer has produced a coverstock 'envelope' into which the bag is placed and from which it can be easily removed prior to bathing or showering.

Support Systems

It is extremely important that a body-worn bag is properly secured so that it cannot suddenly drop, thereby pulling the catheter and traumatising the urethra. The traditional method for this uses straps which are slotted through either end of the bag and fixed around the leg. However, there are a number of alternative methods and a system should be sought which the patient and carers can manage and in which they have confidence.

Packaging and Markings

Most bags and outer packaging have details on them of the company and product name and prescription details. Some bags also have capacity in millilitres marked on the front of the bag. Sterility is noted on the packaging.

Free-standing Bags

These are constructed in a similar way to the body-worn or leg bags but are much bulkier with capacities ranging from 2 to 4 litres.

At home the patient can re-use the free-standing or night drainage bag and so it requires a drainage tap. In hospital, because of the risk of cross-infection, night drainage bags should not be re-used and cheaper, non-drainable bags should be used.

Free-standing drainage bags only have to be sterile if they are to be attached directly to a catheter and not if they are for use in a 'link' system.

Free-standing bags normally have a cardboard or plastic-covered metal stand which is available on prescription. An appropriate stand should always be used as, when full, the bags are very heavy and the sudden weight of a falling bag could dislodge the 'link' system or cause traction on the catheter in the urethra. Indeed, the failure to use such stands to enhance drainage has been implicated in leakage of urine from around the catheter during periods in bed (Kennedy, 1984).

Catheter Valves

While the wide variety of drainage bags now available helps to ensure maximum freedom and independence, they are nevertheless an encumbrance. The catheter valve, as an alternative to a drainage bag, allows more discreet drainage and maximum freedom of movement. Standard spigots have been used to plug catheters but these are unsuitable because the closed drainage system has to be broken to allow bladder drainage. Catheter valves can be opened without having to break the closed drainage system. Valves are designed for use with two hands or a single hand.

The successful use of a valve depends upon the skills of the user and the nurse needs to be sure that the patient is able to manipulate the valve and empty the bladder regularly and before urine volume exceeds bladder capacity. If bladder distension is allowed to occur the patient may be at risk from urinary tract infection and dilatation of the upper urinary tract. Ideally the patient should be able to sense bladder distension which will prompt drainage. If this is not the case then the bladder should be emptied every 3–4 hours unless fluid intake is excessive when the frequency of drainage may need to be increased.

A sterile catheter valve should be connected each time the junction between catheter and valve is broken.

MANAGEMENT OF THE UDS

Management of a UDS is based on the prevention of complications. Some of the complications of catheterisation are inevitable but, with careful management, the effects of these can be minimised.

Urinary Tract Infection

The incidence of urinary tract infection is disproportionately high amongst catheterised patients and accounts for a large proportion of nosocomial infections. The incidence of infection has been shown to be directly proportional to the number of days that a catheter is left in situ (Castle, 1974; Crow et al, 1986).

Organisms most commonly found in the urine are *Escherichia coli*, *Streptococcus faecalis*, *Proteus mirabilis* and *Staphylococcus epidermidis*. Infection related to blockage is caused by organisms which produce the enzyme urease, such as *Proteus*,

Klebsiella, Providencia and *Pseudomonas*. Urease is responsible for splitting urea in the urine which releases ammonia, increasing the pH of the urine. This results in pronounced precipitation of catheter encrustation (Hedelin et al, 1991).

Bacteria may enter the bladder in three ways:

1. *During catheterisation* – contamination of the catheter prior to insertion through poor aseptic technique.

2. *During disconnection of the closed drainage system* – potential ascending infection in the lumen of the catheter.

3. *Ascending infection* – between the urethral epithelium and the external surface of the catheter.

Principles of Management for Reducing Bacterial Access

Closed Drainage

Prior to the use of closed drainage systems, almost 100 per cent of catheterised patients developed urinary tract infections within 96 hours (Kass, 1957). Closed drainage has been shown to reduce this rate of infection substantially (Garibaldi et al, 1974 cited in Wright, 1988).

Urine which leaves the bladder should remain sterile until it passes through the non-return valve of the drainage bag. The non-return valve helps to reduce the risk of bacteria ascending the catheter and gaining access to the bladder. If the catheter and the drainage bag are disconnected the closed drainage system will be broken. This should only occur if absolutely necessary either to change the drainage bag or to perform a bladder washout. Frequent changing of drainage bags and thus manipulation of the closed drainage system has been found to increase the risk of bacterial infection, resulting in more catheter-related problems (Kennedy et al, 1983). It is recommended that drainage bags, attached directly to a catheter, should not be changed more often than weekly. Exceptions to this are after bladder washout or if the drainage bag leaks or becomes odorous.

Gravity Drainage

The free flow of urine through the drainage system is important to prevent areas of stagnant urine collecting in the tubing proximal to the non-return valve. This provides a suitable medium for bacterial multiplication and can also result in unexpected disconnection of the system. Therefore, the drainage bag(s) should always be positioned below the level of the bladder and the catheter and inlet tubing should be secured in a downward position.

The 'Link' System

Overnight drainage may require a larger capacity than a body-worn bag can offer. Before the importance of closed drainage was realised, the connection between the catheter and the body-worn bag would be broken regularly to allow connection of a larger capacity, free-standing night bag.

In order to maintain the closed system, it is now possible to set up a 'link' system whereby the night drainage bag is connected onto the outlet tap of the body-worn bag which is then left in the open position. The outlet taps of most body-worn bags have a universal connection facility. It is important that the large capacity bag is supported on a stand by the bed but that it can move if the patient turns and tugs it. If the bag is tied to the bed this cannot occur and may thus traumatise the urethra (Lowthian, 1989).

Meatal Cleansing

Increased urethral secretions, due to irritation of the urothelium by the catheter, collect at the meatus and may form crusts which, when removed, expose areas of damaged tissue susceptible to bacterial colonisation which may then ascend to the bladder. The practice of using antiseptic agents for meatal cleansing has been shown not to reduce bacterial infection (Burke et al, 1981 cited in Roe, 1989b) and to predispose to the emergence of multi-resistant bacterial strains (Dance et al, 1987). Despite these findings, observation of meatal cleansing procedures has shown that there is still confusion and inconsistency in practice (Crow et al, 1986). It is recommended that secretions are removed using soap and water and clean wash cloths (Roe, 1989b). The frequency of this procedure is dependent upon the amount of secretions produced and, therefore, will vary between individuals although once or twice a day should normally be sufficient.

Treatment of UTI during Periods of Catheterisation

Eradication of bacteria from the bladder during periods of indwelling catheterisation is extremely difficult as bacteria colonise the surface of the catheter. Where urine is in direct contact with the catheter a biofilm (a collection of microorganisms and their extracellular products bound to a solid surface) will form. Organisms seem particularly resistant to antimicrobial agents in this state (Mulhall, 1991) and thus short courses of antibiotics have not been found particularly useful against catheter-associated urinary tract infections.

Despite having large numbers of bacteria in the urine, the patient may remain asymptomatic and not require treatment. It is only when symptoms occur that active treatment should be considered after removal of the catheter. If the reason for catheterisation is urinary retention a period of intermittent catheterisation will allow drainage to continue.

Urine Specimens

The type of antibiotic used will depend upon the organism implicated. However, this may not be determined for up to 48 hours and so a broad-spectrum antibiotic may be prescribed initially.

A catheter specimen of urine should be collected from the aspiration port of the drainage bag. Urine for analysis should never be collected from the drainage bag as it should be fresh and uncontaminated. The specimen should be clearly labelled and sent immediately to the microbiology laboratory for analysis. If this is not possible, a specimen may be kept in a fridge designated for specimens overnight.

The laboratory will culture the organisms and examine them under light microscope and the antibiotics to which the organisms are sensitive will be determined.

Detrusor Spasm

Spasmodic contraction of the detrusor muscle is a common response to the presence of a foreign body in the bladder. It may also occur secondary to blockage of the catheter, and the rate of flow of urine into the drainage bag should be observed. Large catheters with large-capacity balloons can cause contractions (Kennedy et al, 1983; Kunin et al, 1987).

Often referred to as 'bladder spasm', these contractions can cause considerable discomfort to the patient and lead to bypassing of urine from the space between the urethra and the catheter and occasionally are strong enough to cause expulsion of the catheter from the bladder. Catheterisation of an already unstable bladder is likely to worsen the situation so, if time permits, treatment of the detrusor muscle instability should commence prior to catheterisation and may need to continue after catheterisation.

Management is based on removal of the cause of the spasm whenever possible and by ensuring that the catheter is not blocked. Oxybutynin and propantheline bromide are two drugs used to treat detrusor instability for their anticholinergic effect on the detrusor muscle. For some people, however, the spasm may be very resistant to treatment, and removal of the catheter may have to be considered. Spasm occurring immediately after catheterisation may be a temporary response and may settle down after 24–48 hours.

Blockage of the UDS

There are a number of ways in which the UDS can become blocked and these can be hard to correct. The result is a build-up of urine proximal to the blockage which may lead to detrusor spasm and bypassage of urine. High-pressure bladder distension may compromise vascularity and leave the bladder vulnerable to infection (Lapides et al, 1972). In the event that urine does not leak around the catheter, the risk is of high-pressure dilatation of the ureters and renal pelvises resulting in pyelonephritis and hydronephrosis or both (Lowthian, 1989). If urine is prevented from entering the drainage bag the result may be disconnection from the catheter.

A blockage in the drainage bag may be due to either a design fault, in which case the manufacturers should be informed and the bag changed, or large amounts of debris or blood clots. This type of obstruction can often be shifted by repeatedly squeezing and releasing or 'milking' the tubing distal to the blockage. However, this technique should not be used on a regular basis as it may damage the urothelium. If blockage is persistent, other methods should be used to deal with it.

If there does not appear to be a problem with the drainage bag and the blockage is intermittent, it is possible that the inlet tubing is becoming kinked and this should be observed during a range of movements. The patency of the inlet tubing can easily be disrupted if metal clamps or toothed forceps are applied. If it is necessary to disrupt the flow of urine then either non-toothed forceps should be used or gauze wrapped around the jaws of the forceps first. Clamping of the catheter itself should be avoided as compression of the inflation channel may lead to difficulty with balloon deflation prior to removal.

Blockage of the lumen of the catheter is very common, affecting 25 per cent of patients in one series (Kennedy, 1983b). Clues as to the nature of the blockage may be found in the urine if it contains debris or clots. Ammonium magnesium phosphate and calcium phosphate deposits can build up around the portion of the catheter in the bladder in the presence of alkaline urine, blocking the eyes of the catheter and making deflation of the balloon difficult. If milking the inlet tubing of the drainage bag does not improve the flow, a bladder washout will be necessary. A physiological blockage may occur during strong detrusor contractions which compress the catheter temporarily.

Bladder Washouts

After certain urological operations which involve heavy blood loss, the bladder will require continuous irrigation. This is facilitated by the insertion of a three-way Foley catheter usually made out of plastic for extra rigidity and the bladder is continuously flushed with isotonic saline (0.9 per cent).

More commonly, the bladder is washed out on an intermittent basis at a frequency determined by the degree of blockage. This should be an aseptic technique and can be performed using a 60 ml bladder syringe with a tip that fits the funnel end of a catheter. This method allows active flushing of the bladder using a push–pull action which, when repeated, disturbs the debris so it can drain. However, by withdrawing the plunger too forcefully urothelium may be sucked into the eyes of the catheter, preventing drainage of the irrigation fluid as well as the debris. This practice can also cause discomfort, pain and trauma which may predispose to infection. Therefore, once the fluid has been instilled, the syringe should be removed and the catheter allowed to drain freely into a sterile kidney dish and input and output measured. The amount of debris obtained and subsequent urinary flow should also be noted.

In recent years, the use of prepacked, sterile solutions has gained popularity. The advantages of these are that fewer items of equipment are required, they are available on prescription and they allow bladder washout to be performed using an aseptic technique.

Once the connection with the catheter has been made, the clamp is removed and the bag elevated to allow gravity drainage of the irrigation fluid into the bladder. The bag is then lowered to allow the irrigation fluid to drain out. This method does not allow active flushing of the bladder and thus may be more use for prophylactic washouts.

The following solutions are produced:

1. *Saline 0.9 per cent* – recommended for mechanical flushing to remove tissue debris and small blood clots.

2. *Suby G* – a citric acid solution (3.23 per cent) aimed at preventing and dissolving crystallisation in the catheter or bladder.

3. *Mandelic acid 1 per cent* – aimed at preventing the growth of urease-producing bacteria through acidification of the bladder.

4. *Solution R* – a citric acid solution (6 per cent) aimed at dissolving persistent crystallisation in the catheter or bladder.

5. *Chlorhexidine 0.02 per cent* – aimed at preventing or reducing the growth of bacteria in the bladder and particularly contamination with *E. coli* and *Klebsiella*.

Susceptibility to catheter encrustation may be related to various individual factors as encrustations have developed in the absence of urease-splitting organisms (Hedelin et al, 1991). Solutions 2, 3 and 4 may reduce crystallisation through acidification of the urine as well as providing a mechanical flush. However, dilute acid solutions can remove the surface layer of mucus in the bladder (Parsons et al, 1979 cited in Getliffe and Mulhall, 1991) and increased exfoliation of bladder mucosal cells has been observed to follow washouts (Elliot et al, 1989).

Chlorhexidine has been shown not to be effective against a number of commonly occurring pathogens but may be active against some bacteria in the normal urethral flora (Stickler et al, 1987), removal of which may allow colonisation by resistant organisms.

Bladder washouts should only be performed when absolutely necessary as they involve breaking the closed drainage system. However, the use of regular, prophylactic bladder washouts in patients whose catheters are prone to encrustation and regularly block is recommended (Roe, 1989b). Bladder washout is an aseptic procedure and a sterile drainage bag should be connected to the catheter at the end of the procedure.

If used inappropriately, bladder washouts can be hazardous and expose the patient to increased risk of urinary tract infection. Therefore, the current lack of knowledge of nurses about the use of individual solutions and the technique of bladder washout (Roe, 1989b; Bailey, 1991) must be corrected.

If bladder washout does not relieve the blockage it may be necessary to change the catheter. When the catheter has been removed, it should be inspected to ascertain the nature of the blockage. This may not be evident from external examination and it may be necessary to dissect the catheter.

If blockage is an ongoing problem, thought should be given to the type of catheter used and the lumen size. The hydrogel and the all-silicone catheter are recommended as providing a surface more resistant to stone formation and the uncoated, all-silicone catheter will provide a slightly larger lumen relative to the Charrière size than a coated catheter. Whether or not a catheter blocks and after how long depends on the individual and the catheter. The frequency of recatheterisation in the long-term situation will thus be determined by the life-span of a catheter and this should be determined as soon as possible to prevent blockage occurring. If a catheter continues to block, cystoscopy may be required to identify the nature of the blockage.

Vitamin Intake

The use of high doses of ascorbic acid to reduce debris formation in the bladder is not new although it is unclear what actual role it plays. Ascorbic acid acidifies the urine, reducing the formation of mineral deposits, although a bacteriostatic effect remains unproven (Kunin, 1989). Cranberry juice has been recommended but is expensive and not always easily obtainable.

Catheter Expulsion

The simplest reason for a catheter leaving the bladder unexpectedly is that the retention balloon has become deflated. It may not have had the correct amount of water inserted in the first place and this should always be recorded in the patient's notes. Also, it has been shown that the water is gradually lost from retention balloons and at different rates according to the catheter material but most rapidly from 100 per cent silicone catheters (Studer et al, 1983; Barnes and Malone-Lee, 1986).

Occasionally, a catheter will be expelled with the balloon fully inflated. This may be due to detrusor spasm which should be dealt with as above. If the catheter is not fully expelled, the retention balloon should be deflated and the catheter removed. No attempt should be made to reinsert the catheter without deflating the balloon as this would cause urethral trauma.

If the support system for the catheter and drainage bag is inadequate the catheter may accidentally be pulled out. A more secure system should then be set up prior to recatheterisation. Occasionally the catheter will be removed deliberately by the patient. This is most likely to happen when the patient is confused and recatheterisation should not be attempted while the confusional state remains. The chronically confused patient may repeatedly remove the catheter which is a traumatic event. Complaints of discomfort, therefore, should never be ignored, because, if severe enough, may drive even the most rational patient to remove the source if he does not feel he is being listened to.

Pain

Catheter-related pain is varied and may be felt in the suprapubic region or be referred to the tip of the penis or the labia. Temporary discomfort may be experienced immediately after catheterisation and should settle in 24–48 hours with mild analgesics.

Severe pain immediately after catheterisation should arouse suspicion that the catheter was not properly sited in the bladder and that the retention balloon had been inflated in the urethra. If not corrected immediately, this can lead to pressure necrosis of the surrounding urethral tissue. Therefore, the catheter should be inserted up to the bifurcation in men and a further 1 inch after urine has drained in women.

The pain of detrusor spasm can range from a dull ache to severe pain. The spasm should be dealt with and the patient given analgesics. If this situation continues and cannot be controlled, it may be necessary to remove the catheter.

If the drainage bag is allowed to drag on the catheter, this in turn will pull on the bladder neck and the urethra, causing urethral pain. Pain is always a warning that something is amiss and, particularly when it cannot be felt, as with some neurological lesions, it is vital that the nurse checks that the drainage bag and catheter are well supported.

Phimosis and Paraphimosis

For the purpose of catheterisation or cleansing, the foreskin must be retracted. After these procedures, it should be replaced over the glans or else it may become oedematous and fixed in the retracted position, constricting the penis. This condition is known as paraphimosis. Phimosis is a condition where the foreskin cannot be retracted and the glans exposed. Both these states require surgical correction.

LONG-TERM COMPLICATIONS OF URETHRAL CATHETERISATION

Urethral strictures are the most serious of the late complications. The commonest cause of stricture formation is instrumentation of the bladder and the early complications of trauma, bleeding and inflammation may result in their formation. Inflammation may also be caused by infection, chemical irritation or ischaemia (Burkitt and Randall, 1987). Too large a catheter will cause blockage of the paraurethral glands, resulting in paraurethral abscesses. These will either heal with scar tissue formation or burst outside the urethra, allowing urine to escape into the surrounding tissues and thus causing urinary fistulae.

Too large a catheter can also cause blockage and infection in the ejaculatory ducts, resulting in epididymitis. Similarly, blockage and subsequent infection of the prostatic ducts can result in prostatitis or prostatic abscesses (Blandy and Moors, 1989).

An unsupported catheter will traumatise the urothelium which will heal to form scar tissue. In severe cases, pressure can result in complete destruction of the urethra.

Perhaps a less obvious complication relates to self-perception of the catheterised patient. Alteration of body image and a feeling of dependence may result. It is very important that the nurse listens to the anxieties of the patient and takes into account life-style when planning a UDS. It may be appropriate to include the patient's partner in this discussion (see later).

GENERAL CARE

Lack of mobility, particularly in the community, has been found to be of major significance in catheter-related problems. Immobile patients may be on their own all day without access to fluids and unable to change their position and improve the flow of urine (Kennedy et al, 1983).

Close proximity of the bowel to the bladder means that constipation can affect it by worsening instability and possibly resulting in bypassage of urine and catheter expulsion.

Maintaining an adequate fluid intake can be difficult, particularly for elderly people. However, the aim should be 1500–2000 ml per day to replace fluid lost and ensure adequate hydration. It has been suggested that diuresis may assist in voiding microorganisms from the bladder although it may not reduce encrustation (Getliffe and Mulhall, 1991).

CATHETER REMOVAL

For most people, catheterisation will be temporary and the timing of removal will depend on the general condition of the patient or the healing time after a specific urological operation. The increased risk of urinary tract infection with time means that the need for the catheter should be reassessed on a daily basis during the initial period post-catheterisation.

If the catheter has been inserted for permanent bladder drainage, the decision to decatheterise may not be so easy. Catheterisation is normally seen as a last resort and, therefore, when all other attempts at management have failed to eradicate persistent problems, the decision to remove the catheter may be difficult.

There are a number of options to urethral catheterisation including suprapubic and intermittent catheterisation. If the initial bladder dysfunction was of urinary retention, one of these alternatives will be required. However, if the bladder empties completely and incontinence was the initial reason for catheterisation, management with an aid or appliance might be preferable (Association of Continence Advisors, 1988).

Catheters have traditionally been removed at 6 a.m., thereby allowing the whole day for normal voiding to resume. However, removal is often followed by a period of urinary frequency and urgency which can be stressful to the patient. Removal of catheters at midnight compared with 6 a.m. has shown a significant increase in the time to the first void post-removal and, consequently, a greater initial volume. This has been shown to result in a faster return to a regular voiding pattern which has the added advantage of allowing earlier discharge (Noble et al, 1990).

Retention Balloon Deflation

Actual removal of the catheter is a straightforward procedure although occasionally problems will be experienced when trying to deflate the balloon. It should be remembered that there is likely to be less water in the retention balloon than was initially inserted.

Once the syringe has been attached to the valve of the inflation channel, the pressure of the water draining from the balloon should push the plunger out. Thus it should be unnecessary to pull on the plunger and this additional suction can result in the inflation channel collapsing, thereby preventing further water from being withdrawn.

If water does not drain out, the insertion of a further 1–2 ml of water and its subsequent withdrawal will indicate patency of the inflation channel, thus indicating that the water has been lost from the balloon, and the catheter can be safely removed. If there is resistance when trying to withdraw the catheter, the inflation arm of the catheter should be cut in case the problem lies with the valve. The catheter can be left for 24 hours like this during which time it may drop out (Blandy and Moors, 1989).

If the catheter remains in situ, there are a number of methods which can be used by urologists to burst the balloon. A fine, ureteric catheter stilette can be passed up the inflation channel and the balloon punctured from within. An alternative method has been described where a needle is introduced transvesically into the balloon, causing it to burst (Moisey and Williams, 1980). This may also be achieved using a perineal approach.

One method that should not be used is the insertion of ether up the inflation channel to dissolve the balloon. Ether is harmful to the urothelium and vaporization may expand the balloon to a point at which the bladder ruptures. Stones may then form around the fragments of balloon left in the bladder.

The Clamping Issue

Periods of catheterisation may result in the loss of detrusor muscle tone resulting in poor bladder emptying after decatheterisation. One method used to overcome this involves the clamping and periodic release of the catheter. A review of the research on this practice suggests that it may result in the earlier resumption of normal voiding after short periods of catheterisation only (Roe, 1990).

The current trend is to remove the catheter immediately using intermittent catheterisation and drainage of residual urine after each attempt to void. Voided volumes should increase and residual volume decrease. A hazard of this type of decatheterisation programme is that the patient may be forgotten and left in urinary retention. Therefore, the patient should be made aware of the timing for voiding and measurement of residual volume and the timing may need to be adjusted so that the amount of urine voided plus the residual does not exceed 400–500 ml. It should be remembered that intermittent catheterisation carried out in the hospital setting is an aseptic procedure and requires a sterile catheter.

Catheter/Inlet Tube Fixation

Various references have been made throughout this chapter to the problems encountered when the catheter and drainage bag inlet tube are allowed to hang unsupported.

There are two ways in which this can be remedied, both requiring fixation to the leg. Traditionally, this has involved the use of adhesive tape. While this may be a relatively cheap alternative in the short term it can be unsatisfactory for a number of reasons. The most important of these is that adhesion is often short-lived especially when the skin is moist from sweat. Where the catheter is silicone or silicone-elastomer coated, adhesion is thought to be reduced as these materials are used as 'release systems' for medical adhesive tapes (Pomfret, 1991). Allergy to any of the tapes used will cause further discomfort. The use of a catheter support may be more appropriate especially where there is a long-term requirement for support.

Whichever method is used, it is important that there is no restriction to the free flow of urine from the bladder. This may occur more easily where the support is applied to the relatively soft catheter rather than the inlet tube. The comfort of the patient is always of paramount importance and thus his/her preference should be taken into account. For males, there should be enough 'slack' in the system to allow for penile erection. Finally, the method used must be one that the patient can manage.

Potential Problems Post-Removal

Urinary retention can be dealt with using intermittent catheterisation. Occasionally retention continues and the patient should be taught intermittent self-catheterisation (see section on CISC). This is preferable to a further episode of indwelling catheterisation which does not provide an opportunity for the bladder tone to improve.

Slight bleeding may occur, particularly if the catheter tip has become calcified. The patient should be warned to expect some blood loss when next passing urine. If the bleeding persists or becomes heavy, cauterization of the bleeding vessels will be required.

Similarly, slight pain may be experienced during and after removal, particularly when the bladder starts to fill. This may be due to reduced detrusor compliance and the patient may also experience urinary frequency and urgency. This usually subsides as the bladder becomes used to holding increased volumes of urine. The patient can speed up this process by attempting to extend the time intervals between voids. If the pain is due to trauma on removal, mild analgesia should be used until it subsides.

PREPARATION FOR DISCHARGE

As the numbers of patients cared for in the community grows and non-professional carers are expected to provide more care, it is increasingly important that both groups are provided with adequate instruction on various aspects of catheter care. However, it has been found that many patients are being discharged to the community with little idea about how to care for their catheters and that this results in frequent telephone calls to the ward and may result in increased admissions (Kennedy, 1983a).

Studies of what information is in fact given by nurses to patients and their carers have shown that it is neither comprehensive nor consistent with research literature (McCullough, 1989; Roe, 1989a).

Further work has shown that patients do benefit from education programmes and that these should be consistent and continued after discharge (Roe, 1990). To aid education, some manufacturers of urinary drainage equipment produce illustrated booklets written specifically for patients.

Although much of this literature is also useful for staff, it has been recognised that they need information which is more technical and research-based (Wright, 1989). Thus it may be useful to have written guidelines for nurses and staff which act as an adjunct to practice policies and procedures.

Information patients require include the following:

- Simple anatomy of the urinary tract
- The position of the catheter in the bladder in relation to function
- Emptying and changing the body-worn bag
- Setting up the 'link' system and caring for the free-standing bag
- How to recognise the onset of problems such as blockage and infection
- How to deal with specific problems
- Where and when to seek further advice (names and telephone numbers).

Some patients will also need to be taught how to recatheterise themselves and how to perform bladder washouts. This process cannot be completed overnight and discharge planning should reflect this. Only when the patient is confident and support from the community nursing staff has been arranged should the patient be sent home.

The patient should be discharged with 2 weeks' supply of the correct equipment. Prescription details should be given so that further supplies can be obtained. The community nurse should be sent details of the system and informed of any problems encountered with it.

The date for recatheterisation should be arranged and, if the patient is male, it should be established if the community nurse is able to do this and the out-patient appointment adjusted as necessary.

SUPRAPUBIC CATHETERISATION

Bladder drainage by suprapubic catheterisation involves the insertion of a catheter into the bladder via an incision through the anterior abdominal wall. This artificial entrance into the bladder is known as a cystotomy.

As an alternative method of bladder drainage, suprapubic catheterisation has some distinct advantages over urethral catheterisation:

1. It allows sexual intercourse to take place with less impediment and should be the method of choice for sexually active people.

2. It may reduce the risk of UTI as it does not compromise the urethral defence mechanisms (Norton, 1986).

3. It allows the resumption of normal voiding after urological/major surgery. The suprapubic catheter can be clamped to allow urethral voiding and released if voiding does not occur.

Also, access to the site of catheter entry is easier for cleansing purposes. There are a number of different types of suprapubic catheter available. Some are specifically designed for this purpose and require a suture to secure them in place, although, for long-term use, a Foley catheter is adequate.

In some instances, urethral closure may be performed after insertion of the suprapubic catheter if urethral leakage is a problem.

Care of the Suprapubic Catheter

The nursing care is the same as for urethral catheters and exactly the same principles of management apply. Secretions which often occur around the catheter site can be removed during bathing or just with soap, water and a clean cloth. A dressing may be required if secretions soil clothing but this is not essential.

Changing the catheter is a simple procedure which can be easily undertaken by nursing staff on the ward or in the patient's home and according to local policy. In some cases, the patient or carers may be taught to change the catheter.

After removal of the catheter, the channel should heal rapidly under a dressing.

SEXUALITY AND BODY IMAGE

The problems resulting from permanent catheterisation are not only physical but also invade emotional well-being. Although this form of urinary drainage may provide increased freedom, it can also severely interfere with self-esteem and dignity. However, when the alternative is the constant need for pads to control incontinence, a UDS can be a very positive form of management. Attending to individual needs and life-style will go a long way to ensuring optimum quality of life for the catheterised person.

Many able-bodied people have complexes about how their partners view them and so it is perfectly natural for the catheterised patient to have anxieties about whether or not his/her partner still finds him/her sexually attractive. Involving the partner in the management of the UDS may not only be necessary but can also help the partner demonstrate that the UDS does not affect a deep and loving relationship.

It is a common misconception that the presence of a urethral catheter precludes sexual intercourse. If the bladder dysfunction coexists with a physical disability, the patient may feel that sex is no longer a viable prospect. This belief has been compounded by the fact that little, if any, sexual advice is given to patients with urethral catheters. A study of 36 catheterised males and females found that no professional had voluntarily discussed sex with any of the patients fitted with a catheter and the patients did not know that intercourse was possible with a catheter in situ (Roe and Brocklehurst, 1987). Fifty per cent of the males questioned stated that they no longer experienced erections and, of those that did, pain was a common experience.

Sexual behaviour encompasses a range of activities from caressing, kissing and masturbation to penetration of the vagina by the penis. Therefore, it should be remembered that many people enjoy active and fulfilling sex lives without penetration taking place.

It is possible for the patient or his/her partner to be taught to remove the catheter and replace it after intercourse has taken place. Women can tape the catheter onto the abdomen where it will come to no harm. Men can tape the catheter along the erect penis and secure it under a condom. The drainage bag, once emptied, can be positioned out of the way in the bed although care should be taken that the drainage tubing does not become compressed, preventing urine from draining from the bladder. Alternatively, the drainage bag can be disconnected from the catheter and a spigot attached during intercourse. A water-based lubricant can be used to facilitate insertion. Oil-based lubricants should not be used as these will rot the rubber condom.

The patient should be counselled about position during intercourse. While a comfortable position, in which the patient can relax, should be sought, some positions can cause increased traction on the catheter. An example of this is the missionary position and a 'side-to-side' position may be preferable.

These more intimate problems need to be addressed in the early stages of catheterisation before inter-relationship problems have a chance to develop. Some health authorities have a sexual counsellor who will be able to offer advice and practical suggestions. The patient's GP or local Relate branch should be able to suggest other local facilities that offer this type of service.

Mutually reading a book such as *Treat Yourself to Sex – A Guide to Good Living* by Paul Brown and Carolyn Faulder or *How to Improve Your Sex Life* by Dr David Devlin can help to establish sexual needs and promote discussion. The Association to Aid the Sexual and Personal Relationships of People with a Disability (SPOD – Sexual Problems of the Disabled, 286 Camden Road, London, N7 0BJ) is a useful educational and informative resource for carers and clients.

CLEAN INTERMITTENT SELF-CATHETERISATION (CISC)

CISC is an alternative method of bladder drainage whereby a catheter is passed intermittently into the bladder and removed immediately drainage has ceased. It is a relatively simple procedure which can easily be taught by a nurse.

The increasing popularity of CISC over the last 20 years is largely due to the work carried out by Lapides and his colleagues in the United States. They suggested that 'most cases of urinary tract infections are caused by some structural or functional abnormality of the urogenital tract, which leads to a decreased resistance of tissue to bacterial invasion' (Lapides et al, 1974). They postulated that high intravesical pressures caused by a build-up of residual urine would compromise the vascular supply to the bladder and render the patient more vulnerable to infection. Thus they emphasised the importance of regular bladder drainage.

Lapides' studies have shown that intermittent catheterisation markedly reduces the complications associated with permanent indwelling catheterisation (see section on Management) and that there is no advantage to be gained from the use of sterile intermittent self-catheterisation over the clean technique in terms of increased urinary tract infection or renal damage. These findings have been based on follow-up over a number of years and have been corroborated by a number of researchers (Lapides et al, 1972, 1974, 1976; Champion, 1976; Webb et al, 1990).

Indications

The technique of CISC is suitable for draining residual urine from the bladder resulting from most causes. It is most commonly used in the presence of an upper or lower motor neurone lesion but is also appropriate in cases of diabetic neuropathy and mechanical outflow obstruction if surgery is not indicated or does not relieve the retention completely. It may be used for postoperative retention and can be used on a temporary or permanent basis.

CISC is equally suitable for males and females although location of the urethra is generally easier for males. Children of 4 years and older can be taught the procedure with parental supervision (Eckstein, 1979).

Criteria for Successful Use of CISC

Probably the most important criteria for the success of CISC are motivation and cognitive skills. If the patient is unwilling to perform the procedure or does not understand the importance of regular bladder drainage, then the complications of urinary tract infection and upper tract dilatation are likely.

Frequency of Catheterisation

One of the aims of CISC is to allow increased freedom and the chance to return to a more normal life-style than that offered by permanent catheterisation. Therefore, it is important that CISC does not have to be performed at an unacceptable frequency. Assessment of the functional capacity of the bladder either by cystometry or through the use of a frequency chart will give this information. It is usually felt that every 2 hours is the maximum frequency which is acceptable during waking hours and that sleep should be undisturbed.

It is commonly believed that catheterisation should be carried out at a frequency which maintains the sum of the voided volume plus the residual volume at below

400–500 ml (Alderman, 1988). However, of 240 patients using CISC, many of whom are unable to void unaided, a number catheterise only once or twice a day without any apparent harmful effects. In practice, CISC is a means by which the patient can control bladder emptying and symptoms, thus regimens should be encouraged to suit individual needs. For example, an extra catheterisation before a period in which reaching a toilet would be impossible or prior to sexual intercourse is perfectly acceptable.

If the patient is also experiencing symptoms of a hyper-reflexic bladder, such as frequency of micturition, urgency, urge incontinence, nocturia and nocturnal enuresis, anticholinergic drugs can be used. In some cases, high bladder pressures or small bladder capacity can be remedied using the surgical procedure known as clam cystoplasty.

Learning CISC

Manual dexterity may prohibit some people from learning CISC although those with the use of only one hand, if highly motivated, can still learn the technique. Use of the Rosenbaum device may assist some patients, particularly those with a tremor, because it aims to allow alignment of the catheter with the urethra without requiring fine hand movements. Also available are plastic 'handles' which the patient with a poor grip may find easier to hold than the catheter itself.

Poor eyesight or even complete blindness does not preclude this form of management. Providing the patient is able to identify the urethral meatus without contamination of the catheter tip and is able to clean the catheter afterwards, deficient eyesight should not present any problems.

Some people find it easier to learn CISC by touch from the outset thus giving them an advantage when catheterising over the toilet. This method of learning is useful when teaching elderly females with reduced spinal flexion coupled with poor eyesight which prevents them identifying the meatus using a mirror. However, many women learn CISC by lying or sitting in a comfortable position either on the bed or floor. With the legs apart, a magnifying mirror and a good light source will allow identification of the meatus and passage of the catheter. Gentian violet may be used to highlight the meatus. A small dish or bowl can be used to collect the urine drained. Alternatively, there are catheters manufactured with an integral collecting bag to prevent the problem of spillage.

For some people, the effort of getting into a suitable position for CISC will be impossible or impracticable on a regular basis (Henderson, 1989). The Deavin–Hunt device has been specifically designed to enable identification of the meatus using a mirror while in a wheelchair (Hunt and Whitaker, 1990).

Whichever technique is used for learning CISC, it is always important that the patient is as relaxed as possible and has had plenty of time to discuss with the nurse or doctor the advantages and disadvantages of the technique. All questions should be answered as comprehensively as possible using terminology appropriate to the individual. Patients catheterising at home should have easy access to their nurse and doctor and should receive as much support as they require. This will help to reduce the number of people who abandon the technique when they feel unable to cope with problems to which there is often a simple solution. If being taught in hospital, thought should be given to how the patient will manage at home and whether adequate support can be given.

Hygiene

Hands should be thoroughly washed before and after catheterisation. After the catheter has been withdrawn it should be washed using soapy water and the outside dried. Care should be taken to ensure that globules of lubricating jelly are flushed out from around the tip of the catheter. The catheter should then be placed in a small plastic bag. Where the catheter is kept will depend on individual needs. As discretion and normality are so important, catheters are kept in various everyday-type containers such as a pencil case, make-up bag or knitting-needle holder. When at home, keeping the catheter in the fridge helps to maintain its rigidity and reduce bacterial multiplication. Most of these types of catheter can be re-used for up to a week although this practice must be based on the recommendations of the company manufacturing the catheter.

Different Types of Catheter

Because CISC does not require the catheter to be retained in the bladder, it need not have a retention balloon. There are two types of catheter commonly used, the Nelaton and the Scott catheters. The Nelaton catheter is made from soft plastic with two drainage eyes at one end and a funnel at the other and comes in a standard length for males and a shorter length for females. The Scott catheter is made of harder plastic which provides a more rigid catheter to aid insertion and does not have a funnelled end. It is not unknown for patients to cut off the funnelled end of the catheter and this has resulted in the catheter disappearing into the bladder (Morgan and Weston, 1990). The Scott catheter is only suitable for negotiating the female urethra and thus is only manufactured in the shorter length. Silver catheters are available and can be cleaned by washing and drying as above followed by baking in a preheated oven at 180°C (350°F) for 10 minutes.

Most catheters require lubrication to aid insertion. However, there is now available a self-lubricating catheter which, when dipped into water, becomes extremely slippery. These catheters are not recommended for re-use as handling can reduce the lubricant effect.

Potential Problems with CISC

UTI

The reduced incidence of UTI associated with CISC has been discussed. However, the patient should be able to identify the onset of a UTI, recognising the signs and symptoms of cloudy, offensive or blood-stained urine, a sudden increase in bladder symptoms, pain on passing urine and feeling generally unwell with an associated temperature. During periods of treatment with antibiotics, it is important that CISC continues to ensure that residual urine does not further contribute to urine infection.

Bleeding

Blood may be evident on the outside of the catheter during initial catheterisation and is usually due to slight trauma during insertion. Insertion can be made easier by using a water-based lubricant jelly or a self-lubricating catheter. Blood in the urine may also be due to the trauma of insertion but could indicate a UTI if it occurs in association with any of the above signs or symptoms. If the bleeding becomes heavy or is persistent, medical help should be sought.

Pain

Pain is often experienced during early catheterisation and can be worsened by tension and anxiety. Good lubrication and, for men, the use of an anaesthetic jelly, can reduce the discomfort. Men should be shown how to position the penis during insertion of the catheter to minimise trauma experienced as the catheter passes through the curved portions of the urethra. Postmenopausal women may experience discomfort from trauma to de-oestrogenised tissue particularly when they are not skilled at identifying the urethral meatus immediately. Hormone replacement therapy can improve the quality of the urethral tissue and reassurance that it often takes a lot of practice to be able to insert the catheter easily can help to relax the patient.

Why Should CISC be Considered

Being able to dispense with the burden of a catheter or the need to wear incontinence pads has revolutionised the lives of many people:

> 'Words cannot express how different I feel. No more pads, it is marvellous. Nobody knew what I was going through. I was too ashamed and embarrassed to talk to anybody about it, not even my own mother.'
>
> 'I now feel far more confident in myself. I look forward to going out and getting dressed up. I wish I had known about self-catheterisation 2½ years ago, then I wouldn't have had 2½ years of utter misery.' (Sibley, 1988).

INTERMITTENT CATHETERISATION (IC)

There are a number of people for whom self-catheterisation is impossible. This may be due to physical handicap such a quadriplegia or a psychological inability to accept the technique. In these instances, IC can be performed by a carer who may be a friend, relative or nurse. If a nurse is doing IC it should be an aseptic technique whether in the hospital or the patient's home and a fresh catheter should be used for each catheterisation.

When embarking on a programme of IC or CISC in hospital, it is extremely important to consider whether it will be practical in the home situation. It is often useful to teach another person IC as a back-up during times of reduced ability.

Acknowledgements

The Association for Continence Advisors for allowing representation of pictures from the *Directory of Continence and Toiletting Aids*.

Petra Britton for her assistance in the formulation of the chapter.

References

Alderman C (1988) DIY catheters freedom. *Nursing Standard* **2**: 25–26.
Association of Continence Advisors (1988) *Directory of Continence and Toiletting Aids*, 3rd edn. London: Association of Continence Advisors.
Bailey S (1991) Using bladder washouts. *Nursing Times* **87**: (24): 75–76.
Barnes K and Malone-Lee J (1986) Long-term catheter management: minimising the problem of premature replacement due to balloon deflation. *Journal of Advanced Nursing* **11**: 303–307.
Blandy JP and Moors J (1989) *Urology for Nurses*. London: Blackwell Scientific Publications.
Blannin JP (1982) The selection and management of catheters. *Geriatric Medicine* **12**(6): 57–58.
Burke JP, Garibaldi RA, Britt MR et al (1981) Prevention of catheter associated urinary tract infections. *American Journal of Medicine*, **70**: 655–658.
Burkitt D and Randall J (1987) Urethral trauma. *Nursing Times* **83**(43): 59–63.
Castle M (1974) Urinary tract catheterisation and associated infection. *Nursing Research* **23**(2): 170–174.
Champion VL (1976) Clean technique for intermittent self-catheterisation. *Nursing Research* **25**(1): 13–18.
Crow R, Chapman R, Roe B and Wilson J (1986) *A Study of Patients with an Indwelling Catheter*. Guildford: University of Surrey Nursing Practice Research Unit.
Crummey V (1989) Ignorance can hurt. *Nursing Times* **85**(21): 67–68.
Dance DAB, Pearson AD, Seal DV and Lawes JA (1987) A hospital outbreak caused by a chlorhexidine and antibiotic-resistant *Proteus mirabilis*. *Journal of Hospital Infection* **10**: 10–16.
Eckstein HB (1979) Intermittent catheterisation of the bladder in patients with neuropathic incontinence of urine. *Zeitschrift für Kinderchirurgie und Grenzgebiete* **28**(4): 408–412.
Elliot TSJ, Gopal Rao G, Rigby RC et al (1989) Bladder irrigation or irritation? *British Journal of Urology* **64**(4): 391–394.
Garibaldi RA, Burke JP, Dickamn ML et al (1974) Factors predisposing to bacteriuria following indwelling urethral catheterisation. *New England Journal of Medicine* **291**: 215–219.
Getliffe KA and Mulhall AB (1991) The encrustation of catheters. *British Journal of Urology* **67**: 337–341.
Hedelin H, Bratt CG, Eckerda G and Lincoln K (1991) Relationship between urease-producing bacteria, urinary pH and encrustation on indwelling urinary catheters. *British Journal of Urology* **67**: 527–531.
Henderson JS (1989) Intermittent clean self-catheterisation in clients with neurogenic bladder resulting from multiple sclerosis. *Journal of Neuroscience Nursing* **21**(3): 160–164.

Hunt GM and Whitaker RH (1990) A new device for self-catheterisation in wheelchair bound women. *British Journal of Urology* **66**: 162–163.

Kass EH (1957) Bacteriuria and the diagnosis of infections of the urinary tract. *Archives of Internal Medicine* **100**: 709–714.

Kennedy A (1983a) Incontinence advice: long-term catheterisation. *Nursing Times* **79**(17): 41–45.

Kennedy A (1983b) Care of the elderly catheterised. *British Journal of Geriatric Nursing* **2**(6): 10–15.

Kennedy A (1984) An extra hot water bottle? *Nursing Times* **80**(17): 57–61.

Kennedy A, Brocklehurst JC and Lye MDW (1983) Factors related to the problems of long-term catheterisation. *Journal of Advanced Nursing* **8**: 207–212.

Kunin CM (1989) *Detection, Prevention and Management of Urinary Tract Infection*, 3rd edn. Philadelphia: Lea and Febiger.

Kunin CM, Chin QF and Chambers S (1987) Formation of encrustations on indwelling urinary catheters in the elderly. A comparison of different types of catheter material in blockers and non-blockers. *Journal of Urology* **138**: 899–902.

Lapides J, Ananias CD, Silber SJ and Lowe BS (1972) Clean intermittent self-catheterisation in the treatment of urinary tract disease. *Journal of Urology* **107**: 458–461.

Lapides J, Ananias CD, Lowe BS and Kalish MD (1974) Follow-up on unsterile intermittent self-catheterisation. *Journal of Urology* **111**: 184–187.

Lapides J, Ananias CD, Gould FR and Lowe BS (1976) Further observations on self-catheterisation. *Journal of Urology* **116**: 116–119.

Lowthian P (1989) Preventing trauma. *Nursing Times* **85**(21): 73–75.

McCullough J (1989) Catheter care at home. Community outlook. *Nursing Times* **85**: 4–8.

Moisey CU and Williams LA (1980) Self-retained balloon catheters – a safe method for removal. *British Journal of Urology* **52**: 67.

Morgan JDT and Weston PMT (1990) The disappearing catheter – a complication of intermittent catheterisation. *British Journal of Urology* **65**(1): 113–114.

Mulhall A (1991) Biofilms and urethral catheter infections. *Nursing Standard* **5**(18): 26–29.

Noble JG, Menzies D, Cox PJ and Edwards L (1990) Midnight removal: an improved approach to removal of catheters. *British Journal of Urology* **65**: 615–617.

Norton C (1986) *Nursing for Continence*, p. 293. Beaconsfield: Beaconsfield Publishers Ltd.

Parsons CL, Mulholland SG and Anwar H (1979) Antibacterial activity of bladder surface mucin duplicated by exogenous glycosaminoglycan (heparin). *Infection and Immunity* **25**: 552–554.

Pomfret I (1991) The catheter debate. *Nursing Times* **87**(37): 67–68.

Roe B (1989a) Long-term catheter care in the community. *Nursing Times* **85**(36): 43–44.

Roe B (1989b) *Catheter Care: Meatal Cleansing, Bladder Washouts and Catheter Removal*. London: HG Wallace Ltd.

Roe B (1990) Do we need to clamp catheters? *Nursing Times* **86**(43): 66-67.

Roe B and Brocklehurst JC (1987) Study of patients with indwelling catheters. *Journal of Advanced Nursing* **12**: 713–718.

Roe B, Reid FJ and Brocklehurst JC (1988) A comparison of four drainage systems. *Journal of Advanced Nursing* **13**: 374–382.

Sibley L (1988) Confidence with incontinence. *Nursing Times* **84**(46): 42–43.

Stickler DJ, Clayton CL and Chawla JC (1987) The resistance of urinary tract pathogens to chlorhexidine bladder washouts. *Journal of Hospital Infection* **10**: 28–39.

Studer UE, Bishop MD and Zing EJ (1983) How to fill a silicone catheter balloon. *Urology* **22**(3): 300–302.

Webb RJ, Lawson AL and Neal DE (1990) Clean intermittent self-catheterisation in 172 adults. *British Journal of Urology* **65**(1): 20–23.

Wright E (1988) Catheter care: the risk of infection. *The Professional Nurse* **3**(12): 487–490.

Wright E (1989) Teaching patients to cope with catheters at home. *The Professional Nurse* **4**(19): 191–194.

5

Urinary Tract Stones

Urinary calculi are among the most common urological problems. It is estimated that 2–3 per cent of the UK population suffer with stones in the urinary tract, with 20–40 per cent of these requiring hospitalisation for pain, obstruction or infection.

CAUSES OF RENAL STONE FORMATION

Many patients with a stone-forming tendency have abnormal crystallisation in the urine. Diseases which result in excessive urinary excretion of solutes such as calcium, oxalates, amino acids (e.g. cystine) or urates exacerbate this tendency to crystallisation. If there is any nucleus on which the crystals can grow, for example:

- Another fragment of stone
- Sloughed renal papillae
- A foreign body, e.g. J–J stent, surgical suture, urinary catheter

then they will precipitate and form stones, especially if there is some urinary obstruction, stagnant pockets of urine (as found in medullary sponge kidneys, for example) or if the patient has inhibited mobility.

Many renal calculi have a nucleus made up of microcrystals of precipitated solute embedded in a substance known as **matrix**, which is a mucoprotein/protein complex probably secreted by renal tubular cells. Eighty-five per cent of stone-forming patients have matrix substance A which develops calcium-binding properties in the urine. As substance A is not found in the urine of patients free from renal stone disease, it is thought that matrix deposition may be the precursor of stone formation.

All patients having treatment for renal stones, either surgical or medical, should undergo evaluation to identify specific metabolic abnormalities that can sometimes be corrected and thus prevent or minimise further stone formation.

On admission to the ward, the patient with stone disease needs a full assessment using the ward's nursing model. This provides a valuable opportunity for the nurse to establish a rapport with her patient and to commence an education programme regarding the further prevention of renal stones. (Details given below are only of the particular titles relevant to renal stones.)

Present State of Health

Present medication and effects/side-effects should be investigated; for example, is the patient with calcium stones taking phosphate-binding antacids? If the patient suffers from pain, the type, locality and severity of pain and how it is relieved should be assessed. How well does the patient actually feel?

Breathing and Circulatory State

Signs of hypertension may accompany idiopathic hypercalciuria or primary hyperparathyroidism, and may also be indicative of deteriorating renal function which could be due to renal calculi.

Maintaining Fluid and Electrolyte Balance

Particular attention should be paid regarding the patient's usual daily fluid intake, and advice given as appropriate. A ward urinalysis should be performed and the specific gravity, presence of protein, blood, etc. recorded. If a 24-hour urine collection for metabolic studies has not been collected within the last 6 months, then one should be commenced. Blood chemistry is checked for urea, calcium, phosphorous, uric acid, creatinine, etc.

Nutritional status

The nurse should be aware of any present dietary restrictions/requirements, e.g. an excessive intake of vitamin C can be a cause of hyperoxaluria, as can excessive consumption of calcium or foods high in oxalates, etc. The dietician should be consulted as necessary. It is important to assess what the patient normally eats while at home. Any signs of nausea and vomiting which could be secondary to renal colic, should be noted.

Eliminating Body Waste

Signs of urinary frequency, dysuria, haematuria or urgency of micturition should be noted. The nurse should assess urinary stream and look for signs of urinary incontinence. She should check for signs of urinary tract infection and collect a midstream urine specimen for microscopy and culture. She should enquire whether any gravel or stone fragments have been passed. Bowel actions should be assessed – chronic diarrhoea and malabsorption syndrome can both be causes of hyperoxaluria. Menopausal women are at risk of osteoporosis.

Level of Independence

The nurse should look for signs of mobility impairment, as immobilization and skeletal disease can be signs of gout. She should check type of occupation, as urinary calculi are more common in professional groups and those working in raised environmental temperatures than those with active physical employment. (Doctors are the most common professional group to suffer from stones.)

Attitudes to Hospitalization

The nurse should look for signs of anxiety which could be due to loss of independence, financial worries, particularly if the patient has had several hospital admissions, or fears of identity loss.

The patient will be clerked and examined by the doctor, and radiological investigations, such as a kidney, ureter and bladder X-ray (KUB), will be performed and an intravenous urogram or ultrasound scan may be performed to identify urinary obstruction. If the patient is pyrexial, blood cultures may be taken and the patient will be commenced on a course of antibiotics. Any inherited metabolic disorder will be discussed and if stones have been passed or retrieved, a stone analysis will be performed and discussed. If the patient requires surgical removal of stones, such as percutaneous nephrolithotomy or lasertripsy or extracorporeal piezo-electric lithotripsy, then preparations will be made.

TYPES OF RENAL STONE

There are four major types of renal stone: struvite, uric acid, calcium-containing and cystine. Figure 5.1 illustrates the likely areas of stone formation within the urinary tract.

Struvite Stones

Struvite stones are composed of calcium, magnesium and ammonium phosphate, known as 'triple phosphate'. They occur only when the urinary pH is > 7.5 and they form only in the presence of chronic urinary tract infection. They are formed by the action of many microorganisms, especially *Proteus mirabilis*, which produce the enzyme urease which hydrolyses urea (which the kidneys excrete in large amounts), to form ammonium ions with the result that the urine becomes intensely alkaline. The phosphates which are normally present in urine are insoluble in alkaline urine, resulting in the growth of struvite stones. Struvite stones continue to grow as the bacteria multiply. These stones tend to be soft and crumbly, and grow very rapidly, often forming large irregular staghorn calculi. They can grow to fill each calyx and the renal pelvis and cause obstruction, damage to the kidney and can lead to renal failure.

Once formed, no matter how dilute the urine, struvite stones cannot be dissolved and need lithotripsy or surgical removal. All the fragments must be removed as any that are left are infected and will regrow. After complete removal of the stone, antibiotics, such as trimethoprim 200 mg b.d., must be administered for 2–4 weeks, to prevent recurrence of infection in the urinary tract. Patients who suffer from recurrent urinary tract infections are often treated with a long-term, low-dosage antibiotic, such as trimethoprim 100 mg nocte, to maintain sterile urine.

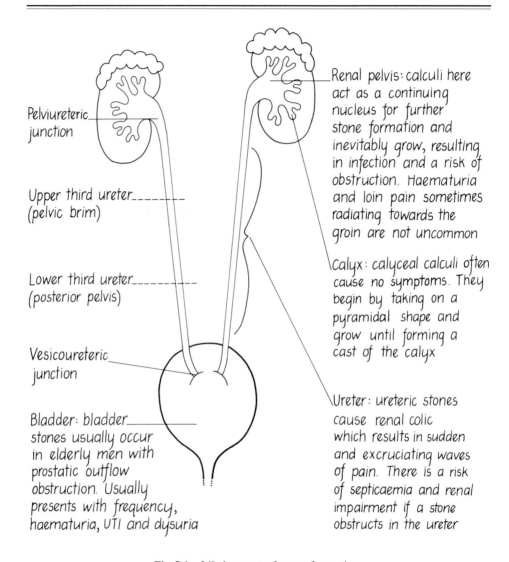

Pelviureteric junction

Upper third ureter (pelvic brim)

Lower third ureter (posterior pelvis)

Vesicoureteric junction

Bladder: bladder stones usually occur in elderly men with prostatic outflow obstruction. Usually presents with frequency, haematuria, UTI and dysuria

Renal pelvis: calculi here act as a continuing nucleus for further stone formation and inevitably grow, resulting in infection and a risk of obstruction. Haematuria and loin pain sometimes radiating towards the groin are not uncommon

Calyx: calyceal calculi often cause no symptoms. They begin by taking on a pyramidal shape and grow until forming a cast of the calyx

Ureter: ureteric stones cause renal colic which results in sudden and excruciating waves of pain. There is a risk of septicaemia and renal impairment if a stone obstructs in the ureter

Fig 5.1   Likely areas of stone formation

Uric Acid Stones

Uric acid is a normal urinary solute, but is almost insoluble in acid urine; therefore, those patients who habitually produce acidic urine are at risk of developing uric acid stones. Uric acid stones can grow very large and fill the whole of the collecting system, forming staghorn calculi.

In most cases, the cause of uric acid stones is a urine pH persistently less than 5.5, due to impaired renal ammoniagenesis. Other predisposing factors are:

- Hyperuricosuria (up to 40 per cent of patients with uric acid stones have this condition)
- Excessive purine in diet – meat, fish, poultry, yeast, etc.
- Gout
- Malignancy
- A metabolism error, e.g. Lesch–Nyhan syndrome
- Alcohol ingestion

Patients with ileostomies suffer from alkaline losses in the upper gastrointestinal tract which results in a persistently acid and concentrated urine that also predisposes to the formation of uric acid stones.

Uric acid stones are radiolucent and are only seen on X-ray if they also contain calcium.

The normal range of urate present in urine varies with age, diet and sex and is between 250 and 1000 mg daily. The higher the dietary purine intake, the greater the urinary urate excretion. About two-thirds of urate is excreted in urine and the remainder is lost via bile and intestinal and gastric secretion.

Initial treatment consists of advising patients to restrict purine in their diets, and limit their total daily meat and fish ingestion to 5–7 ounces daily. If this fails, allopurinol is indicated for patients with hyperuricosuria.

Patients without hyperuricosuria but who have persistently acid urine are advised to increase their urine volumes by drinking at least 3 litres of fluid daily and by taking sodium bicarbonate 10–20 mg daily as prescribed in order to maintain a constant urinary pH over 7.

Hypercalciuria

Calcium-containing stones are the most common type and have the largest array of potential metabolic causes. Hypercalciuria is the most common abnormality in patients with calcium-containing renal calculi, and the condition has many causes. Hypercalciuria is identified by urinary calcium excretion of more than 300 mg/day in men and 250 mg/day in women.

Hypercalciuria can be caused by:

- Idiopathic hypercalciuria
- Hyperparathyroidism
- Malignancy, associated with bony metastases/multiple myeloma
- Sarcoid
- Excessive dietary ingestion of calcium and vitamin D
- Renal tubular acidosis
- Prolonged recumbency

Most patients with first-time calcium stones are treated conservatively. A fluid intake of over 3 litres daily is recommended to reduce the chance of calcium precipitating in the urinary tract. Patients should be advised to check their domestic tap water, for example, in London, tap water is 'hard', containing about 2.5 mmol/l (10 mg/100 ml) of calcium.

A moderate intake of calcium of two or three servings daily should be maintained to keep the daily calcium intake to 800 mg. If calcium consumption is too restricted, an increased urinary excretion of oxalate results and this leads to a negative calcium balance which can cause osteoporosis.

Those patients with primary hyperparathyroidism may require surgery in the form of a partial or total parathyroidectomy.

If hypercalciuria persists, despite a calcium restriction of 800 mg maximum daily, normal levels are often achieved by the administration of sodium cellulose phosphate 5 g t.d.s. half an hour before meals. Sodium cellulose phosphate is an agent that binds intestinal calcium. It is unsuitable for use with some patients due to its possible side-effects of sickness and diarrhoea. Thiazide diuretics are often beneficial, as they lower urinary calcium excretion by increasing calcium reabsorption in the renal tubules. Bendrofluazide is the drug of choice, and a dosage of 5–10 mg is often effective.

Cystinuria

Cystinuria is an autosomal recessive disorder of the proximal tubules. A defect of amino acid transportation by the brush border membranes of the proximal tubule results in a failure of tubular reabsorption of the amino acids cystine, ornithine, arginine and lysine (note: can be remembered by abbreviations C–O–A–L). Cystine is poorly soluble and although in cystinuria, urinary lysine excretion is twice that of cystine, lysine stones do not form; this is because cystine is much less soluble than lysine in urine with a pH of less than 7. Therefore, cystine stones form in the urinary tract whilst lysine remains inconspicuously in solution.

Cystinuria is frequently diagnosed in the late teenage years and early twenties and is inherited by a recessive gene. Most cases do not require treatment, but 3 per cent, if left untreated, tend to develop into progressive renal failure.

Cystinuria is diagnosed by either a nitroprusside test of the urine which is used as a qualitative screen, or by demonstration of cystine crystals in urine, which are of a typical hexagonal shape. A cystinuric may excrete over 200 mg daily. A normal urinary cystine excretion is up to 40 mg daily. Cystine stones have a low radio-opacity, but they can be detected on a plain abdominal radiograph, especially when coated with calcium phosphate which increases their radiodensity. Cystine stones can grow large enough to form staghorn calculi and sometimes cystine forms a sludge-like substance in the renal tract.

Large volumes of fluid decrease the cystine concentration in the urine and increase its solubility; therefore, the first line of treatment is fluid therapy. If the urine volume can be maintained at over 3 litres in 24 hours, cystine stones can be dissolved or their formation discouraged. Total cystine excretion is measured by testing a 24-hour urine collection, and a urine volume is then aimed for which is high enough to maintain the final cystine concentration at less than 250 mg/day. For example, in a patient with a cystine excretion of 1000 mg/day, a urine volume of at least 4000 ml/day should be achieved. The fluid intake should be spread out over 24 hours, and it is particularly important that the patient drinks at night when the urine is more concentrated and the volume generally decreased. Ideally, the patient should drink 800 ml before going to bed, and then when the patient gets up in the night to pass urine he should drink another 800 ml and this should be continued throughout the night. It is perhaps of little surprise that most patients are reluctant to follow this advice, but nevertheless, it should be encouraged.

When cystine excretion persists at too high a concentration for an increased fluid intake to be effective (e.g. if the 24-hour urinary cystine were 2000 mg, the urine volume would need to be at least 8 litres per day!), then an alternative form of treatment is needed. The drug D-penicillamine is effective in reducing the concentration of cystine, but it is reserved for use as a last resort as it has many side-effects. Penicillamine is nephrotoxic, can cause Goodpasture's syndrome, haemolytic anaemia, systemic lupus erythematosus, rheumatoid-like disorders, thrombocytopenia and myasthenia gravis, and is known to be teratogenic in rats. Obviously, because of these severe side-effects, the patient should be carefully observed, particularly for signs of nephrotic syndrome.

Hyperoxaluria

Oxalate salts are extremely insoluble and even mild hyperoxaluria may significantly increase the rate of calcium oxalate stone formation. The underlying cause in most hyperoxaluric patients is acquired enteric hyperoxaluria, which occurs as a secondary abnormality in conditions associated with fat malabsorption, e.g. inflammatory bowel disease, small bowel resection, intestinal bypass, etc.

Primary hyperoxaluria has a poor outlook, and end-stage renal failure is common by the teenage years. At post-mortem, oxalate crystals are often found in the renal parenchyma, blood vessels, epiphyses, the heart and testes. Primary hyperoxaluria is a hereditary condition and often causes more than 100 mg of oxalate excretion daily.

Mild to moderate hyperoxaluria (40–80 mg/day) can be caused by an excessively high intake of foods rich in oxalates, such as: grapefruit, cola, tea, strawberries, nuts, chocolate, tomatoes, rhubarb and spinach. As ascorbic acid is metabolized to oxalate, the foods rich in vitamin C are therefore also contributory factors to the formation of oxalate stones.

Treatment consists of the patient taking a low oxalate, low-fat diet with an increased consumption of foods with a high calcium content. If this is unsuccessful, calcium supplements 1–4 g daily in divided doses with meals are prescribed. This does result in increased urinary calcium, but apparently the benefits far exceed the risks. Cholestyramine is sometimes used as it binds both bile salts and oxalates so they do not injure the colon. It is effective, but most patients do not like it because of its odour and the bulky stools it causes. It also causes vitamin K depletion, which must be treated prophylactically.

PERCUTANEOUS NEPHROLITHOTOMY (PCNL)

PCNL is a recent development in renal surgery whereby calculi are removed through a narrow track under X-ray vision. The track is established by gradual dilatation following an initial needle puncture of the kidney. The track, passing through the skin, muscle and parenchyma is dilated to a size of 26–30 Charrière (CH), large enough to allow the introduction of a nephroscope enabling inspection of the interior of the kidney. The procedure requires the close cooperation of the radiologist and urologist.

The stone is extracted by grasping forceps or disintegrated by ultrasonic lithotripsy (USL) or electrohydraulic lithotripsy (EHL). Remaining stone fragments are flushed out through the nephroscope or pass spontaneously down the ureter.

During the procedure the patient is intubated under general anaesthetic and fluid is given intravenously to replace intraoperative blood loss. In most cases a urethral catheter is inserted at the outset of the procedure as haematuria with clots may result. Following extraction of the stone, the kidney is screened to ensure that no fragments remain in the collecting system. A whistle-tipped nephrostomy is left in the track to facilitate drainage of blood and urine and reduce the risk of formation of an intrarenal haematoma. Stone fragments are sent for biochemical analysis and in certain cases advice may be given to the patient to reduce the risk of stones re-forming.

History

The percutaneous route was first used in 1941 when Rupel and Brown (1976) used a cystoscope and forceps to remove a stone which was obstructing a single kidney. A number of similar procedures were performed in the following years but the most significant development took place in 1976 in Sweden when Fernstrom and Johansen (1976) combined the use of a percutaneous track and the extraction of stones under X-ray guidance using stone-grabbing forceps.

In 1981 Wickham reported the successful removal of stones via the percutaneous route at the Institute of Urology in London (Wickham and Kellett 1981). He was the first to use the procedure in Britain in association with radiologist Dr M. J. Kellett.

Indications

The indications for PCNL are the same as for open renal surgery and are as follows:

- Persistent or intermittent loin pain
- Haematuria
- Recurrent urinary tract infection
- Obstruction of a kidney by a stone
- Rapid growth of an existing stone
- Asymptomatic patients found to have stones on routine screening whose profession precludes the presence of stones, e.g. airline pilots – due to the risk of renal colic

Contraindications

There appears to be only one major contraindication to PCNL and that is the presence of a blood clotting disorder – this naturally precludes this type of surgery unless remedial treatment is undertaken.

Preoperative Investigations

Preoperative investigations are shown in Table 5.1.

Table 5.1 Preoperative investigations for PCNL

Procedure	Rationale
Midstream urine samples (MSU)	To exclude urinary tract infection/commence appropriate antibiotic therapy
Plain abdominal X-ray (KUB)	To show current position of stone
Serum urea and electrolytes	To establish status of renal function
Serum full blood count	To exclude anaemia
Serum clotting screen	To exclude clotting abnormalities
Intravenous urography (IVU)	To show anatomy of kidney
Cross-match 2 units of blood	In case of haemorrhage

Advantages of the Percutaneous Route

Advantages of PCNL are as follows:

1. It allows direct access to the renal pelvis with clear vision of stones, particularly those in the pelvis and upper part of the ureter; removal is therefore simpler.

2. The procedure may be carried out under light general anaesthesia thus enabling patients who would be at risk during a long procedure under general anaesthesia (e.g. patients with spinal injuries, cardiac arrhythmias, obstructive airways disease, spina bifida) to undergo PCNL and be relieved of painful symptoms.

3. Reduced trauma at the time of operation: a small wound and reduced postoperative hospital stay result in early recovery and resumption of work. This in turn has economic benefits, i.e. savings on payment of sickness benefits, faster turnover of hospital in-patients.

4. Reduced risk of wound infection – the nephrostomy drain site does not require sutures and is healed within 48 hours.

5. Reduced postoperative pain following minimally invasive surgery, generally managed with oral analgesia.

6. Low patient morbidity.

7. Reduced risk of postoperative complications associated with prolonged immobility following open surgery (e.g. chest infection, thromboembolic problems).

Complications of Surgery

Haemorrhage

This risk increases with the prolonged operation time required to remove large or multiple stones. Intravenous fluids are increased to maintain the blood pressure, the nephrostomy tube is spigotted to tamponade the track.

In rare cases persistent bleeding may need to be investigated by arteriogram to identify and embolise the vessels involved.

If haematuria persists the urethral catheter remains in situ until the urine clears; a bladder washout may be required to remove clots. The patient is asked to maintain a high intake of oral fluids, 3 litres/24 hours at least.

Bacteraemia

Postoperative pyrexia is not uncommon though less than 5 per cent of patients have been found to have developed bacteraemia and these have been caused by the presence of infective stones. Intravenous antibiotics are given prophylactically on induction of anaesthesia in all cases (e.g. cefuroxime 750 mg and at 8-hourly intervals thereafter for 24–48 hours postoperatively).

Paralytic Ileus

This has been noted in 4 per cent of patients and is managed conservatively with intravenous fluid replacement. The patient is given nil by mouth and a nasogastric tube is passed if nausea and vomiting persist.

Pneumothorax

The risk of pneumothorax increases if the kidney lies high and puncture is above the level of the 12th rib. A chest drain may have to be inserted.

Nursing Management

On Admission/Preoperatively

Nursing management on admission and preoperatively is shown in Table 5.2.

On Return to the Ward

The patient returns with an intravenous infusion (IVI) in progress. This is maintained until he/she is able to resume oral intake of fluid.

In most cases a nephrostomy drain is left in the track. The volume of drainage is recorded on the fluid balance chart along with bladder urine and fluid intake. It is not a cause for concern if the nephrostomy does not drain a significant amount as long as the patient remains comfortable. The drain may have slipped out of the collecting system; this is confirmed by X-ray.

Table 5.2 Preoperative nursing management

Procedure	Rationale
Record temperature, pulse, respirations and blood pressure	Establishes baseline observations, identifies abnormalities
Routine urine test	Excludes diabetes and other underlying disease
MSU for microbiological assessment	Excludes infection, ensures results are current, determines appropriate antibiotic cover is prescribed
Record patient's weight	Enables accurate dosage of premedication, antibiotic and anaesthetic to be prescribed
Complete nursing assessment document (current health status, activities of daily living)	Ensures patient details are correct, identifies special needs and ensures they are met
Complete preoperative care-plan	Provides opportunity for patient to receive information about pre- and postoperative care
Patient has nil by mouth for 6 hours preoperatively	Reduces risk of aspiration of vomit
Premedication is given as prescribed	Reduces patient's anxiety

A urethral catheter may remain in situ if urine drainage is heavily blood-stained. Drainage is observed closely and the urine bag tubing may be gently 'milked' manually to encourage the passage of blood clots or debris.

The patient's pulse and blood pressure are recorded on return and at half-hourly intervals for a period of 2 hours. The temperature may be recorded less frequently, e.g. 2–4 hourly, unless the patient shows signs of pyrexia. The nurse should also be aware of the respiratory rate and record any abnormalities. The frequency of observations may be increased or decreased as the patient's condition dictates.

Following the operation day the patient generally requires little in the way of nursing care as he/she is able to get up when the patient recovered from the anaesthetic. The patient may need assistance with manoeuvring the catheter and nephrostomy if they are present but they do not greatly impede mobility.

First Postoperative Day

IVI is discontinued if:

● Normal diet and fluid have been resumed with no nausea or vomiting
● Patient is apyrexial; if pyrexia is low grade, i.v. cannula may be left in situ for administration of i.v. antibiotics

TPR and BP are recorded 4-hourly unless:

● Heavy haematuria persists
● Pyrexia persists
● Recovery has not been straightforward

KUB X-ray is performed. If no stone fragments remain the nephrostomy may be clamped (on the Resident Surgical Officer's instructions).

Second Postoperative Day

Nephrostomy is removed if:

- No pain has been experienced since clamping
- No leakage has occurred at the nephrostomy site

Possible Problems

Leakage of Urine from Nephrostomy Site

Leakage can persist if oedema is present in the kidney or ureter following the trauma of surgical intervention. It may also indicate the presence of stone fragments not seen on X-ray which obstruct the normal flow of urine. The nephrostomy site will normally close within 24 hours with a firmly applied pressure dressing.

If persistent leakage causes distress to the patient and the skin becomes sore, a urostomy bag can provide accurate measurement of drainage and also help prevent excoriation. This measure should only be taken as a last resort, however, as some urologists believe that the bag encourages the track to continue draining. However, in practice, as the internal oedema decreases, urine drainage via the track diminishes and the bag can usually be removed 24–48 hours later and a light dressing is applied.

Pain

Patients generally experience very little pain postoperatively. Pain is managed with oral analgesics and more severe pain can be managed effectively with diclofenac suppositories 100 mg once daily (a non-steroidal anti-inflammatory drug).

Infection

The nephrostomy site itself rarely becomes infected but urinary tract infections can persist. Oral antibiotics are prescribed according to the sensitivities obtained with the MSU result.

Discharge from Hospital

The patient may be discharged from hospital on the third postoperative day if:

- He/she is afebrile
- He/she has a normal urine output, i.e. colour and volume
- He/she has a dry nephrostomy site

Advice and discharge

Rest and Activity

If the patient has a sedentary occupation he/she may return to work as soon as the patient feels well enough. If he/she is involved in more active or manual labour he/

she should allow 1–2 weeks to convalesce. Any patient with children and/or a household to look after may find it useful to arrange for help in the home to be available for the first week or so.

Sexual Relations

This is very much up to the individual but there are no contraindications to resuming usual relations after recovering from PCNL. Women using the contraceptive pill should seek medical advice about when to start taking it again.

Eating and Drinking

Normal diet can be taken unless advice to the contrary is given. An increased intake of fluid is advised to 'flush' the kidneys and help prevent recurrence of stones; 2.5–3 litres per 24 hours is the aim. A moderate amount of alcohol can improve the appetite and is not thought to be harmful, though it may be contraindicated by certain drugs and this should be ascertained before discharge.

Bowels

Irregular bowel habits may follow a period in hospital after surgery but this usually corrects itself with the resumption of normal diet and exercise. A mild laxative may be required in the short term.

Urine

The patient should be advised that he/she may continue to have blood in the urine after being discharged home. This is not a cause for concern as long as the patient is able to pass urine without difficulty and no blood clots are present. However, if the bleeding is heavy and persists with accompanying discomfort he/she should contact his/her general practitioner who may refer the patient back to the hospital for investigations. Any urinary symptoms e.g. frequency, burning pain on micturition, urgency should not be ignored as they may indicate the presence of a urinary tract infection which should be treated with the appropriate antibiotic.

Wound Healing

The nephrostomy site should be kept covered with a light, sealed-edge dressing until a dry scab forms over it. The scab should form by the third or fourth day after removal of the tube. The dressing need only be changed in the unlikely event that oozing or bleeding occurs once the patient is at home. Dressings should be provided for a further two changes or information should be given on purchasing a suitable alternative from the chemist.

The patient should be advised that he/she may experience itching, tingling or numbness at the nephrostomy site and the tissue may feel hard and lumpy as the healing process progresses. Help should be sought if:

● Pain in the wound increases
● Redness or swelling in the wound increases
● Any discharge occurs

Driving

All patients should ensure that their insurance policy covers them to drive after a general anaesthetic. A time limit to allow for full recovery may apply. The individual must then decide when he/she is strong enough to cope with the various road and traffic conditions likely to be encountered, e.g. emergency stops.

Follow-up

The patient should attend the out-patient clinic for review by the urologist 6 weeks after discharge. At this time a KUB X-ray will be performed, an MSU is sent for microbiological assessment and a blood sample is sent for biochemical assessment to ascertain that renal function has not been impaired. The results of the stone analysis should be available and advice is given on what measures should be taken to reduce the risk of recurrence. In the majority of cases the simple step of increasing fluid intake to 2.5–3 litres/24 hours may be all that is required.

Persistent stone-formers with underlying metabolic causes should be kept under review every 3–6 months to monitor renal function.

NEPHROSTOMY TUBES

A nephrostomy tube is a temporary method of draining the renal pelvis. There are two types:

● Needle nephrostomy tube which is very fine, inserted under local anaesthetic and is used to relieve hydronephrosis caused by ureteric obstruction.
● 28FG nephrostomy tube which is used as a drainage tube following percutaneous nephrolithotomy and can be very uncomfortable.

Care of Nephrostomy Tube

There is a high risk of infection occurring, so the tube must have an occlusive dressing at all times which should be changed if it is soiled, becomes detached or if the patient complains of discomfort. With a needle nephrostomy tube, it is important that it is coiled round and taped securely as it can kink very easily and the suture can come out. A large nephrostomy tube should be taped round to the patient's side so that it does not become occluded while sitting.

The patient should be advised to drink 3 litres of fluid per day.

Night catheter bags can be attached to the nephrostomy tube and a closed-circuit drainage system should be maintained at all times. Leg bags with long tubing can be used if the patient is mobile.

Complications

Haemorrhage

If used postoperatively, the tube may drain large amounts, e.g. 500–1000 ml of blood immediately postoperatively. If so, the tube can be clamped for 1 hour and then released.

Leakage around the Tube

Sometimes urine will leak out continually from around the tube, requiring repeated changing of the dressing. To prevent the patient having an uncomfortable wet dressing, it is possible to apply a 28 mm drainable urostomy bag and combihesive flange. The catheter bag should be detached from the nephrostomy tube and inserted into the night bag outlet of the urostomy bag. The hole in the flange is then cut so that it is just big enough to take the nephrostomy tube, and is then applied firmly to the skin, ensuring it will not leak. The nephrostomy tube can then be manipulated through the flange and into the bag. This procedure requires an aseptic technique and the use of sterile gloves. (This technique can also be used if, once the nephrostomy tube is removed, the site is leaking through dressing pads, and usually after 24 hours the site will have healed enough for a dressing to be adequate.)

Pain

Changing the dressing often makes the tube more comfortable. The tube should be checked for any obstruction and if blocked with clots or debris in the urine, it can be gently flushed with 5–10 ml sodium chloride 0.9 per cent using an aseptic technique. Analgesics, e.g. co-proxamol 2 tablets, may be required to relieve the discomfort.

Infection

The patient should be advised to drink 3 litres/day. A closed-circuit drainage system should be maintained at all times. A specimen should be obtained for microculture and sensitivity if there are signs of urine infection present.

PERCUTANEOUS CHOLECYSTOLITHOTOMY (PCCL)

Percutaneous cholecystolithotomy (removal of gall stones) has been included in this chapter as the procedure is often performed by urologists experienced in percutaneous surgery. Urology nurses therefore need to be familiar with the procedure and the nursing care.

Preoperative Preparation

On the evening prior to surgery, the patient should eat a fat-free meal (see Table 5.3), then take 12 Biloptin capsules which contain a total of 3.68 g of iodine in 6 g of sodium ipodate and is an oral contrast medium (do not give if patient is allergic to iodine). The patient may drink fat-free drinks freely until he/she is to be starved in preparation for the general anaesthetic. Prophylactic intravenous antibiotics, e.g. metronidazole 1 g, gentamicin 80 mg and cefuroxime 750 mg, are given on induction as a tract will be made through the peritoneal cavity.

Table 5.3 Example of a fat-free meal

Fruit juice
White bread
Lean meat
Salad – no dressing
Grilled fish (no added fat or oil)
Fruit jelly
Black tea/coffee

Procedure

Ultrasound is used to locate the gall bladder. A 1 cm puncture is made and a guidewire is then passed into the gall bladder which is aspirated and diluted contrast is flushed in. The tract is then dilated and an Amplatz dilator is inserted, through which the nephroscope is introduced. Small stones are removed under direct vision with alligator forceps and larger stones are disintegrated using an electrohydraulic probe or ultrasound lithotripter. Once the gall bladder is cleared of all visible fragments, an X-ray is taken to exclude residual calculi. A 14CH Foley catheter is inserted and the balloon inflated under fluoroscopic control to check the position of the balloon.

Postoperative Procedure

The patient is discharged with the catheter in situ as soon as he/she is well enough (1–3 days postoperatively) and is competent to look after the tube. One week postoperatively the patient is admitted as a day-case. A tubogram is performed to check that:

● No calculi are present
● No extravasation of contrast has occurred into the peritoneal cavity
● There is free flow of contrast into the common bile duct and duodenum and no evidence of calculi in the common bile duct

The catheter can then be removed and a dry dressing applied to the site which will heal over by the next day.

A care plan for PCCL is shown in Table 5.4.

Table 5.4   Care plan for specific problems following PCCL

Patient's problem	Aim of nursing action	Nursing action
Pain following surgery and due to presence of T-tube	Patient will state that his/her pain is relieved/reduced to a tolerable level so he/she can move around	1. Ensure tube is taped securely and is not pulling 2. Assist patient to adopt a comfortable position supported by pillows 3. Give analgesics as prescribed and required and monitor effect 4. Ensure T-tube is not obstructed
Potential infection due to operation and presence of T-tube	Patient's temperature will be 36–37°C Patient's wound will not be red and swollen Patient will state that he/she he/she does not feel feverish	1. Monitor temperature 4-hourly and report to doctor if > 38°C. 2. Give antibiotics as prescribed 3. Redress T-tube as required, i.e. if dressing is soiled, has come loose or if painful
Potential obstruction of T-tube	Maintain free flow of bile through T-tube, i.e. tube will drain continuously	1. Empty T-tube 4-hourly and record on fluid balance chart 2. Ensure tubing is not kinked, and redress if necessary 3. Flush tube with 5–10 ml sodium chloride 0.9% using an aseptic technique if T-tube is blocked
Patient has a knowledge deficit regarding care of T-tube at home	By date of discharge, patient will state that he/she feels competent regarding care of T-tube	1. Teach how to redress tube 2. Teach patient how to change night bag and how to clean it 3. Refer district nurse and arrange visit

LASERTRIPSY

LASER = light amplification by stimulated emission of radiation
Lasertripsy = fragmentation of ureteric calculus

Procedure

The patient is positioned in the lithotomy position (on his/her back with legs apart and feet held up in stirrups). A ureteroscope is passed along the urethra into the bladder, through the vesicoureteric opening and into the ureter. When the calculus is visualised, the 'Q'-switched dye laser is fired using 100–1000 shocks. The calculus is broken into tiny fragments which the patient can then pass urethrally. The procedure can take 0.5–2 hours.

Lasertripsy is usually a retrograde procedure. However, if the calculus is at the top of the ureter, the procedure can be antegrade. For antegrade, a needle nephrostomy tube is inserted under local anaesthetic 5 days preoperatively. The patient is then discharged and readmitted one day preoperatively.

Preoperative Preparation

A midstream specimen of urine (MSU) is obtained. The patient is prepared for a general anaesthetic; however, premedications are only given if necessary so that an X-ray of the kidneys, ureter and bladder (KUB) can be performed immediately (ideally) preoperatively. The patient is then asked to rest quietly before going to theatre.

Postoperative Complications

Postoperative complications and their nursing requirements are as follows:

1. *Obstruction of urinary tract*
   a. Urinary output is monitored.
   b. Patient is assessed for pain on treated side.
   c. Urine is sieved for calculi and sent for chemical analysis.
   d. KUB is performed to check fragments have been passed.

2. *Haematuria*
   a. Urine is observed for degree of haematuria and patient warned so he/she is not alarmed.
   b. Once patient has recovered from anaesthetic, ensure he/she is encouraged to drink 3 litres fluid/day.

3. *Pain*
   a. Co-proxamol is usually adequate; however, if the calculus was stuck in the ureteric wall, Voltarol 100 mg p.r./orally twice daily may be required.
   b. If a double-J stent is inserted, the patient may experience discomfort and will be reassured once he/she knows the cause.

4. *Infection*
   a. Prophylactic antibiotics are given on induction, e.g. gentamicin 80 mg i.v.
   b. Temperature is monitored and doctor informed of pyrexia as this may be indicative of an infection which needs treating with antibiotics, or is a sign of obstruction.

5. *Risk of perforation of ureter causing extravasation of urine*
   This is characterised by severe pain and tenderness. An ultrasound is needed and a double-J stent may be required (see Figure 5.4).
   If the stone cannot be fragmented by laser, the alternatives are:

1. The calculus is flushed up into the renal pelvis with saline, a double-J stent is inserted and extracorporeal piezoelectric lithotripsy (EPL) is used.

2. If the stone is in the lower third of the ureter, it is retrieved using a Dormia basket (Figure 5.2).

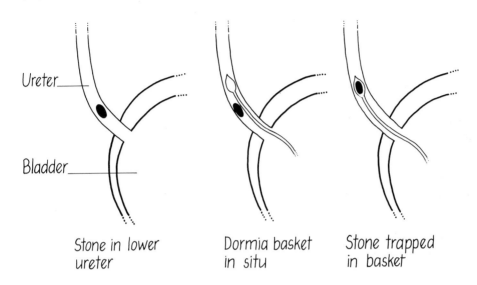

Ureter

Bladder

Stone in lower
ureter

Dormia basket
in situ

Stone trapped
in basket

Fig 5.2   Diagram to show use of the Dormia basket

Discharge from Hospital

The patient is usually discharged 1 day postoperatively. Follow-up depends on whether there are any remaining stones, e.g. EPL may be required. Otherwise, the patient will be seen in the out-patients clinic in 6 weeks and will have a KUB.

LAPAROSCOPIC SURGERY

Laparoscopic surgery is one of the latest advances in urology. Laparoscopic varicocele repairs can now be performed as day-case surgery. Further, major laparoscopic surgery, e.g. nephrectomies and reimplantation of ureters into the bladder, are also now being performed, though they remain extremely recent surgical innovations.

Laparoscopic Nephrectomy

Procedure

Nephrectomy generally involves a large, painful incision, close to or involving the 12th rib pair. For this reason, a very recent innovation in urology has been the development of percutaneous (or laparoscopic) nephrectomy, which utilises essentially the same method as that employed for percutaneous nephrolithotomy. To be considered for the technique, patients must be non-obese and the kidney to be removed both small in size and also free of any malignancy.

Patient preparation is very similar to that of percutaneous nephrolithotomy, and the postoperative care also involves the same essential priorities of care. Prior to the procedure, angiographic embolisation of the kidney is performed. Some 24–36 hours later, a tract is made down onto the kidney, but instead of a nephroscope then being employed, a modified surgical liquidiser/blender is inserted.

This is then used to sequentially liquify the renal substance, and each liquidised segment is then removed by aspiration, and/or the use of forceps. The method is clearly still experimental and the procedure can be very prolonged when compared to that of conventional nephrectomy e.g. 4–6 hours is not uncommon.

However, percutaneous nephrectomy offers a significant advantage in that no large, permanent scar is left, and the tract utilised to remove the kidney heals rapidly. The average patient stay in hospital is approximately 3–4 days.

Clearly, a nephrostomy tube is left in situ for the first 48–72 hours, both to allow adequate wound drainage and to observe for any signs of significant postoperative haemorrhage.

Specific Postoperative Problems

1. *Breathing*   At present the procedure entails a long anaesthetic; however, this will become less of a problem as the procedure is perfected.

2. *Haemorrhage*   The patient should be monitored closely for signs of haemorrhage. A wound drain is left in situ for 24–48 hours or until there is minimal drainage.

3. *Pain*   This is mainly due to abdominal gas which is relieved by movement. The patient should be encouraged to move about in bed as much as possible, and as soon as he/she is able, he/she should be assisted out of bed.

The patient is more critically ill during the first 24 hours postoperatively. However, after this initial period he/she recovers quickly and is discharged after 4–5 days. This procedure is obviously advantageous from a cosmetic point of view, and also eliminates the possible complications of chronic wound pain, which may be a result of open nephrectomy.

Ison et al (1989) and Ikaro et al (1990) provide an overview of both the surgical method and also the equipment used. It remains to be seen if the technique becomes more widely established within urology.

PERCUTANEOUS PYELOLYSIS

This procedure is a treatment for pelviureteric junction (PUJ) stenosis, and is particularly effective in secondary PUJ obstruction following scarring from calculus disease.

Preoperative Preparation

The patient is prepared for major surgery (as for PCNL).

Procedure

A guidewire is passed retrogradely up into the ureter. A percutaneous puncture to the kidney is then made and the tract dilated to 24FG. Through this, the ureteric guidewire is grasped and pulled through the PUJ to the surface.

From the top, a urethrotome is passed alongside the guidewire to the PUJ. A 5 cm length of the ureteric wall is incised in a posterolateral direction. (This direction is important so as not to transect the lower pole vessels.)

A 16Fr Payne drain (a tapered splint nephrostomy tube which has holes that lie in the renal pelvis) is passed down the ureter over the guidewire and urine drains to the surface and into a nephrostomy tube drainage bag.

Postoperative Care

A nephrostogram is performed 48 hours postoperatively, to check that the Payne drain is in a good position. If so, it is spigotted and strapped down under a dressing. The tube is left in situ for 4–6 weeks when a further nephrostogram is performed and if this shows good drainage, it can then be removed.

A care plan is shown in Table 5.5

Table 5.5 *Care plans for specific problems following percutaneous pyelolysis*

Patient's problem	Aim of nursing action	Nursing action
Pain following surgery and due to presence of Payne drain	Patient will state that his/her pain is relieved/reduced to a tolerable level so he/she can move around freely	1. Ensure that Payne drain is taped securely and not pulling 2. Ensure that Payne drain is not blocked and is draining freely 3. Assist patient to adopt a comfortable position supported by pillows 4. Give analgesics as prescribed and required and monitor effect
Potential infection following operation and presence of Payne drain	Patient's temperature will be 36–37°C. Patient's wound will not be red and swollen. Patient will state that he/she does not feel feverish	1. Monitor temperature 4-hourly and report to doctor if above 38°C 2. Give antibiotics as prescribed 3. Redress Payne drain as required, i.e. if dressing is soiled, has come loose or if painful 4. Ensure patient is aware he/she should drink 3 litres/day

Patient's problem	Aim of nursing action	Nursing action
Potential obstruction of Payne drain	Maintain free flow of urine through Payne drain, i.e. continuous urine drainage	1. Empty Payne drain 4-hourly and record on fluid balance chart 2. Ensure drain is not kinked, and redress if necessary 3. Flush drain with 5–10 ml sodium chloride 0.9% using an aseptic technique if drain is blocked
Knowledge deficit regarding care of Payne drain at home	By date of discharge, patient will state that he/she feels competent regarding care of Payne drain	1. Teach patient to redress Payne drain 2. Refer to district nurse and arrange visit 3. Teach patient to recognise problems which require further advice

EXTRACORPOREAL LITHOTRIPSY

Extracorporeal Shock-wave Lithotripsy (ESWL)

History

The 'first-generation' Dornier lithotripter was developed at the University of Munich, Germany by Professor E. Schmidt and Professor Eisenberg and came into use in 1981. The Dornier aircraft company had observed that shock-waves induced by high-speed aircraft flying in stormy weather conditions had caused damage to internal equipment while the exterior of the craft remained intact. As a consequence, research was carried out into the effects of focusing shock-waves onto hard objects, e.g. renal calculi, to bring about their destruction. Since this machine has now been superseded by the 'second generation' the treatment is briefly described below.

Outline of Treatment

Shock-waves are generated by underwater discharge of a high-voltage spark. Shock-waves are transmitted to the stone through de-ionised, de-gassed water heated to 37°C (the efficiency of shock-waves is adversely affected by air bubbles). The stone is located by two diagonally directed X-ray beams. The patient is supported in the water in a computer-controlled hydraulic chair. The chair is positioned so that the stone is at the focus of the shock-waves.

Up to 4000 shocks may be required to disintegrate a stone. Treatment is painful; therefore, the patient needs a general or epidural anaesthetic with its attendant risk.

Temporary haematuria is caused by the shocks and a urethral catheter is inserted in case of clot retention. It is removed when the urine is clear.

Cardiac arrhythmias can occur. The heart beat is monitored throughout the treatment and the shock-waves are synchronised to the refractory phase of the cardiac cycle on the R-wave.

The patient is observed as is usual following a general anaesthetic. Oral fluids (3 litres/24 hours) are encouraged to promote the passage of stone fragments out of the system. This can take anything from 24 hours to 2 weeks. X-ray (KUB) confirms the position of remaining fragments 2 days after treatment. The patient is discharged at this time if he is:

- Apyrexial
- Pain-free
- Taking normal diet and increased fluids without nausea or vomiting
- Passing clear urine without difficulty

Extracorporeal Piezoelectric Lithotripsy (EPL)

The 'second-generation' lithotripters are now in use. The Wolf lithotripter has been operative in the St Peters' Hospital's Lithotripter Centre since 1988.

With this system the stone is disintegrated by shock-waves generated by the piezoelectric effect – this is the vibration which results from high voltage passing across the piezoelectric ceramic crystals. Approximately 2000 crystals form a mosaic in a concave dish and the shock-waves produced from each crystal are collected at the focus, i.e. the kidney stone. This focus is much more accurate than in the Dornier machine and this results in more efficient delivery of shocks to the stone in a shorter period of time. Consequently the treatment is not so painful and the patient does not need an anaesthetic although children and anxious adults may need sedation. Again the shock-wave is transmitted through de-gassed, preheated water which is contained in a closed bath. The patient lies over the bath with only the loin area in contact with the water. The stone is located by ultrasound probe which is fixed within the dish; an image of the stones' position can be seen on the ultrasound monitor.

Up to 4000 shocks can be given in one session and this lasts 45 minutes on average. There is no risk of induction of cardiac arrhythmias so cardiac monitoring is not necessary.

The majority of patients may be treated as out-patients but hospital admission is necessary if the patient needs to be observed closely after treatment, e.g. in cases of single kidney, renal impairment, ileal conduit or other urinary diversion, and in cases of obstruction or deterioration of renal function. Hypertensive patients may experience raised blood pressure, which should be monitored, as should patients with cardiac or respiratory problems. Such problems may be exacerbated by stress rather than the treatment itself. Patients with reduced mobility as a result of spinal injury, spina bifida, multiple sclerosis, etc., are admitted as repeated journeys to hospital are time-consuming and difficult. To avoid inconvenience and possible financial hardship, hostel accommodation is provided for those travelling long distances for treatment.

The introduction of the Wolf lithotripter has significantly reduced the medical and nursing needs of patients with renal stones as 85 per cent are now treatable by lithotripsy.

Pretreatment Investigations

The patient attends a pretreatment clinic where a detailed clinical history is taken; the following investigations are carried out routinely:

1. Blood pressure is recorded.
2. Blood is screened for clotting abnormalities.
3. Blood urea and electrolytes are checked to assess renal function.
4. MSU is microbiologically screened.
5. Urine is tested for glucose, ketones, blood, protein, etc.
6. KUB X-ray and IVU are performed if indicated.
7. 24-hour urine collection for 'stone-screen'.
8. Suitability for treatment as an out-patient is assessed.
9. Special needs are identified, arrangements made for admission to ward or hostel after treatment.

Advantages of Treatment

The advantages of treatment by EPL include the following:

1. EPL reduces in-patient stay. Only those who meet previously mentioned criteria need be admitted.

2. Most patients can resume normal activities the next day and can return to work within 1 week.

3. There is minimal morbidity – world-wide 80 000 patients had been treated up to 1986 with no deaths.

4. There is minimal pain following treatment, most patients being treated with oral analgesics.

5. Eighty-five per cent of renal stones can be treated by EPL, including those previously considered unsuitable for open or minimally invasive surgery, e.g. spinal injury patients, those with cardiac and obstructive airway conditions.

6. Repeated treatments may be carried out with no ill-effects discerned as yet. It is possible to keep those with metabolic calculus disease free from stones, thus preserving their renal function.

7. There is reduced exposure to X-rays – ultrasound is used to monitor progress during treatment.

8. Although the initial cost of the machine is high, the procedure is more cost-effective than open or minimally invasive surgery. One patient per hour is treatable, allowing high patient turnover.

Disadvantages of Treatment

Disadvantages of EPL include the following:

1. EPL cannot be used initially on staghorn calculi.

2. EPL cannot be used on cystine stones as they are too hard.

3. Large stones (more than 2 cm in diameter) need repeat treatments and patients incur travelling expenses for repeated journeys to hospital. It can also prove inconvenient for those who have to arrange time off work.

4. Admission to hospital has to be arranged for insertion of ureteric stent prior to treatment of large stones and removal of stent on completion of treatment.

Lithotripsy Treatment

The introduction of the Wolf lithotripter (Figure 5.3) has significantly reduced the medical and nursing needs of patients with renal stones. No special preparation is required for the treatment.

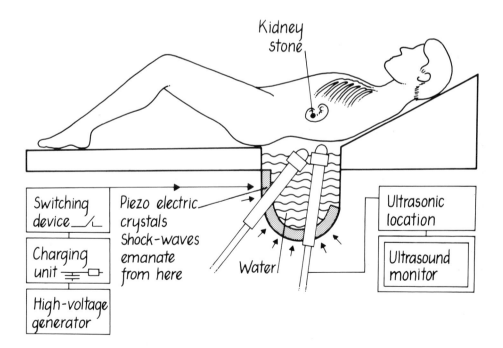

Fig 5.3 Diagram to show patient's position on the Wolf lithotripter

On Attending the Lithotripter for Treatment

The patient attends the X-ray department for KUB X-ray to check the stone's position 30 minutes prior to treatment except on the first visit as an X-ray would have been taken at the pretreatment clinic attendance. The patient is introduced to lithotripter staff who will explain the procedure. After putting on an open-backed gown (and disposable paper pants if preferred) the patient's stone is located manually by ultrasound probe and its position is marked on his/her back.

The patient is helped on to the lithotripter, where he/she lies in a supine position with the marked loin sagging into the water close to the ultrasound probe. The dish and probe are moved electrically until the stone is aligned in two planes at the focus of the shock-waves. Shock-waves are then generated, building up to maximum rate and intensity as tolerated by the patient. These are reduced if the patient experiences pain.

The position of the stone is monitored throughout on the ultrasound screen and the patient may be repositioned as required during the procedure (position may be changed if pain is experienced).

On completion of the treatment, the patient is helped down from the lithotripter, towels are provided and he/she can change back into his/her clothes.

A recovery area is provided where patients may sit and relax before their journey home. Patients are encouraged to begin their increased fluid intake at this stage. If an in-patient, they may return to the ward with or without an escort as their condition dictates. There is no reason why patients may not leave for home as soon as the treatment is over if they feel able.

Patients are advised to drink large amounts of fluid to encourage diuresis and flushing out of stone fragments from the kidney. Approximately 3 litres/24 hours minimum is recommended (at least 6 pints).

Initially two appointments for treatment are given with dates approximately 1 week apart with an X-ray prior to treatment. Further sessions are booked as necessary and progress is reviewed after four treatments to evaluate the effectiveness of the treatment. If the stone is broken into fragments of less than 2 mm no further treatment is necessary as these should pass spontaneously.

Patients are given co-proxamol tablets x 10 to take home in case of pain and trimethoprim 200 mg twice daily for 3 days (prophylactic antibiotic).

The average number of treatments required is four to five. Patients are reviewed in the out-patient client 6 weeks after completion of treatment.

Patients are admitted to the ward for observation following lithotripsy if they experience any of the following:

- Loin pain, ureteric or renal colic
- Pyrexia
- Fainting
- Nausea or vomiting

Table 5.6 shows a typical advice sheet for lithotripsy.

Table 5.6 Typical advice sheet for lithotripsy

---

1. ADVICE TO PATIENTS FOR LITHOTRIPSY
Treatment is generally carried out on an out-patient basis but sometimes a patient may need to be admitted overnight. This is usually planned before treatment.

Lithotripsy is a comparatively painless procedure; however, occasionally patients have experienced some discomfort or pain during treatment. If you experience pain during treatment inform the surgeon and he will adjust the shock-wave.

2. INSTRUCTIONS TO PATIENTS POST-LITHOTRIPSY
2.1. Some patients experience pain after treatment. This is mostly caused when stone fragments pass from the kidney to bladder.
2.2. You will be given pain-killing tablets with instructions.
2.3. Most stones are infected. In order to prevent infection spreading you will be given a course of antibiotics to take for 3 days. It is very important that you complete this course even if you feel quite well.
2.4. If you develop a temperature, feel generally unwell or are having a lot of pain, you should contact your local doctor who will have been informed about your treatment.
2.5. After treatment you may pass blood-stained urine. You should not worry as this is normal after the treatment. However, if the urine remains heavily blood-stained on the day following treatment contact your local doctor.
2.6. After treatment you should drink plenty of fluid – about 4 pints in the first 24 hours after treatment. This will help to clear the urine of stone fragments and blood.

If you have further queries ask the surgeon or the nurse in the Lithotripter Centre.

Complications following Lithotripsy

'Steinstrasse' (German; literally translated = stone street)

This describes obstruction of the ureter by impacted stone debris. It can be avoided by positioning a double-J stent (see section on Stent Insertion) in the ureter where the stone is over 2–3 cm in diameter prior to the commencement of a course of treatment.

Signs of steinstrasse are:

- Severe loin pain
- Pyrexia
- Nausea and vomiting

Treatment of steinstrasse involves the use of analgesia and opioid if pain is severe; otherwise, oral analgesics or non-steroid anti-inflammatory suppositories (e.g. diclofenac 100 mg) are prescribed.

Antibiotics are prescribed prophylactically or as appropriate to urine cultures. Intravenous fluid replacement is commenced if indicated and an antiemetic given.

Renal ultrasound is performed to determine the degree of obstruction. If the tract is dilated a percutaneous nephrostomy drain is inserted and attached to a drainage bag to relieve hydronephrosis. The gradual dispersal of debris is effected by continued ureteric peristalsis. The patient is kept under X-ray review and the nephrostomy is removed when the steinstrasse has dispersed.

Dispersal of debris may be achieved more speedily if the patient undergoes endoscopic insertion of a ureteric stent as the ureter dilates around the stent, allowing stone fragments to pass down more easily.

Ureteric Colic

There is reduced incidence of colic after treatment on the Wolf lithotripter as the stones are broken into small pieces. However, if it does occur the patient may have to be admitted to hospital for observation and administration of analgesics parenterally, orally or rectally as dictated by the degree of discomfort.

Pyrexia

This may indicate a urinary tract infection. An MSU is taken for microbiological assessment and the patient commences a suitable antibiotic, e.g. trimethoprim 200 mg twice daily, until the laboratory report indicates the appropriate drug. If the pyrexia persists blood should be sent for culture and antibiotics given intravenously.

Inadequate Fragmentation

This is confirmed by X-ray after treatment. If the ureter is not obstructed repeat treatments can be arranged.

Haematuria

Patients are warned before treatment that this may occur and it is not a cause for alarm as long as they are able to void urine without difficulty. An increased intake of fluids is recommended as mentioned previously.

Combined Techniques

Staghorn Calculi

A combined approach is used to 'de-bulk' large staghorn calculi with percutaneous nephrolithotomy and EPL is used to disintegrate residual stone fragments when the patient has recovered from the initial procedure.

'Push–Bang' or 'Push–Pull' Procedure

This technique is used for stones in the middle and upper third of the ureter which are not accessible to ureteroscopic removal or lasertripsy. During ureteroscopy, a narrow catheter is passed into the ureter through which saline is flushed rapidly, dislodging the stone back into the kidney where it can be treated with EPL. Stent insertion is often carried out at this time to prevent the stone from falling back into the ureter.

An antegrade approach can also be used to retrieve stones in the upper third of the ureter. A nephroscope is introduced into the ureter via a percutaneous track and the stone is disintegrated with a flexible lithotripsy probe. The laser may also be used via this route.

Stent Insertion

Indications

Indications for the insertion of a stent are:

● Prelithotripsy, where the stone is larger than 2 cm in diameter
● To relieve ureteric obstruction/stricture, e.g. calculi, tumour, retroperitoneal fibrosis
● To facilitate drainage of urine when ureteric trauma has occurred, e.g. perforation of ureter during endoscopic removal of stone

Stent insertion takes place under general anaesthesia and the patient may be treated as a day-case. A cystoscopy is performed, the appropriate ureteric orifice is identified and the stent is inserted into the ureter over a guidewire (see Figure 5.4). When the guidewire is removed the stent remains positioned between the kidney and bladder. Patients are warned that they may experience some disturbances to their normal voiding pattern but these should resolve within 24–48 hours.

Possible problems

Possible problems following stent insertion include:

● Frequency of micturition
● Urgency of micturition
● Haematuria
● Suprapubic pain, particularly on finishing voiding

These symptoms resolve spontaneously in most cases but some patients may have to be given oral analgesics. Again a high fluid intake is advised to flush out the haematuria and relieve suprapubic discomfort, which is more acute when the bladder is empty.

Stent Removal

This can be done under general or local anaesthetic as a day-case if a flexible cystoscope is available. Cystoscopy is performed, and the end of the stent is grasped and withdrawn through the bladder and urethra. If local anaesthetic is used, lignocaine gel is inserted into the urethra and in males a penile clamp is applied for 20 minutes. Sedo analgesia should be used, as the procedure can be uncomfortable.

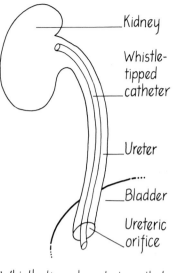

Whistle tipped ureteric catheter is introduced via the ureter into the renal pelvis cystoscopically

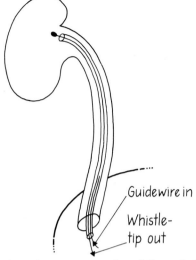

A guidewire is introduced through the lumen of the ureteric catheter which is then withdrawn leaving the tip of the guidewire in the renal pelvis

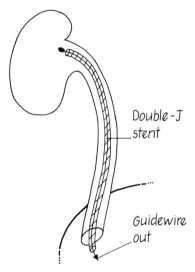

Double-J stent is inserted over guidewire and positioned correctly, guidewire is then removed

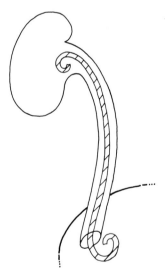

When guidewire is out, both ends of the stent curl into a 'J'-shape in the kidney and bladder, thus securing it in place

Fig 5.4   Double-J stent insertion

Table 5.7 shows a summary of guidelines for patients undergoing various procedures in the radiology department.

Table 5.7   Suggested guidelines for preparation of patients undergoing procedures in the radiology department

Intravenous Urogram

Examination in morning:	No food after midnight.
	Fluids permitted up to 4 hours prior to procedure
Examination in afternoon:	No food after 9.00 a.m.
	Fluids permitted up to 4 hours prior to procedure

Additional preparation is required for the following patients:

(a) Diabetic patients:
    Examination to be arranged for morning.
    Fluids allowed.
    Patient to recommence diet and hypoglycaemic agents after examination.
(b) Patients in renal failure:
    Fluids allowed within patient's individual restriction.
(c) Patients with coronary heart disease or cardiac failure. Inform X-ray staff. This ensures a non-toxic contrast medium is administered.
(d) Children under 12 years:
    A biscuit may be given 2 hours prior to examination.

Needle Nephrostomy

Examination in morning:	No food allowed after midnight.
	Fluids permitted up to 4 hours prior to procedure
Examination in afternoon:	No food allowed after 9.00 a.m.
	Fluids permitted up to 4 hours prior to procedure

Shave loin area if necessary.

No premedication required. (Patients usually administered intravenous midazolam in department if necessary).

Arteriogram

No food or fluid allowed for 4 hours prior to examination.

Shave right groin.

Ask Doctor if premedication required.

Ultrasound of Bladder and Kidneys

Patient instructed to drink plenty of fluid to fill bladder and not to empty bladder prior to examination.

Ultrasound of Liver or Gall Bladder

No food or fluid for 4 hours prior to examination.

Cholecystogram

Day before examination: Patient attends for X-ray.
                                 Is given packet of Biloptin capsules.
Evening: Patient instructed to eat a fat-free meal – about 6.00 p.m.
                                 Swallow Biloptin capsules afterwards.
                                 Nothing further to be eaten until after examination.
                                 Fluids allowed, which must be without milk or fat-free.
Fat-free foods allowed:
Tea/coffee without milk. Fruit juice. White bread. Lean meat. Salad (without dressing).
Grilled fish (without added fat/oil). Fruit jelly.

Patients in Renal Failure, on Restricted Fluids or Diabetic

Follow instructions on sheet except those regarding extra fluids, which may be harmful.

BLADDER STONES

Primary stones of the bladder are uncommon in both children and adults, within
Europe. However, it is commonplace to find children with bladder stones in parts of
India, Indonesia, the Middle East and China. These stones usually occur in urine
which is sterile, and are more common in males (Tanagho and McAninch, 1992).

In such countries, the mechanism of stone formation would appear to be related to
a diet low in protein and phosphate, which may then be compounded by dehydration
(due to the ambient temperature) and also diarrhoea. In areas where such stones are
endemic, they are usually ammonium and/or urate based (Tanagho and McAninch,
1992).

Bladder stones among Europeans, in contrast, are commonly the result of bladder
outflow obstruction, although stones can form within diverticulae of the bladder
mucosa (especially if the diverticulum does not drain effectively, and therefore
contains a pool of stagnant urine), or upon a foreign body within the bladder (e.g. a
catheter), which thus acts as a nidus for calcium deposition and stone formation.

Bladder calculi may also be the result of stones which have successfully passed
down the ureter, but then lodged and subsequently enlarged within the bladder
lumen. Bladder stones, within a European context, are nearly always seen in men,
and are frequently associated with urinary stasis and/or chronic urinary tract
infection. The exact composition of these stones varies, according to the urinary pH
and also the concentration of stone-forming elements within the urine. In the USA,
calcium oxalate is the most common stone constituent, whereas in European
populations, uric acid and urate stones predominate (Tanagho and McAninch,
1992).

Presenting Problems

The 'classical' presentation appears as the sudden loss of urinary stream during
voiding, along with the acute onset of pain radiating into the penis or perineum.
Small amounts of blood may also be passed.

Pain radiating down and along the penis may be present when the stone intermittently obstructs the bladder neck, in much the same way as would a ball-valve. Pain resulting from bladder calculi is relieved when the patient lies down, as the stone will then clearly fall backwards, away from the trigone, thus relieving the obstruction.

Urinary infection is also common when bladder stones and outflow obstruction co-exist, particularly as bacteria can lodge within the stone matrix, which then serves to partially (or completely) protect such pathogens from antibiotic agents within the urine. Thus patients with bladder stones frequently give a history of hesitancy, frequency, dysuria, haematuria, dribbling and poor urinary stream, or of a chronic urinary tract infection unresponsive to antibiotic therapy.

Treatment

Bladder stones can be removed endoscopically, or via an open procedure, or can be treated with lithotripsy (EHL or ultrasound) or laser. Small bladder stones may be removed via transurethral irrigation, under either general or local anaesthetic.

Larger stones need to be broken into fragments, to facilitate their removal. This fragmentation can be achieved using either lithotripsy or laser (which is more recent). Laser would clearly require the passage of an endoscope, and is thus performed under general or local anaesthetic, with appropriate precautions (e.g. eye protection, etc.).

Patient Care

The nursing management of these patients is the same as that of any patient undergoing lithotripsy or lasertripsy, though clearly haematuria is less likely, as the stone is not tightly held within the substance of the bladder.

The patient must be reassured that the passage of small stone fragments is normal, following the procedure(s), and encouraged to drink an adequate amount of fluid to facilitate removal of such fragments (i.e. at least 3 litres/day, if there is no medical contraindication).

LITHOLAPAXY

The historical and still commonly employed method for bladder stone removal is lithalapaxy. A manual lithotrite is used. This is an instrument which resembles an adjustable set of 'jaws' which can be controlled from the exterior. Once inside the patient's bladder the jaws of the lithotrite are closed, with the stone between them, resulting in fragmentation of the stone.

The lithotrite is introduced via the urethra, and the stone gripped. It is then crushed into pieces small enough to be evacuated from the bladder via cystoscopy and irrigation. Originally, the procedure was performed 'blind'. Nowadays, however, this has been replaced with the optical lithotrite (incorporating a fibre-optic light source and telescope) which allows the stone to be visualised and crushed under direct vision, reducing the risk of bladder damage. Stone fragments are then removed via irrigation, and the bladder lumen rechecked. The procedure is usually performed under general or spinal anaesthetic and the postoperative care centres upon observing for excessive haematuria, and ensuring that the patient maintains an adequate oral fluid intake, to facilitate the removal of any small stone fragments that remain. Clearly, appropriate advice and reassurance are important.

Cystolithotomy

Stones that cannot be crushed safely (e.g. stones which are very large) may need to be removed surgically, via a suprapubic incision. The bladder wall is opened, and the stone removed.

Patient Care

Such patients will return from theatre with a urinary catheter in situ. Some units will use both a suprapubic and a urethral catheter, especially if the patient has a history of outflow obstruction. There will also be an intravenous infusion. Some form of wound drainage may also be present.

The patient can eat and drink as soon as they feel able, and clearly some form of analgesia will be required.

The catheter remains in situ until the bladder wall has healed (between 7 and 10 days) and a cystogram may then be performed to check that there is no leakage from the bladder wall. The catheter will then be removed.

If the bladder stone has resulted from chronic outflow obstruction, this will also need to be treated. An open removal of the stone may be combined with either retropubic or transvesical prostatectomy. Some units prefer, on the basis of safety, to resect the prostate first, via a transurethral approach, and then to open the bladder simply to remove the stone.

Occasionally long-standing bladder calculi may cause sufficient urothelial irritation/inflammation as to induce squamous metaplasia and then carcinoma of the bladder. In such cases, the stone is removed, any outflow obstruction relieved and the tumour managed according to its staging and histology.

URETHRAL STONES

Urethral stones are rare, and usually represent stones which have formed elsewhere and then 'lodged' in the urethral lumen.

Most small stones (i.e. < 1 cm) will pass down the urethra (though often with pain) but larger stones can impact, causing pain, bleeding and actual retention.

Primary urethral stones are usually found in association with lower tract abnormalities that may then induce urinary stasis or chronic urinary tract infection.

Patients with urethral diverticulae, strictures, urethral foreign bodies, chronic fistulae and meatal stenosis, as well as benign prostatic hyperplasia, are all more prone to urethral stone development.

Most urethral calculi (approx. 60 per cent) are located in the anterior urethra and up to 10 per cent at the fossa navicularis. However, up to 40 per cent impact at the membranous urethra or external urinary sphincter (Tanagho and McAninch, 1992).

In females, such stones can often be seen in the urethra, or are evident on trans-vaginal urethral palpation.

In males, retrograde urethrography will identify the presence and location of the stone.

Treatment

In females, such stones can be removed directly, or pushed back into the bladder and then evacuated (e.g. via litholapaxy). In males, the stones can usually be pushed back into the bladder via a cystoscope (i.e. under direct vision) and then evacuated. However, in some male patients, impaction of the stone may be so severe as to prevent any attempt to push the stone back up into the bladder. In this situation, the stone is retrieved via a direct incision into the urethra, via the underside of the penis. The incision is then closed, and a urethral catheter left in situ for at least 7 days, to allow closure of the incision line.

Patient Care

Patients may return from theatre with both a suprapubic and a urethral stent catheter (though this may vary with individual units) which then remain for 7–10 days. Patients may, however, resume both diet and fluids, and begin to mobilise, as soon as they are able.

Urethrography will then be performed, prior to the removal of the catheter(s), to ensure that healing has occurred. If any underlying pathology is present (e.g. a diverticulum) then this may also need to be repaired at the time of surgery.

Prostatic Calculi

Prostatic calculi are very common. They usually form just within the prostatic capsule in cases of benign prostatic hypertrophy and are unable to migrate into the urethra. During prostatectomy such stones will usually be removed, to prevent them from subsequently impacting into the urethra.

References

Fernstrom I and Johansen B (1976) Percutaneous pyelolithotomy. *Scandinavian Journal of Urology and Nephrology* **10**: 257–259.

Ikaro O, Netto N Jnr, Palma PC and D'Ancona CA (1990) Percutaneous nephrectomy in non-functioning kidneys: a preliminary report. *Journal of Urology* **144**(4): 966–968.

Ison KT, Copcoat MJ, Timoney A and Wickham JE (1989) The development and application of a new surgical device – the endoscopic liquidiser and surgical aspirator (ELSA). *Journal of Medical Engineering and Technology* **13**(6): 285–289.

Rupel E and Brown R (1976) Nephroscopy with removal of stone following nephrostomy for obstructive calculus. *Journal of Urology* **46**: 177–182.

Tanagho EA and McAninch JW (eds) (1992) *Smith's General Urology*, 12th edn. London: Prentice Hall International.

Wickham JEA and Kellet MK (1981) Percutaneous nephrolithotomy. *British Journal of Urology* **53**: 297–299.

6

Reconstructive Surgery for
Urinary Tract Defects

This subspeciality has been developed in order to repair anatomical defects in the urinary tract that result from congenital deformity, trauma or tissue damage. Surgery of this type requires not only a skilled surgeon, but nursing care delivered by nurses who are able to empathise with the patient and his family, as many of these patients have already had protracted hospital stays.

Damage can occur to any area of the urinary tract. In this chapter we will look at the treatment and nursing care for repairing defects in the kidney, the ureters, the bladder and the urethra.

THE KIDNEY

Trauma

The kidney, by virtue of its anatomical position, surrounded by the ribs, the vertebral column and the paravertebral musculature, is relatively well protected from trauma. However, certain events can cause damage to the kidney, and when this occurs it is often a serious situation. Depending on the nature of the injury different types of damage will occur. A penetrating wound such as that resulting from a gun shot wounds or a stabbing, will result in severe blood loss and damage to the kidney. A non-penetrating wound may occur as a result of a sports injury or following a direct blow to the loin. A severe injury of this type may cause the kidney to shatter within its capsule. Due to the highly vascular nature of the kidney any injury is always associated with some degree of haematuria; more severe damage will be accompanied by hypotension and loin swelling.

Diagnosis

The following considerations form the basis for diagnosis:

● History of injury to loin area
● Haematuria
● Loin pain
● Swelling in the loin area
● Hypotension and tachycardia

Confirming Diagnosis

To assess the extent of the damage the following investigations will be performed:

- An IVU
- A renal ultrasound
- A renal arteriogram

Treatment

If the damage is major and accompanied by severe hypotension, emergency surgery is indicated. If attempts to repair the kidney fail then either partial or total nephrectomy is performed. The damage may also extend to the renal artery.

If the injury is more minor then conservative management is indicated. This consists of the following:

1. Bed rest.

2. Observations in order to detect shock – half-hourly blood pressure and pulse, observations of urine volume.

3. Observation of urine colour.

4. Pain relief.

5. Measurement of abdominal girth, an increase in which will indicate continued bleeding.

6. Replacement of lost fluid by either an increased oral input or by intravenous replacement. Blood products may be required to replace lost blood volume.

7. Antibiotic therapy will be given in order to prevent infection as a result of the extravasation of urine.

8. The patient must continue to rest for at least 2 weeks following the injury as the risk of secondary haemorrhage is high. The patient should be warned to look for renewed bleeding at 10–14 days after the injury.

The patient should be seen in the out-patients department and a repeat IVU performed after 6 weeks.

Nephrectomy

Nephrectomy refers to the surgical removal of a kidney. This is performed for a variety of reasons, including the arrest of uncontrollable haemorrhage following renal trauma.

Other common reasons for removing a kidney are:

- Renal cancer (see Chapter 10)
- Chronic infection, which has led to renal scarring and loss of function
- Renal calculi, which have destroyed most of the viable renal substance, and which continue to cause recurrent urinary infection
- Live donor renal transplant
- Significant renal trauma, with uncontrollable bleeding

The kidney is removed via one of three approaches

- Flank approach
- Lumbar approach
- Thoraco-abdominal approach

Traditionally, the thoraco-abdominal approach has been reserved for cases of renal cancer, as it would appear to allow earlier clamping of the major renal blood vessels, prior to mobilisation of the kidney (thereby reducing the risk of systemic, tumour dissemination).

However, this is not universal, and some centres may only consider a thoraco-abdominal approach in cases where the tumour mass is very large. However, such an incision may cause significant postoperative problems relating to both respiration and also possible involvement of the peritoneal cavity.

The loin incision is most commonly employed, as it offers a retroperitoneal approach.

Unfortunately the operative incision (whatever 'open' approach is used) is usually large and extremely painful postoperatively. For this reason, and because of the risk of possible complications, some centres are now experimenting with endoscopic nephrectomy, as described in chapter 5. However, this remains an experimental procedure, at the present time.

Preoperative Care

The preoperative care of patients undergoing nephrectomy is fairly simple and centres upon the following considerations:

Safety Aspects

As for any patient undergoing surgery.

Adequate Explanation and Information

The teaching of postoperative breathing exercises (the physiotherapy department is involved in this).

Routine Blood Assay

The cross-matching of at least two units of blood.

Assay (and/or culture) of Urine

To ensure that no preoperative urinary infection is present.

Prior to the removal of a kidney, it is essential to ascertain that there is a contralateral, functional kidney present.

In emergency cases, this would usually be done by a single film IVU (see Chapter 2), taken at 20 minutes, which would display both the size and number of kidneys present.

In cases where nephrectomy is an elective procedure, more detailed estimation of renal function will be performed. This will usually involve isotopic study of the kidney(s) using some form of renogram. In addition, in cases where the kidney is being removed because of cancer, renal arteriography may also be utilised, to display the nature and extent of the blood supply to the tumour mass.

Postoperative Care

The nursing management of patients undergoing nephrectomy, due to the nature of the incision, centres upon the following priorities:

Effective Pain Management

Aggressive pain control, post-nephrectomy, is crucial, as the patient will not breathe effectively (or cough) if pain control is neglected.

An intravenous or subcutaneous opioid infusion, via a pump, is an excellent management option. Also, an intercostal catheter may be sited into the line of the incision (during wound closure) and analgesic agents such as Marcaine then injected into this.

Other alternative strategies may be used as required (e.g. localised heat, transcutaneous electronic nerve stimulation, appropriate relaxation methods, etc).

Positioning of the Patient

To enhance comfort and maximise chest expansion on the affected side. This will usually involve either a semi-recumbant position, well supported with pillows, or a high up, side-lying position (on the unaffected side) to maximise chest expansion on the side where the operative incision has been made.

Observation for Signs of Possible Haemorrhage

At least two suction drains are normally inserted in theatre, because of the risk of bleeding postoperatively. Any blood loss from the wound site is observed, and marked if appropriate.

Observation of Postoperative Urine Output

Postoperative output is important, and some units may catheterise the patient in order to measure urine volumes more accurately.

Assisting the Patient with Deep Breathing and Coughing

To attempt to minimise the risk of postoperative chest infection all patients will receive physiotherapy. This aspect of care will only be effective if the patient's pain is adequately controlled.

Effective Wound Management

Wound dressings are usually removed after approximately 48 hours (or sooner if they are heavily blood stained) and an appropriate dry dressing then applied.

Intravenous Fluids

Are given until bowel sounds are present and the patient is tolerating small amounts of fluid without adverse effect. The exact time scale for re-introducing the patient to food and fluids will vary with individual patients.

Early Ambulation

Again, this is only realistic if pain control is effective. Also, the use of thrombo-embolytic deterrent (TED) stockings, in association with subcutaneous heparin, forms a common postoperative strategy to help reduce the possible risk of deep-vein thrombosis and/or pulmonary embolism.

Adequate Information and Explanation

This should aim to reinforce preoperative teaching.

Suture Removal, if Appropriate

The suture(s) may be sub-dermal, traditional skin sutures or clips. If removal is required, this will normally be performed at approximately 10 days following surgery.

If the patient has undergone removal of a kidney because of cancer, the ureter is also likely to be removed, along with surrounding perinephric fat, the adrenal gland and associated lymph nodes (so called radical nephrectomy). As this will then require the wall of the bladder to be sutured (at the previous point of ureteric entry) these patients may return from theatre with a urethral catheter in situ, which aims to prevent pressure being placed on the anastomosis by bladder filling. The catheter is then removed between 48 and 72 hours following surgery. This practice is not, however, universal.

Possible Complications

These include:

Shock

Caused by loss of circulating volume.

Chest Infection

As a result of poor chest expansion postoperatively (often as a result of inadequate pain control).

Pneumothorax

Can occur, because the loin incision is very close to the 12th rib. Further, in cases where it is very difficult to mobilise the kidney (e.g. if there has been previous renal infection with subsequent fibrosis and scarring) it may be necessary to actually remove the 12th rib, in which case pneumothorax becomes more likely. Patients may therefore return from theatre with underwater seal chest drainage in situ.

Pulmonary Embolism

This is a result of compression on the venae cavae and other large vessels, during surgery. It is, however, a very rare occurrence.

Wound Infection

Is more common in cases where renal infection has been present.

Subphrenic Abscess

This is again more likely if pre-existing renal infection has been present.

Urinary Tract Infection

This is more likely to occur if a urinary catheter is present or if the patient's mobility is poor postoperatively.

Pyeloplasty

A structural defect of the pelvis of the kidney can exist at its junction with the ureter, resulting in obstruction (pelvi-ureteric junction obstruction). This may be a congenital problem, as a result of repeated infection or following injury either from surgery or external trauma. There is a narrowing of the ureter, causing an obstruction to the free flow of urine.

Diagnosis

There is a history of colicky-type loin pain, which may be accompanied by vomiting, especially after the consumption of large volumes of fluid.

Confirming Diagnosis

The following investigations may be performed:

- An IVU; this may be performed with a diuretic challenge
- A renogram
- A Whitaker's test

Preoperative Care

In addition to basic preoperative needs the patient should be protected from postoperative infection. A midstream specimen of urine should be obtained at the time of admission, in order that any pre-existing infection can be treated appropriately. Prophylactic antibiotics are usually given at the time of surgery. The risk of postoperative chest infection is high due to the location of the surgical incision, the pain from which can inhibit deep breathing. The patient should be discouraged from smoking and be seen by the physiotherapist for instruction in deep-breathing techniques.

Postoperative Care

In addition to the basic postoperative needs the patient should be observed for potential chest infection/difficulties with breathing. The patient should be positioned in such a way as to promote deep breathing. This is usually the position that the patient finds most comfortable. The patient should be well supported with pillows. The physiotherapist should be involved and regular physiotherapy given. In order to help facilitate deep breathing, early mobilisation should occur.

Postoperative Pain

The successful relief of pain is of paramount importance to the prevention of complications, i.e. chest infection and deep-vein thrombosis. High doses of opiate analgesia are given in regular doses intramuscularly or continuously subcutaneously or intravenously via a pump, with careful observation being made for signs of respiratory depression. When the patient is tolerating food oral analgesia should be given regularly, and the dose of opiate analgesia gradually reduced. The patient should also be taught how to support himself or when moving coughing.

Potential Haemorrhage

Due to the highly vascular nature of the kidney the risk of haemorrhage is high. Blood pressure and pulse should be recorded in order to detect shock; initially this will be quite frequently at half-hourly intervals. This can be reduced as the patient's condition allows. The wound site should be observed for blood loss and the wound drainage measured. Excessive blood loss should be reported. Urine output should be measured and the degree of haematuria assessed.

Prevention of Potential Blockage to Urinary Output

In order to protect the surgical anastomosis and prevent extravasation of urine the patient will either have a double-J stent from the kidney to the bladder or have external drainage of urine via a nephrostomy tube. If there is a nephrostomy tube it is important that it is kept patent; if it becomes blocked the patient will experience increased pain and the resultant collection of urine will damage the repair. If the tube becomes blocked it should be gently flushed using 10–20 ml of sterile normal saline. The tube should be dressed in such a way as to avoid any kinking of the tube and to prevent accidental dislodgement.

At 10–14 days post-surgery a nephrostogram may be performed in order to establish the patency of both the repair and of the ureter. If all appears to have healed then the tube can be removed. Some units do not perform a nephrostogram but simply clamp the tube and if the patient experiences no pain or increase in temperature then the tube is removed. Following removal of the tube the patient can be warned to expect some leakage of urine from the site for up to 24 hours. If this is troublesome a stoma bag can be used in order to promote comfort.

If the patient has a double-J stent this should be removed in the out-patient's department after 2–3 months.

Potential Inability to take Normal Diet and Fluids due to Nausea and Possible Paralytic Ileus

On return from theatre if bowel sounds are absent the patient should only be allowed 15–30 ml of fluid orally per hour. As bowel sounds return fluids and diet can be gradually reintroduced. Initially fluid will need to be given intravenously as directed. Nausea should be controlled using an appropriate antiemetic, since vomiting will be painful.

Prevention of Possible Wound Infection

The wound should be kept clean and redressed as necessary. The clips or sutures should be removed 10–12 days post-surgery.

Advice on Discharge

Patients should be advised not to return to work for between 2 and 6 weeks depending on their occupation.

THE URETERS

Trauma

Injury to the ureters from external violence or from penetrating wounds seldom occurs. Most commonly any injury to the ureter occurs as a result of iatrogenic damage during abdominal surgery.

Diagnosis

Extravasation of urine will occur. This may be either intraperitoneal or extraperitoneal. It often remains unrecognised for some time. If the urine is sterile at the time of injury its presence in the peritoneal cavity will cause few symptoms, apart from increasing abdominal distension as a result of it collecting. Eventually urine may begin to drain either via a wound or from the vagina. If the urine is infected at the time of injury, peritonitis will occur and the patient will complain of abdominal pain in the lower abdominal quadrant. Vomiting may also occur due to paralytic ileus.

Injury may also occur due to accidental ligation of the ureter during surgery. This results in complete blockage to the passage of urine from the kidney on that side, resulting in hydronephrosis. The presence of the ligature will also cause local tissue necrosis and possible formation of a fistula which leads to delayed extravasation.

The diagnosis can thus be summarised as follows:

- Pain in lower abdominal quadrant
- Vomiting and paralytic ileus
- Peritonitis
- Leakage of urine from wound or vagina

Confirming Diagnosis

A specimen of any leaking fluid should be sent to biochemistry for urea and electrolyte analysis to confirm diagnosis. If complete occlusion is present serum creatinine will be raised. A plain abdominal X-ray may show the presence of extravasated urine. An intravenous urogram and isotope scanning tests should be done.

Treatment

If Recognised at the Time of Operation

1. End-to-end anastomosis The ends of the severed ureter are rejoined, and a double-J stent inserted. This will allow free passage of urine whilst healing occurs. This type of surgery may result in stricture formation.

2. Transureteroureterostomy The damaged ureter is anastomosed to the other ureter.

3. Implantation of ureter into bladder (ureteroneocystostomy) If the upper length of the ureter is significantly long to reach the bladder without undue tension, it can be implanted directly into the bladder wall. The anastomosis at the bladder must be tunnelled. A double-J stent is inserted and the patient should have a urethral catheter.

4. *Boari flap procedure*   If the upper length of the ureter is not sufficiently long to reach the bladder a Boari flap can be created. A rectangular flap is cut into the bladder wall and rolled to create a tube into which the ureter can be secured. A double-J stent should be inserted and the patient should have a urethral catheter.

5. If a bladder flap cannot be made long enough a segment of ileum with its blood supply can be used to replace it.

6. *Conservative management*   If the patient is unfit for major surgery, a nephrostomy tube can be inserted into the affected kidney to provide external drainage and maintain renal function.

Nursing Care

Preoperative

In addition to basic preoperative needs, there is the need to establish correct diagnosis. The nurse should observe for leakage of urine via the wound, wound drainage system or vagina, sending a specimen, if possible, for estimation of urea and electrolyte levels. The nurse should also check for possible septicaemia and shock. Blood pressure, pulse and temperature should be recorded, observing for shock.

Postoperative

The postoperative care will be dependent on the procedure employed. In addition to basic postoperative needs the patient has the following requirements.

1. *Maintain urinary drainage*   Depending on the surgical technique used, either double-J stents or ureteric splints will be used to facilitate healing of the anastomosis. Ureteric splints are commonly brought out through the abdominal wall. This enables the drainage from each kidney to be assessed. The patient should also be observed for the development of loin pain, indicating obstruction. If a blockage occurs it may be gently flushed out using 10–20 ml of sterile normal saline. The bladder may be drained by catheterisation and this should be kept patent. Fluid input should be maintained at a level of 2–3 litres per day in order to maintain urine output. Splints and catheters are normally removed 10 days postoperatively. Double-J stents can be retained in place for up to 3 months and removed under local anaesthesia.

2. *Observations for haemorrhage*   Urine should be observed for the presence and degree of haematuria. The wound site should be observed for blood loss and wound drainage measured. Excessive blood loss should be reported.

3. *Control discomfort/pain*   Relief of pain should be achieved by the administration of suitable analgesia to allow mobility.

4. *Prevent wound infection*   The wound should be kept clean and redressed as necessary. Prophylactic antibiotics may be given in order to render any urine that leaks through the anastomosis sterile.

5. *Possible nausea and paralytic ileus resulting in inability to take normal diet and fluids* On return from theatre if bowel sounds are absent the patient should be allowed no more than 15–30 ml of fluid per hour orally. Fluids should be given intravenously and reintroduced orally when bowel sounds return. Nausea should be controlled using appropriate antiemetics.

THE BLADDER

Trauma

The bladder can be injured in a number of different ways:

1. *External force* – this is commonly seen as a result of a road traffic accident especially if the bladder was distended with urine.

2. *Perforation* – this can occur as a result of a fractured pelvis in 10 per cent of cases. It may also occur during surgery as a result of accidental incision, e.g. during laparoscopy or cystoscopy.

3. *Penetrating wounds* – these may occur as a result of stabbing etc.

4. *Following radiotherapy of the pelvic organs.*

Diagnosis

The diagnosis may be difficult to make as often the patient presents with multiple injuries. Injury to the bladder will result in leakage of urine. This may be extraperitoneal or intraperitoneal.

Extraperitoneal Rupture

Extravasation of urine occurs into the perivesical space:

- There will be increasing abdominal tenderness
- The pulse will rise
- Only small quantities of urine will be passed

Intraperitoneal Rupture

Signs of intraperitoneal rupture are:

- Abdominal distension occurs
- Bowel sounds decrease
- Peritonitis may occur if urine is infected or if diagnosis is delayed
- There is failure to pass urine

Confirming Diagnosis

The following tests are used:

● Cystoscopy
● Cystogram
● IVU

Treatment

Extraperitoneal Rupture

Catheterisation over a period of 7–10 days will normally be sufficient to allow the rupture to heal.

Intraperitoneal Rupture

Surgical repair of the defect is necessary The defect is sutured and the patient left with a suprapubic catheter for 10–14 days until the defect has healed.

If the defect results from damage due to radiotherapy, tissue damage may be widespread and defects are normally excised and a substitution cystoplasty performed (see Chapter 7).

THE URETHRA

Damage to the urethra can occur in a number of ways:

1. *Trauma* – due to a direct blow or a straddle injury or bypassage of a stone.

2. *Iatrogenic* – injury to the urethra is a complication of many treatments, including catheterisation, instrumentation of the urinary tract, and can also follow prostatectomy.

3. *Infection*, e.g. non-specific urethritis.

4. *Childbirth and gynaecological procedures.*

Urethral Trauma

Damage to the male urethra by trauma usually affects the bulbar and membranous portions of the urethra. The anterior urethra is rarely affected.

The Bulbar Urethra

Bulbar injuries normally result from direct trauma, for example falling astride a crossbar.

Diagnosis

Diagnosis is based on the following:

- History of injury
- Bruising of the external genitalia
- Blood at the urethral meatus

Treatment

The patient should be given the opportunity to void normally. If he fails to do so a suprapubic catheter should be inserted. A urethral catheter should not be passed because this may aggravate the injury and increase the risk of infection. Prophylactic antibiotic treatment should be given.

A urethrogram should be performed on those who fail to void to assess the degree of the injury, that future treatment can be planned.

All patients should have urological follow-up, as progression to stricture is common.

The Membranous Urethra

Injury to the membranous urethra occurs in approximately 10 per cent of men with a pelvic fracture. Injuries to this area have a high morbidity associated with stricture formation, incontinence and impotence. This area is surrounded by sphincter-active tissue, and held in place by the pubovesical and pubourethral ligaments. The dislocation of the symphysis pubis can lead to a complete rupture of the urethra, resulting in extravasation of urine, haematoma formation, and the upward dislocation of the bladder and prostate.

Diagnosis

Diagnosis is based on the following:

- History of injury
- Bruising of the external genitalia
- Blood at the meatus
- Retention of urine
- Signs of extravasation
- High riding prostate with bladder displacement

Treatment

Associated injuries often require life-saving treatment and therefore must take precedence over the urethral injury. However, catheterisation is generally required for the monitoring of fluid balance. Urethral catheterisation should only be attempted if there is no blood at the meatus. A small catheter may be gently introduced without the use of force. If urethral catheterisation fails or there is blood at the meatus, a suprapubic catheter should be passed.

An IVU should be performed with an ascending urethrogram when the patient's condition allows, in order to assess the degree of damage, which may be partial or complete rupture of the urethra.

1. *Partial rupture*   Urethroscopy should be performed with suprapubic exploration undertaken in order to drain any haematoma or extravasated urine. A small catheter should also be passed.

2. *Complete rupture*   Suprapubic exploration should be performed in order to drain any haematoma or extravasated urine and under direct vision a urethral catheter passed to act as a splint to keep the urethra in alignment. Fixation of the prostate should be performed along with fixation of the fracture. These patients usually require reconstruction in the long term.

Urethral Strictures

Damage to the urethra by whatever cause invariably results in stricture formation. The management of strictures is very variable from centre to centre. Treatment options will depend on the following factors: the patient's general condition; the location of the stricture; the length of the stricture; previous treatment given; the patient's wishes; and the surgeon's skill.

Diagnosis

Diagnosis is based on the following:

- History of predisposing factor
- Thin/forked stream
- Post-micturition dribble
- Incontinence of urine
- Frequent infections
- Retention of urine

Confirming Diagnosis

- Urinary flow rate
- Urethrogram
- Cystourethroscopy
- Midstream specimen of urine for culture

Treatment

Urethrotomy

Urethrotomy is a technique used in both the primary and long-term management of urethral strictures. It involves cutting the stricture along its length under direct vision, commonly with an Otis urethroscope. Ideally, following this, new epithelial tissue grows to fill the deficit, widening the narrowed urethra. The complications of this technique are the high incidence of stricture recurrence and the possible damage to the sphincter mechanism, resulting in incontinence.

Preoperative care   A urinary flow rate should be obtained.

Postoperative care   Urinary drainage should be maintained. Catheterisation is normally performed at the time of surgery. The length of time that this is retained is dependent upon the surgeon.

There is a risk of potential haemorrhage. Haematuria commonly results in the postoperative period and may persist for up to 10 days. Initially the patient will have a urethral catheter which will act as a splint. The colour of the urine should be assessed to determine the degree of haematuria. On removal of the catheter the patient may experience fresh bleeding due to the disturbance of the healing tissues.

There should be adequate pain control. The patient usually experiences minimal pain, but mild to moderate analgesia may be needed. The pain may be more apparent when the patient restarts voiding urethrally, due to the irritation of the urine on the healing tissues.

Dilatation

This technique is used in the long-term management of strictures, and may be performed on an out-patient basis. The treatment aims to stretch the urethral scar tissue by the introduction of a series of urethral dilators (bougies), increasing in size until the urethra has been adequately dilated. Prior to treatment a local anaesthetic is inserted into the urethra and a penile clamp applied, in order to produce local anaesthesia.

Following the procedure the patient will require a mild analgesic. A urinary flow rate should be taken in order to monitor the effectiveness of treatment.

Complications of this procedure include:

1. *Bacteraemia*, possibly due to poor aseptic technique, or introduction of bacteria into the circulation from a pre-existing urinary tract infection.

2. *Haemorrhage*, due to trauma. The patient's urine should be observed prior to discharge, and a high fluid intake advised.

3. *Urethral rupture* The membranous urethra is particularly vulnerable to rupture following instrumentation.

4. *Restricturing* of the affected area is common.

Self-dilatation

The introduction of self-dilatation of strictures has led to a decrease in the number of patients requiring regular surgery. Meatal strictures can be treated by teaching the patient to self-dilate by the introduction of a well lubricated spigot into the meatus.

Dilatation should be performed on a twice weekly or weekly basis. Other strictures have successfully been treated by urethrotomy followed by dilatation using a low friction, hydrophilised disposable catheter, performed twice weekly for 1 month and then at weekly intervals.

Stenting

A stent suitable for use in the urethra was developed in the 1980s. It is made of an inert metal mesh which is placed over the site of the stricture using an introducer, then released. It then springs into position holding open the stricture. The stent is gradually covered by epithelial tissue, rendering it continuous with the urethral tissue. The advantage of this procedure is that it can be performed under local anaesthesia, offering a curative therapy to the medically unfit.

Infection should be eliminated before the operation is performed. Urine should be sent for culture, and broad-spectrum antibiotics given at the time of operation.

Infection should be prevented postoperatively. Temperature should be monitored and a course of antibiotics given. Pain or discomfort should be controlled. Perineal pain may be a problem initially. Suitable analgesia should be given.

Complications of this procedure include:

1. *Stenosis* The overgrowth of epithelial tissue has been reported, particularly following placement for strictures caused by trauma. This leads to the stent being removed.

2. *Misplacement of the stent* Incorrect placement may lead to the development of incontinence.

3. *Encrustation* can also occur if the stent protrudes above the bladder neck.

4. *Perineal pain* may persist after the initial postoperative period. If this cannot be controlled, removal may be necessary.

The patient with a stent should not undergo urethral catheterisation as this may lead to displacement.

Long-term Catheterisation

Catheterisation, usually suprapubic, can be considered for the management of a stricture in the severely debilitated and in those not wanting further surgery.

Urethroplasty

The type of surgery undertaken to reconstruct the male urethra is dependent upon the following factors:

● Length of the defect
● Location of the injury within the urethra

The Length of the Defect

A defect of up to 1.5 cm in length can be repaired by excising the strictured tissue and creating an end-to-end anastomosis. Any stricture longer than this will require a 'substitution' urethroplasty, where the defect is repaired by grafting.

The Location of the Injury

1. *The glans meatus* (see Chapter 13).

2. *The penile urethra* This area is amenable to the whole variety of treatment methods.

3. *The bulbar urethra* This area is best repaired by skin grafting, as end-to-end anastomosis can result in chordee of the penis.

4. *The prostatic, membranous urethra* This area is sphincter active, and surgery normally consists of grafting by an experienced surgeon.

Surgical Techniques

End-to-end Anastomosis

The strictured part of the urethra is excised and the continuity of the urethra restored by the anastomosis of the ends.

Substitution Urethroplasty

This can be performed in either one or two stages (Figure 6.1). The urethra is exposed via a midline perineal incision and if the stricture occurs high in the urethra an abdominal incision is sometimes also required. Once the strictured area is exposed it is excised and replaced by grafted skin.

If the procedure is complex and hair-bearing skin is used for the graft, it may be decided not to close the wound but to have a two-stage procedure. This allows for inspection of the graft prior to closure, and an opportunity for epilation of the graft. If this is the case the patient will void via a perineal urethrostomy.

The second stage of the urethroplasty involves closure of the new urethra. If the procedure can be done in one stage the graft is closed and a urethral catheter inserted.

Skin Grafting

Types of Skin

1. *Wet* – epidermal skin, which is adapted for a moist environment such as urethra, oral mucosa, vagina, labia.

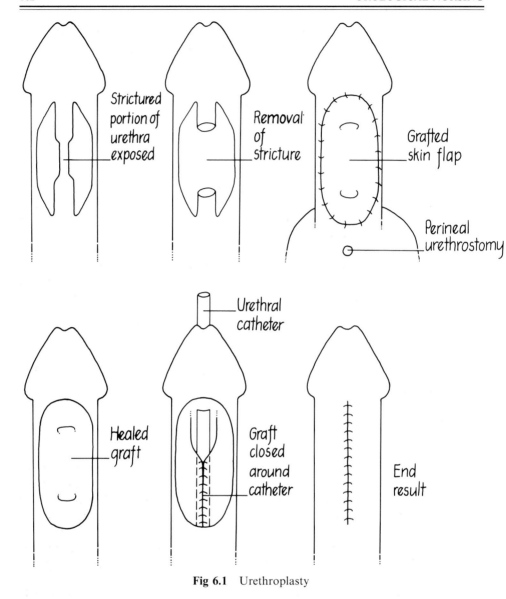

Fig 6.1 Urethroplasty

2. *Dry* – scrotum, thigh, abdominal skin, which in a moist environment becomes inflamed.

3. *Penile* – this is moisture-resistant skin, and relatively hairless.

Types of Grafting

1. *Free grafts* – use full thickness skin.

2. *Mesh grafts* – skin is perforated prior to grafting.

Free grafts and mesh grafting are very dependent upon survival of the whole graft. In pedicle grafting the skin is taken along with its blood supply.

Preoperative Care

Preoperative nursing care should encompass the following:

1. *Postoperative constipation* should be prevented to avoid straining and painful evacuation of the bowels postoperatively. If there are signs of constipation two glycerin suppositories should be given the night before the operation.

2. *The perineal skin* should be prepared. Skin should not be routinely shaved, as the surgeon will need to know what skin is hair-bearing. However, some surgeons do like the hair to be removed – a depilatory cream is ideal for this area. Routine skin preparation should be carried out immediately prior to surgery.

3. *Postoperative infection* should be prevented. Prophylactic antibiotics should be given prior to surgery. The close proximity of the anus to the incision can lead to infection from anaerobic organisms.

4. *Postoperative deep vein thrombosis* should be prevented. The patient should be taught leg exercises and measured for anti-embolism stockings.

5. The patient should be reassured and any anxieties allayed by a complete explanation of what to expect.

Postoperative Management

Postoperative management includes the following:

1. *Urinary drainage* should be maintained. The patient will have a urethral catheter and possibly a suprapubic catheter. It is important that the catheters are not allowed to block. Fenestrated catheters should not be 'washed out' as this will cause damage to the graft. The patient should have a fluid input of at least 3 litres a day in order to prevent stasis.

The catheters stay in place for 10–14 days, at which time a urethrogram is performed, with the contrast being put down the suprapubic catheter to test for extravasation. If there is no leakage, the urethral catheter is removed. If it is fenestrated, removal is achieved by cutting the stitch attached to the abdominal wall. If the catheter is a balloon type it is essential that the balloon is fully deflated prior to attempted removal. Failure to do this may lead to damage of the graft.

2. *Haematoma formation/excessive swelling of the scrotal/penile area* should be prevented. This is not only a source of discomfort but also can lead to failure of the graft to 'take'. There is often some form of compression applied to the penis. This may be in the form of a foam dressing or alternatively achieved by the application of a semi-constrictive piece of tape around the shaft of the penis. The whole of the scrotal area should be well supported with bulky padding secured with elastonet pants.

There might also be some type of wound drainage, either via a corrugated drain or via a vacuum system. It is usual to leave the initial dressing in place for 3 days until the incidence of swelling is reduced. However, padding should be changed if it is blood-soaked. The drain is normally removed 2–3 days postoperatively.

In the initial postoperative period the patient's activity should be limited to moving from bed to chair, as greater exertion could lead to further swelling.

3. *The perineal wound* should be protected from infection. Due to the close proximity of the incision to the anus, the wound is at risk of infection from anaerobic microbes.

If the procedure is a 'one-stage' one, the patient should be allowed to bathe once any wound drain has been removed and should be encouraged to do so daily and after any bowel motion. If the procedure is the first of a two-stage repair, bathing should not occur until 4–5 days postoperatively. After a bath the wound should be cleansed with sterile saline and a supportive dressing applied. The urethral catheter should be taped in such a way as to elevate the penis on the abdominal wall. This helps to reduce swelling. Care must be taken not to put too much traction on this catheter. Antibiotic therapy is usually given until the catheters are removed. Initially this will be intravenously.

4. *Deep vein thrombosis* must be prevented. This is achieved by the wearing of antiembolism stockings, performing leg exercises whilst immobile, early mobilisation and by giving heparin subcutaneously as prescribed.

5. *Straining* will result in pain and discomfort to the patient and so constipation should be prevented as far as possible. If the patient is usually constipated a gentle laxative should be given prophylactically.

6. The patient experiences quite a lot of discomfort in the early postoperative period and opioid analgesia should be given. An anti-inflammatory drug should also be given regularly, either rectally or orally, as this will help to reduce the pain from the oedema. A supportive wound dressing does much to relieve discomfort.

The patient may also be troubled by bladder spasm resulting from the catheterisation. If this is troublesome an anticholinergic such as oxybutynin should be given regularly. After a satisfactory urethrogram, the urethral catheter is removed. The suprapubic catheter can be clamped and the patient should void normally.

Residual urine volumes can be measured via the suprapubic catheter and if these are low the suprapubic catheter can be removed. A flow rate should be obtained.

Postoperative Advice

The patient should be told never to allow an inexperienced person to catheterise him urethrally – a suprapubic catheter is preferable. The patient should continue to rest for a further month. Prolonged sitting and driving should be avoided. Sexual intercourse should not be resumed for 6 weeks.

7

Reconstructive Surgery for the Promotion of Continence

It is commonly supposed that incontinence is a problem which is exclusive to the elderly. Few people realise that it can affect almost anyone. It is not only confined to the elderly or disabled, but is common in people of all ages, fit and disabled. Incontinence can be defined as the involuntary passing or urine and/or faeces in a socially unacceptable place. The International Continence Society defines urinary incontinence as:

'a condition where involuntary loss of urine is a social or hygienic problem.'

This distressing and socially disabling condition affects 5 per cent of the population, with women affected more than men – 8 per cent of all women in the population are affected as opposed to only 3 per cent of men (Bullock et al, 1989). Many people see incontinence as an inevitable discomfort and embarrassment. The general public's interpretation of the term 'incontinence' is often different from its medical interpretation. Many people use the term to describe a total lack of control and deny being incontinent even though they may admit to 'wetting' or 'leakage' (Norton, 1986). Many sufferers hide their problem from society, their family, friends, and even from themselves. Children are teased by their schoolmates, leading to a dread of going to school, absences, deterioration in school-work and a growing sense of isolation. Hiding the problem, even denying its existence may be their coping mechanism to deal with the ridicule, and help them feel less ostracised and avoided.

Older sufferers also show these feelings. The embarrassment and shame of being wet, the risk of leakage, and having to wear incontinence aids can drive them to cut themselves off from others, having grave repercussions on their educational, working and social lives. Loss of self-esteem and confidence, the conviction that the condition is discernible by and obvious to all those around him or her, the belief that he or she 'smells' and that this cannot be hidden, no matter how much washing or perfume is used all contribute to the incontinent person's negative self-image. He or she will not feel attractive to the opposite (or same) sex, and already existing relationships may suffer and founder as a consequence. It is an insurmountable obstacle for the unattached sufferer who wants to establish a relationship, as the fear of rejection is powerful and restricting.

Incontinence does become more common as one becomes older, though it is not an inevitable part of the ageing process. Older people may find talking about the problem impossible, because it relates to a very personal and 'taboo' area of their bodies. It is also a sign of their loss of 'control' and may indicate that hospitalisation or institutionalisation may result.

The cost of incontinence, both in the practical sense (i.e. the money to buy aids, replace bedding, furniture, laundry bills, etc.) and the emotional sense (i.e. the guilt, and feelings of inadequacy and hopelessness felt by the carers), is almost incalculable. Ignorance about the way the body functions, and the conviction that nothing can be done to improve the condition, lead to the sufferer becoming pessimistic about the prospect of any improvement.

Incontinence creates psychosocial problems for all sufferers, and causes disruptions, big and small, to their life-styles, depending on their ability to cope. It is important that sufferers become aware that help is available, and that if a cure is not possible, then considerable help and support is, and should be attempted. (Norton, 1986).

The Incontinent Patient in Hospital

A patient suffering from incontinence, when admitted to a specialist unit arrives with a mixture of apprehension, hope and relief. Many would have endured their condition for some time, and may have consulted (unsuccessfully) their GP or other specialists for help. Having finally been referred to a specialist unit and undergone tests which show the cause of their problem, the fact that something is finally going to happen which may cure them seems hardly possible. It is always wise to be completely honest with these patients and explain all that they should expect as a result of the surgery they are to have. The idea is not to discourage them, but to give a realistic picture of the positive and negative aspects of the treatment. Many patients may have to undergo more than one surgical intervention until the result is deemed acceptable by themselves and their consultants. A greater understanding of their condition, the expected outcome of the surgery, the possible setbacks which may occur and what they are expected to contribute to their care and recovery, helps give them a sense of control and aids in ensuring compliance with the treatment.

When admitted to the ward, the patient often feels that he/she has found a place where it is no longer 'taboo' to talk about the problem, because all the staff are experienced in the treatment of incontinence. It may be the first time many details of his/her condition will be revealed, and the reassurance he/she receives may alleviate feelings of guilt or disgust at the problem. In our unit, this care starts in the out-patients and urodynamics departments and is continued on the ward. The patient is involved in his/her care from the very start.

What Is Incontinence?

Urinary incontinence is the involuntary loss of urine. It is often a symptom of an underlying problem. This loss of urine may occur via the urethra or from an abnormal extraurethral route.

Classification of Incontinence

Incontinence is classified as follows:

- Stress incontinence
- Urge incontinence
- Neurogenic bladder
- Outflow incontinence
- Incontinence secondary to fistulae or congenital anomalies

(Sökeland, 1989 – according to the International Continence Society)

STRESS INCONTINENCE

This term refers to either a symptom or a medical diagnosis. 'Genuine' stress incontinence refers to incontinence caused by a weak or incompetent sphincter. A rise in intra-abdominal pressure, transmitted to the bladder, exceeds urethral closure pressure in the absence of detrusor activity (Bullock et al, 1989). Stress incontinence as a 'symptom' describes the experience of leaking urine upon physical exertion – such as in patients with cough or strain-induced detrusor instability, where leakage is due to the abnormal detrusor activity and not sphincter weakness. A patient in urinary retention can experience overflow incontinence on exertion. Urodynamic investigations are required to determine the true cause of the leakage.

Sphincter weakness is more common in women than in men. Some of the causes include obesity, mutiparity and childbirth. Men may also suffer sphincter weakness following pelvic fracture injuries or prostatectomy. In postmenopausal women a loss of tone in the urethral mucosa and muscle is the result of an oestrogen deficiency.

Surgery for Stress Incontinence

Before attempting surgery, the patient will be encouraged to try non-invasive treatment by his or her doctor. It is only after trying a whole range of such treatments that surgery is contemplated. The aim of the surgery is to elevate and support the bladder neck so that this will be repositioned correctly above the pelvic floor muscles. The repairs can be done vaginally together with repair to any existing cystocele. Repairs also can be done via a suprapubic approach.

There is no special preoperative physical care for anyone undergoing these types of operation. The important thing is to explain that sometimes the results can vary, and the chances of total cure cannot be guaranteed. However, the results may be **too** good in some cases, and the patient may not be able to pass urine urethrally at all. It is always a good idea therefore, to warn the patient of this and discuss and demonstrate intermittent self-catheterisation as a possible solution should this happen. If the patient has not yet completed her family, she should be warned that vaginal delivery might be difficult, and might also undo the effects of surgery. All patients should be told that even if the surgery is successful, there is a possibility of stress incontinence recurring at a later date.

The Vaginal Repair

There are many variations on this type of repair. The bladder neck and proximal urethra are displayed via the divided anterior vaginal wall. The exposed bladder neck and urethra are then mobilised upwards and held with buttress sutures.

Abdominal Repairs

These are usually via a 'bikini-line' incision. The colposuspension operation is a modification of the Marshall–Marchetti–Krantz procedure where the bladder neck is hitched to the back of the symphysis pubis by sutures placed on either side of the urethra. In the colposuspension, sutures are placed in the lateral vaginal fornices, elevating and supporting the bladder neck. Either organic material (e.g. strips of fascia or muscle) or synthetic slings (e.g. polypropylene or polyethylene) can be used to support and elevate the bladder neck by attachment to ligaments or periosteum. In the Stamey operation, a long needle is passed via a small suprapubic incision and nylon sutures are placed in either side of the bladder neck.

Postoperative Care

The specific postoperative care these patients require involves the care of their newly 'hitched up' bladder necks, to ensure they heal adequately and prove strong enough to give some degree of continence back to the patient. The patient returns to the ward with a vaginal pack in situ (to stem vaginal bleeding), a suprapubic catheter, and sometimes a urethral catheter. Besides the usual immediate postoperative care, it is most important that these patients' catheters are checked frequently to ensure they are patent and urine is able to drain out freely. This might involve flushing the catheters to remove debris and blood clots. The patient's fluid intake should also be monitored. An intravenous infusion is usually in progress for the first 24 hours, and the patient is allowed and encouraged to drink as soon as she can tolerate it. The patient's fluid intake over the remainder of her hospital stay is important and she should be encouraged to drink at least 3 litres of fluid a day to keep her bladder and catheters flushed and patent. The vaginal pack is removed after 2 hours, and usually so is the urethral catheter. The latter sometimes depends on the surgeon's preference.

The patient is encouraged to start mobilising on the first postoperative day and is usually independent again by the second or third postoperative day. The rest of her stay in hospital is really a period of waiting until it is time to clamp the suprapubic catheter. For a Stamey operation this is usually within 7 days. This again depends on the individual surgeon's preference. Once the catheter is clamped, the patient should begin passing urine urethrally. It is at this point that the patient needs maximum support. Sometimes the patient is able to pass good amounts (200–300 ml) of urine every 2–3 hours with no leaking urethrally in between visits to the toilet. Some patients, however, find that they pass small amounts (20–60 ml) every 10–60 minutes. This does sometimes improve over the following few days, and patients should be reassured and supported through this time.

Once the patient has passed urine two or three times after clamping, the catheter can be released and any residual urine in the bladder drained out and measured. This is usually measured two or three times a day. The residual aimed for is an amount between 0 and 50 ml. Again if the bladder is holding more than this, the amount may also improve after a day or two.

Once the residual is 50 ml or less, the catheter is removed, and the patient discharged home. There may be some leakage via the suprapubic catheter site. The patient should be reassured that this usually stops after a day or two, and if the leakage is severe, a stoma bag can be worn over the site to collect the urine, and keep the patient dry. If the residual volumes remain large or the patient continues to pass small frequent amounts of urine, with some leakage, then she may be discharged home with the suprapubic catheter still in place, and she will be shown how to clamp and release this herself and record her progress over a period of 2–3 weeks.

Once the residuals are within acceptable limits the patient is readmitted to have the catheter removed and her micturating pattern monitored. If the residuals remain large, the patient may have to be taught how to empty her bladder completely by using intermittent clean catheterisation (*see* Advice Sheet 1 page 170).

Another surgical option is the endoscopic injection of Teflon paste on either side of the bladder neck to relieve stress incontinence. However, Teflon has been found to migrate from its original position of insertion, and has been found lodged in brain tissue. This makes it dangerous to use in the younger patient. A new substance has been developed which is now being used instead of Teflon. This is called Bio or Uro plastique^{TM}.

In men, operations as described above have not been successful. Implantable mechanical devices, such as a silicone gel (Kaufman) prosthesis, can be implanted in the perineum to provide constant urethral compression. Another option is the insertion of an artificial urinary sphincter. This is covered later in the chapter.

URGE INCONTINENCE

Urge incontinence occurs when there is an involuntary loss of urine following a strong desire to void. This urgency may be extreme, with urine being voided simultaneously with the sensation to void. Sometimes there is a short delay between the sensation and capacity, but the sufferer may still be incontinent even if the toilet is reached in time. Detrusor hyperreflexia is the result of involuntary bladder contractions while the bladder is filling. When the normal inhibiting impulses are not sent from the bladder centre in the cortex the reflex arc is completed. The bladder responds by contracting before micturition is initiated voluntarily. This causes a variety of symptoms which include frequency, urgency, urge incontinence, nocturia and possibly nocturnal enuresis. Detrusor instability may be secondary to bladder outflow obstruction or idiopathic in origin (*see* Figs 7.1 and 7.2). Patients suffering from bladder instability may have no obvious neurological lesion which is causing their inability to inhibit bladder contractions. The condition often presents in the second, third or fourth decades of life, and may have no obvious cause.

ADVICE SHEET 1

THIS ADVICE SHEET IS IN ADDITION TO ANY VERBAL ADVICE
YOU MAY BE GIVEN BY THE MEDICAL AND NURSING STAFF ON
BEING DISCHARGED. PLEASE READ THIS SHEET AND KEEP IT
FOR FUTURE REFERENCE.

**PATIENT GUIDELINES
FOR AFTERCARE OF BLADDER NECK SUSPENSIONS**

PASSING URINE

You may still be passing urine frequently, in small amounts, with some
discomfort on leaving hospital. This is to be expected and should gradually
improve over the following weeks. You should try to hold your urine for 5–10
minutes longer in between visits to the toilet each day, so that eventually you will
be able to pass urine every 2–4 hours, and will be dry and comfortable in-
between times. This may take some time to achieve, but please persevere. You
must not strain to pass urine.

FLUID INTAKE

Drink at least 2 litres of fluid daily. This may help keep infection in your urine
from occurring. You should reduce the amount that you drink up to 2 hours
before your bedtime so that your urine output at night will be reduced too and
so you may not have to pass urine too frequently at night. This frequency will
also improve in time.

WORK, REST AND EXERCISE

Allow yourself plenty of rest. Avoid lifting heavy objects (e.g. shopping,
suitcases, or children) for at least 6–8 weeks, then gradually increase your level
of activity. You should aim to reach your preoperation level by the time of your
first out-patient's appointment (about 6–8 weeks). It is a good idea to take some
gentle exercise during this period too (e.g. a short daily walk) if you can manage
it.

Returning to work will depend on the type of work you do. If your job
involves lifting or standing for long periods of time, you may be advised to take
at least 4–6 weeks off work. Please ask the doctor or nurse on the ward for
advice if you are not certain what to do.

Urge incontinence may also have sensory as well as motor causes. Sensory urgency
may result because of intravesical pathology (e.g. urinary infection, interstitial
cystitis, bladder calculi, bladder tumours); however, some patients have no
demonstrable problem, and psychological factors may be involved.

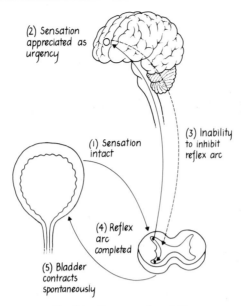

Fig 7.1 Detrusor instability

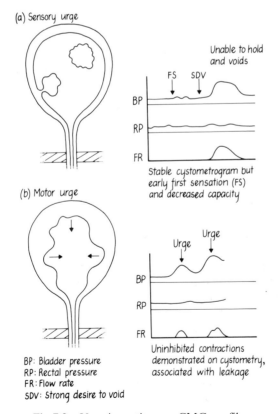

Fig 7.2 Urge incontinence: CMG profiles

Surgery for Urge Incontinence

Hydrostatic bladder distension is one procedure usually performed under general anaesthetic and involves expanding the bladder with fluid, and keeping it distended for 5 minutes. The patient usually stays in hospital for 24 hours after the operation and is discharged once she or he passes clear, haematuria-free urine. A Helmstein distension is a more prolonged distension where a balloon is inflated within the bladder to a pressure between systolic and diastolic blood pressure for 2–4 hours. It is usually performed under epidural anaesthesia. Bullock et al (1989) claim that though improvement occurs in 60–80 per cent of patients, recurrence of symptoms is common. There is also a risk of bladder rupture occurring during the procedure.

Cystoscopic subtrigonal injection of phenol has been used to cause partial denervation of the bladder. Rosenbaum et al (1990) report that this has not been found to be as effective as hoped. This denervation can also be achieved by surgical division or percutaneous ablation of selected sacral nerves (usually S3), or by division and resuturing of the bladder just above the trigone. This is called bladder transection.

If these procedures do not help the only alternative may be that the bladder will have to be enlarged so that bladder capacity is increased. This procedure is known as a cystoplasty. Once again any patient who is to undergo any of the above surgical procedures should be instructed in carrying out self-catheterisation, as there is a possibility of not being able to empty the bladder completely afterwards. Failing a cystoplasty, the patient may have to undergo urinary diversion.

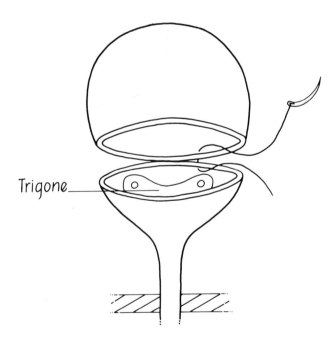

Fig 7.3 Bladder transection

Cystoplasty

A segment of bowel (usually ileum) is used to increase the functional capacity of the bladder. This is known as augmentation cystoplasty. Alternatively the bulk of the bladder can be removed and the bladder refashioned by using caecum. This is known as substitution cystoplasty. The type of operation is obviously decided following tests, and taking the individual patient's condition into consideration. The patient is warned in out-patients that it is a major operation and that he or she will be admitted to hospital 2 or 3 days before the operation itself to be prepared for the operation. He or she is told to expect to be in hospital for a minimum of 2 weeks. Self-catheterisation is also discussed at this point and the patient may require more information about this before deciding to go ahead with the procedure.

The main reason for being admitted a few days earlier is to ensure that the patient's bowel is cleared prior to a portion of it being used as part of the new bladder. The patient is allowed to eat a low residue diet on being admitted 3 days before the

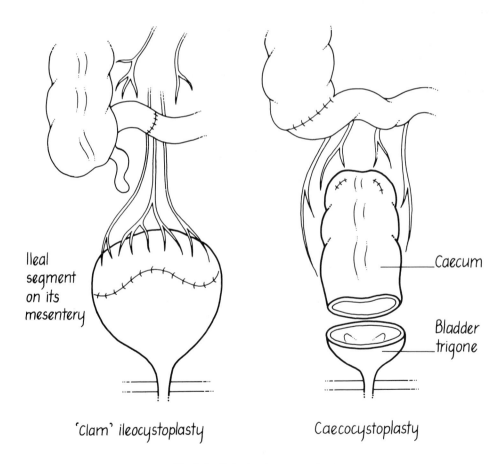

'Clam' ileocystoplasty   Caecocystoplasty

Fig 7.4   Substitution cystoplasty

operation. He is then allowed to drink free fluids on the next day and given oral aperients (our unit uses Picolax). On the day before the operation, he is only allowed clear free fluids which will not form a residue in the bowel, and another dose of aperients. This is a hard period for the patient. It is also embarrassing if any faecal accidents occur. He or she should be well supported and allowance made for tiredness and weakness. Visitors should be encouraged as well as some form of entertainment or distraction to help the patient and ensure his or her compliance with the procedure. Some surgeons favour starting intravenous fluid therapy some hours before the start of the operation to help replace fluid lost by the profuse diarrhoea.

Postoperative Care

The most important part of the postoperative care involves the newly formed bladder. The aim is to keep the bladder deflated so that the new anastomosis heals. The patient usually has a suprapubic and urethral catheter in situ. It is essential that these are kept patent and allow all urine and debris to drain out. The bowel will also form mucus which may cause obstruction. These catheters are kept patent by flushing them. Again this is done as per the surgeon's preference. Some surgeons advocate flushing only if the catheters seem blocked. Some prefer to attach continuous irrigation to flush the bladder out by trickling in fluid via the suprapubic catheter and draining it out via the urethral catheter. This requires careful monitoring to ensure there is no build-up of fluid in the bladder if the urethral catheter blocks. The third option is to flush both catheters with 20–30 ml of sterile saline twice or three times daily. Debris and mucus can be gently washed out after the third or fourth postoperative day without damaging the new anastomosis.

The urethral catheter is sometimes removed after 48 hours. It then becomes vital to ensure that the suprapubic catheter remains patent as it is the only tube draining the bladder. Once the patient commences oral intake again, he or she should be encouraged to drink at least 3 litres of fluid daily to keep the system flushed.

The patient may experience problems with diarrhoea and irregular bowel movements once he or she begins to eat and drink again. The patient should be reassured that this does happen and that it may be some months before bowel movements follow a more normal pattern.

A cystogram is usually performed after the tenth postoperative day. This will show the outline of the new bladder and if no contrast leaks out into the pelvic cavity, it will show that the bladder has healed. The suprapubic catheter is then clamped, the urethral catheter removed and the patient's voiding pattern monitored. Again this may vary. Some patients begin to void small, frequent amounts. This will improve slowly, as the bladder starts to become accustomed to holding urine again, and begins to stretch. Some patients find they do not void until the bladder is full. The suprapubic catheter is unclamped two or three times during the day to measure the residual urine in the bladder. If the residual is 50 ml or less, the suprapubic catheter is removed and the patient discharged home. If the residual is large, the patient will have to empty his or her bladder by intermittent self-catheterisation. It is vital that the possibility of this happening is made known to the patient before the operation, so that though the result of the operation may be a disappointment, he or she will know what to expect. Some patients find that they only have to catheterise for a few months, and after a while can actually cut this down to once or twice a day. Some patients find they have to start catheterising after some months as the bladder will have stretched to hold a large volume and they cannot empty the bladder completely. They complain of feeling uncomfortable and pass urine frequently. The build-up of urinary leads to recurrent urine infections. By self-catheterising, these patients can reverse this process.

Another complication of this operation is that some patients begin to experience spasms of pain in the bladder. These contractions usually originate in the bowel part of the new bladder and if very intense, could lead to urine leaking out of the bladder urethrally because of the increase in pressure. Antispasmodic medication, such as Colofac, which works on the smooth muscle contractions, may help. However, some patients may need another section or patch of bowel added to the original cystoplasty to enlarge the bladder and stop the spasm pattern.

Excess mucus production may lead to recurrent urinary tract infections and bladder stones. The importance of frequent (3–4-hourly) bladder emptying and the intake of at least 3 litres of fluids daily must be reinforced to these patients. Drinking cranberry juice (200 ml) twice a day has been shown to reduce the quantity of mucus produced in some patients (Rosenbaum et al, unpublished). Some patients may have to resort to removing excess mucus by performing bladder washouts via a urethral catheter.

Some patients may have both stress and urge incontinence and so will require a cystoplasty, as already described, but with the insertion of an artificial urinary sphincter to keep them dry (see Fig 7.5).

All compression devices such as the sphincter of the Kaufman's prosthesis mentioned earlier, are prone to complication including urethral erosion, infection and mechanical failure. Preoperative preparation is vital to reduce the risk of these complications. Once again, the specific preparation depends on the individual surgeon's preference. However, all involve some form of bowel preparation to ensure the rectum is empty at operation. The patient is encouraged to have two or three baths using either an antiseptic skin detergent or an iodine-based surgical skin scrub. Some units prefer patients to use the detergent on their hair also. Rectal antibiotics are given as part of the premedication and the patient's pubic area is always shaved in the operating theatre immediately before surgery. These procedures all reduce the risk of infection.

Postoperative care also varies, though a period of bed rest ranging from a few days to 3 weeks is common to all. Patients usually have a suprapubic catheter in situ to drain away urine, though this is usually removed before discharge. The sphincter is not activated until 6 weeks after the operation. The patient must be prepared to be wet during this time, and to watch out for any sign of infection so that this can be treated immediately. He or she is allowed to have a bath, but instructed to dry the area well afterwards.

The patient is usually taught to activate the device in the out-patient department. Some patients with neurogenic bladder problems may have cystoplasty and insertion of the artificial sphincter but actually empty their bladders by self-catheterising. This may sound complicated, but it gives the individual control and it achieves the aim of

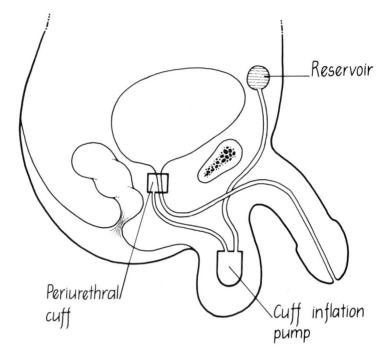

Fig 7.5   Position of artificial urinary sphincter

making the patient continent and improving his or her quality of life (see Advice Sheet 2).

NEUROGENIC BLADDER

Continence is not something we are born with, it is a skill we acquire and retain in childhood. A baby voids on response to a sacral relex arc. With practice, voluntary control of the child's bladder becomes possible, and the reflex arc response to a full bladder can be blocked, and micturition can be prevented (See Figs 7.6 and 7.7).

The bladder and urethra therefore act as a single functional unit, and the storage and expulsion of urine are controlled by a complex neurological system. Lesions at any point in the neurological pathway can disturb the continence voiding mechanism.

Neurogenic bladder disorders resulting from CNS lesions are:

1. *Congential anomalies*
    (a) spina bifida
    (b) myelomeningocele
    (c) spinal dysraphism
    (d) dermoid cyst or fistula of the sacral cord

ADVICE SHEET 2

THIS ADVICE SHEET IS IN ADDITION TO ANY VERBAL ADVICE YOU MAY BE GIVEN BY THE MEDICAL AND NURSING STAFF ON BEING DISCHARGED. PLEASE READ THIS SHEET AND KEEP IT FOR FUTURE REFERENCE.

PATIENT GUIDELINES
FOR AFTERCARE OF BLADDER AUGMENTATIONS

PASSING URINE

You might find this quite difficult at first, and it might take some time for you to establish a normal pattern. You may find that you are passing urine frequently and in small amounts. Try holding your urine for 5–10 minutes longer each time you need to pass urine. This will help expand your bladder, and in time it will be able to hold more urine.

If you find that you are passing less and less urine and feel you have a full bladder and start to get more urine infections, please contact your doctor or the ward for advice.

Do not strain when trying to pass urine.

DIET AND FLUIDS

You may find that you have irregular bowel habits when you are first discharged home. This is because some of your bowel has been used to create the new bladder. Eat a varied diet, with plenty of fruit and vegetables, which should stop you becoming constipated. Your appetite may be smaller than it used to be, so you may prefer to eat smaller, more regular meals, instead of three main meals a day.

Drink at least 3 litres of fluid a day. Drinks which are high in vitamin C and cranberry juice may help to reduce the mucus production of the bowel part of your new bladder. The fluid will dilute the mucus, making it easier to pass out of the bladder, and reduce the risk of you developing a urine infection.

PLEASE CONTACT YOUR GP IF:

(a) Your urine becomes thick and smells offensively, if you suffer fevers, or shivering, feel unwell or your urine contains blood.
(b) Your operation scar becomes hard, or reddened, or inflamed or begins to ooze.
(c) You have abdominal pain which does not get better within 2–3 hours, even after taking pain-killers.

PLEASE CONTACT THE WARD IF:

You begin to pass smaller, more frequent amounts of urine and feel your bladder is still full of urine and never completely empty.

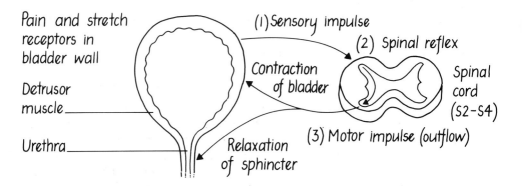

Pain and stretch receptors in bladder wall

Detrusor muscle

Urethra

(1) Sensory impulse

(2) Spinal reflex

Contraction of bladder

Spinal cord (S2–S4)

Relaxation of sphincter

(3) Motor impulse (outflow)

Fig 7.6   Sacral reflex arc

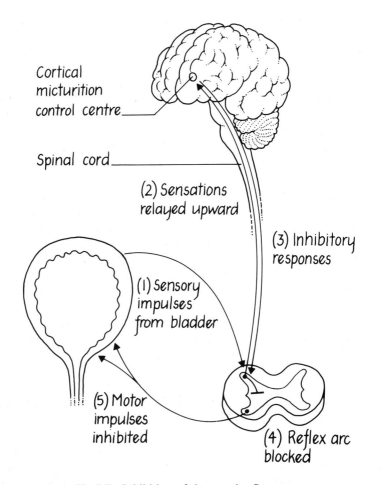

Cortical micturition control centre

Spinal cord

(2) Sensations relayed upward

(3) Inhibitory responses

(1) Sensory impulses from bladder

(5) Motor impulses inhibited

(4) Reflex arc blocked

Fig 7.7   Inhibition of the sacral reflex arc

2. *Acquired CNS lesions*
  (a) trauma with partial or complete damage of spinal cord or bladder innervation
  (b) inflammatory process (poliomyelitis)
  (c) tumours
  (d) degenerative diseases (Parkinson's, diabetes mellitus, encephalomyelitis)

In some cases bladder function is disturbed before symptoms of the neurological disease become manifest (e.g. urinary retention can be the first symptom in multiple sclerosis. The micturition centre is located between the vertebral bodies S1 and S4. The detrusor muscle is innervated by parasympathetic nerves originating from S2–S4 and reaches the bladder wall via the pelvic nerve. Sympathetic fibres from the thoracolumbar plexus at T11–L2 reach the trigonal muscle and the bladder neck via the pelvic nerve. The pudendal nerve (S2–S4) controls the external sphincter. The sensory nerves follow the sympathetic and parasympathetic fibres (S2–S4 and T9–L2).

Since the underlying disease causing the neurogenic bladder is often incurable, medical and/or surgical treatment of the local symptoms originating from the bladder is indicated. See Fig 7.8 for common causes of neuropathic bladder dysfunction.

Lesions which affect the sacral cord or peripheral nerves can result in both the detrusor and urethra becoming underactive. Lesions of the suprasacral cord result in fewer inhibitory impulses, causing detrusor overactivity. The urethra is also overactive and uncoordinated with detrusor contraction (dyssynergia). Lesions which occur above the pons result in the loss of cerebral inhibition. This may produce an overactive detrusor. The detrusor and urethral activity remain uncoordinated.

Besides suffering from bladder disorders, these patients may also suffer from upper tract dilation as a result of high intravesical pressures caused by detrusor hyperreflexia and detrusor sphincter dyssynergia. Vesicoureteric reflex may also occur, especially in children with congenital lesions of the spinal cord.

The management of incontinence in these patients depends on an accurate diagnosis of the cause of the change in the detrusor and urethral function. Some conditions may respond to drug treatment, while some form of surgery (as described previously in this chapter) may be required.

Ultimately, however, the patient may have to undergo a urinary diversion. The field of urinary diversion is expanding and new procedures are constantly being developed. Some patients may have to have a conventional ileal or colonic conduit formed and collect the urine formed using external appliances. Recent developments in this field have resulted in the development of continent urinary diversions. These work on the principle of forming a reservoir for the urine which can then be drained by catheterising a percutaneous non-return valve tunnelled into the reservoir (the Mitrofanoff principle).

The 'reservoir' can be the bladder itself which has had the urethra closed, or a bladder which has been augmented with bowel or indeed completely made of bowel. The catheterisation channel can be the appendix, intussescepted bowel or a piece of

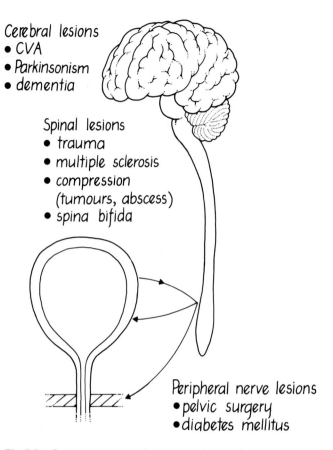

Cerebral lesions
• CVA
• Parkinsonism
• dementia

Spinal lesions
• trauma
• multiple sclerosis
• compression
  (tumours, abscess)
• spina bifida

Peripheral nerve lesions
• pelvic surgery
• diabetes mellitus

Fig 7.8 Common causes of neuropathic bladder dysfunction

ureter or fallopian tube. This is tunnelled into the newly formed reservoir or pouch and brought to the skin's surface to form a nipple. As the pouch fills with urine, pressure is put on the tunnelled end of the channel, thereby closing it off and preventing urine leaking out. When the pouch needs emptying, a catheter is gently inserted into the tunnel until it reaches the pouch and the urine drains out. When empty the catheter is removed, and the patient is once more continent and appliance free. See Figs 7.9–7.12.

This is a major operation and it is vital that the patient is well prepared both physically and psychologically to comply with his treatment and especially the care needed after the operation to maintain the pouch. Just as in the care of a transplanted organ, the patient must be involved and aware of what to expect as normal, and what is not. He or she must be able to recognise and deal with some problems by himself/herself, while being aware of when to call for help. Many patients have been incontinent for years or have worn stoma bags since childhood.

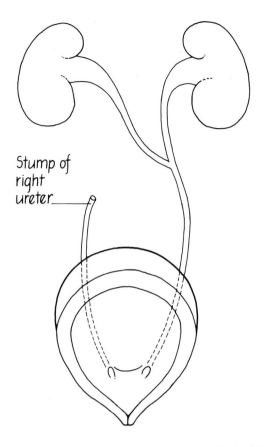

Fig 7.9   Diagram to illustrate the Mitrofanoff principle

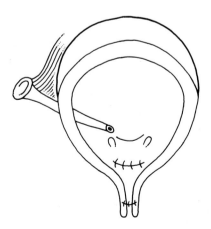

Fig 7.10   System of continence using the Mitrofanoff principle for a patient with sphincter incontinence

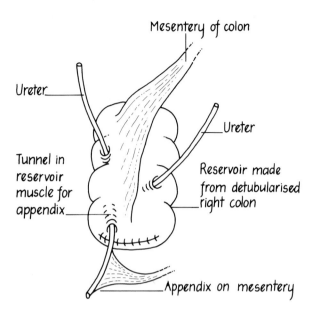

Fig 7.11 Diagram to illustrate a reconstruction using appendix and right colon

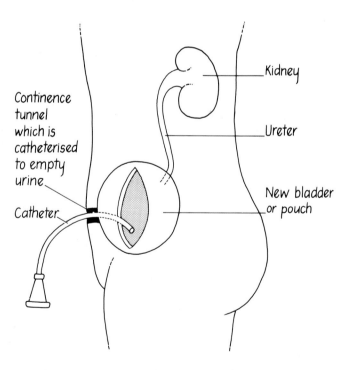

Fig 7.12 Position of neobladder or pouch

The fact that they are going to be free of these sometimes 'blanks out' anything else they are told about the new diversion. They must be prepared for any complication of the surgery, and problems which may occur later, without, of course, making them feel totally negative about the whole procedure. Preparation for this operation therefore starts in the out-patients department. Specific preoperative investigations include glomerular filtration rate studies, and DTPA (Technetium-99m Diethylene-triamine Penta-acetic Acid) scans to ensure the patient's kidneys have adequate function to cope with the change. Urodynamic studies are also carried out to ascertain bladder size, function and pressure, and to test for ureteric reflux.

The patient is admitted to the ward 2–3 days before operation to ensure these tests are complete, and to start bowel preparation. The majority of patients have this bowel preparation even if it is thought that the bladder is going to be used as the reservoir. This is done as a precaution in case, once the operation has commenced, it is felt that some bowel will be needed either to make the bladder larger or to use as part of the channel.

Patients should also be warned about the many drainage tubes they return to the ward with, as many tend to forget what has already been told them in out-patients. Once again they need support and time to ask questions during this period.

Specific postoperative care focuses again on maintaining patency of the drainage tubes, to ensure anastomosis of the new pouch and tunnel, and monitoring urine output. The new bladder usually has a catheter inserted into the new stoma or channel and a 'suprapubic' catheter. If the patient's ureters had to be reimplanted, the patient may also have one or two ureteric stents in situ. He or she will also have one or two wound drains and a nasogastric or gastrostomy tube, as well as a peripheral line and sometimes a central venous pressure line. This is quite an impressive amount of tubing to be confronted with if the preparation has not been adequate.

Careful monitoring of the vital signs and urine output is essential to ensure the kidneys are adequately perfused. There is a danger of patients needing increased amounts of fluid replacement postoperatively, to replace fluid lost during the procedure, and also because of the 2–3 days of bowel preparation before this. An intravenous infusion is sometimes started preoperatively to start the rehydrating process before surgery. The amount of fluid lost is estimated by monitoring weight loss while bowel preparation is in progress.

The 'suprapubic' and pouch catheters are flushed twice a day with 20 ml of sterile saline or water for the first 3 days. The ureteric stents may also be flushed if drainage is not adequate and they are thought to be blocked. As with the cystoplasty operations, after the fourth postoperative day the pouch can be washed out gently twice daily to clear the pouch of debris and mucus produced by the bowel. Once the patient is able, he/she can take over this procedure as he or she will have to maintain the skill of washing out the pouch once discharged.

The ureteric stents are gently 'tweaked' on day 7 after the operation, and generally loosen enough to be totally removed by day 10. After the tenth day the patient may have a pouchogram or cystogram to check if the 'bladder' is intact. If no dye leaks out, the suprapubic catheter may be removed, leaving the pouch urine to drain out via the pouch catheter in the nipple. Patients are usually discharged after this, with instructions to carry on with the bladder washouts at least twice daily, to ensure the pouch urine drains out and that the pouch is not stretched at any time.

The patient is readmitted after 4 weeks (i.e. 6 weeks after the operation). This gives time for the channel to heal and be ready to be catheterised intermittently. The pouch catheter is clamped and the patient is encouraged to drink plenty of fluids. This fills the pouch up with urine and helps the patient to try and establish what sensation is experienced as this happens. Many patients have never experienced the feeling of a full bladder before, and some find it strange, frightening and painful at first. The pouch catheter is released after 3–4 hours, depending on how well the patient can tolerate the discomfort and the amount of fluid drunk. This process is repeated once or twice more to continue expanding the pouch. The volume eventually aimed for is approximately 600 ml. Some patients reach this target easily, while others find that initially they can only tolerate 300 ml or less. It is important to reassure these patients that they will become used to the sensation in time, the pouch will stretch, and they will eventually be able to tell when the pouch needs emptying by the feeling of fullness they experience. However, it is vital that the pouch is not allowed to become too full and in our unit we recommend that the pouch be emptied at least every 3–4 hours. If it becomes too full, there is a danger of trauma and rupture of the pouch, as well as urine leaking out of the tunnel and the tunnel becoming too compressed to let a catheter into the pouch to drain it. If this happens the urine can be released by insertion of a suprapubic catheter percutaneously into the pouch using ultrasound. Alternatively, urine can be aspirated out of the pouch via a needle and syringe, until a catheter is able to be pushed into the channel.

After stretching the pouch, the catheter is removed and the catheterisation procedure explained and demonstrated. The patient is then supervised catheterising the pouch until he is confident about doing this by himself, and his supervisor is happy with his technique. Most patients remain in hospital for 1 or 2 days, and some only require to be admitted as day patients.

Patients are discharged with supplies of catheters and washout equipment, as well as detailed discharge advice to help them through any initial problems. They are encouraged to keep close links with the hospital so that any problems which arise can be dealt with quickly via the phone or by arranging emergency appointments to see the doctor. This is necessary as the procedure is still relatively new and the appropriate care cannot always be obtained via the local hospitals or GP surgeries.

Patients are followed up closely after the operation. Each consultant has a different follow-up regimen, but most include yearly intravenous urograms or kidney, ureter and bladder X-rays, GFR tests, pouch pressure studies and blood tests. Most of the complications patients seem to experience include stone formation in the pouch, urine infections, tightening of the catheterision channel, and leakage of urine via the tunnel. Many of these problems mean further hospitalisation and surgery. However, most patients will put up with this, because having a continent diversion, not having to use appliances and to be dry enhances their self-image. They are in control of their bodies perhaps for the first time in their lives, and the freedom this gives them is immeasurable (*see* Advice Sheet 3).

ADVICE SHEET 3

<u>THIS ADVICE SHEET IS IN ADDITION TO ANY VERBAL ADVICE YOU MAY BE GIVEN BY THE MEDICAL AND NURSING STAFF ON BEING DISCHARGED. PLEASE READ THIS SHEET AND KEEP IT FOR FUTURE REFERENCE.</u>

PATIENT GUIDELINES
FOR AFTERCARE OF CONTINENT URINARY DIVERSIONS

CATHETERISING YOUR POUCH

Please remember that this is a clean procedure, and that it is therefore important to make sure you have everything you need before you begin. Only then should you wash your hands. This avoids unnecessary handling of equipment and potential contamination which could lead to introducing infection into the pouch. Remember that you can catheterise yourself in whatever position is most comfortable or convenient for you (e.g. sitting on the toilet, standing over it, or sitting in your wheelchair or a chair instead).

You may use some lubrication (e.g. KY jelly) on the catheter to make it easier to insert but you may find that this becomes unnecessary in time. The catheter should be inserted gently into the stoma until urine begins to flow out. When the flow has stopped, you should try pushing the catheter in a little further and you may find more urine will flow out. Please do not push it in if you experience any pain. To ensure all the urine has drained out, rotate the catheter gently as you withdraw it. This may dislodge any debris or mucus blocking the tube, and allow urine to flow. Once the pouch is empty withdraw the catheter.

FLUID INTAKE

You must drink at least 3 litres of fluid a day. If your pouch has been made out of bowel or had some bowel added to it, you may find that it can produce a great deal of mucus. This mucus can build up and besides blocking your catheter when you are emptying the pouch, can act as a medium on which bacteria can grow, causing infections. A good fluid intake will keep this mucus diluted, making it easier to flow out of the catheter. Drinks which are high in vitamin C also help keep the urine free of mucus. Cranberry juice, which is available from many large supermarkets or health-food shops, also helps make the mucus less thick, and helps keep the urine infection free. We recommend you drink two glasses of this daily (approximately 200 ml a glass). If you find the taste too sharp, you may dilute it with other fruit juices.

DIET

If you have had your new pouch made of bowel or if you have had some bowel added to your already existing bladder or pouch, you may find it will take some time for your bowels to return to their normal pattern. Try to eat a well-balanced diet with plenty of fruit and vegetables. This will help to prevent constipation. Eventually your bowels will return to normal. If you feel that this has not happened after a few weeks ask your doctor for advice, or ask for advice at your next out-patient's appointment.

WORK, REST AND PLAY

Please allow yourself plenty of time for rest once you are discharged. You should not do anything too strenuous (e.g. gardening) or lift heavy objects (e.g. shopping or children) for the first 4–6 weeks after the operation. It is best to take gentle exercise at first, slowly increasing this as you feel able. You should aim to reach your preoperation level of activity by the time of your first out-patient's appointment.

It is very important that before doing any vigorous activity (e.g. sport or sexual activity), you empty the pouch. This will make you feel more comfortable, and ensure any extra pressure on the pouch will not cause a rupture or trauma.

IMPORTANT

If you find you cannot catheterise your pouch, do not make the stoma sore by repeated attempts. Stop for a few minutes, do not drink any fluids, then try again. If this persists, CONTACT YOUR GP OR THE WARD. YOU MAY HAVE TO GO INTO YOUR LOCAL HOSPITAL TO HAVE A CATHETER INSERTED INTO THE POUCH OR YOU MAY BE DIRECTED BACK TO THE WARD FOR TREATMENT.

FINALLY

Please keep your out-patient's appointments. If the one given to you is inconvenient you should contact your consultant's secretary and a new one will be made for you.

REMEMBER
CONTACT YOUR GP IF:

(a) Your urine becomes thick, smelly, you suffer fevers, or shivering, feel unwell or your urine contains blood.
(b) Your operation scar becomes hard, or reddened, or inflamed or begins to ooze.
(c) You have abdominal or back pain which does not get better within 2–3 hours.

PLEASE CONTACT THE WARD IF:
YOU ARE UNABLE TO PUSH THE CATHETER INTO THE STOMA TO EMPTY THE POUCH

OUTFLOW INCONTINENCE

This occurs when the intravesical pressure in an overdistended bladder exceeds the urethral closure pressure. The bladder becomes overdistended because of increased resistance to the outflow of urine. This may be because of outflow obstruction such as that caused by an enlarged prostate, or urethral strictures. An unobstructed acontractile bladder may also result in the patient suffering from incontinence. Obstruction to the flow of urine from the bladder may occur anywhere along the length of the urethra. This sort of obstruction is more common in men than women.

Causes of Bladder Outflow Obstruction (from Bullock et al, 1989)

Causes of bladder outflow obstruction are:

1. *Congenital*
    Urethral valves
    Urethral polyps
    Urethral stricture

2. *Acquired*
    (a) Structural causes:
        benign prostatic hyperplasia
        carcinoma of the prostate
        bladder neck stenosis
        urethral strictures
        urethral carcinoma
        urethral calculi
    (b) External compression:
        faecal impaction
        pelvic tumour

3. *Functional causes*
    Bladder neck dyssynergia
    Detrusor–sphincter dyssynergia

   The detrusor muscle responds to the increase in pressure needed to empty the bladder by hypertrophy. The bladder wall becomes thick and coarse, and may show increased irritability while filling with urine. This results in detrusor instability and the involuntary or 'unstable' contractions which cause frequency and urgency of micturition, which may lead to incontinence if the obstruction is not removed. The detrusor will eventually fail, becoming inefficient and giving up its contractions before the bladder is empty. The active, hypertrophied detrusor turns into an inert atonic bag, with a huge residual urine. The patient is in chronic retention of urine, and only a small quantity of urine is voided at a time. This chronic obstruction can lead to hydroureter and hydronephrosis. The ureters may also be partially obstructed

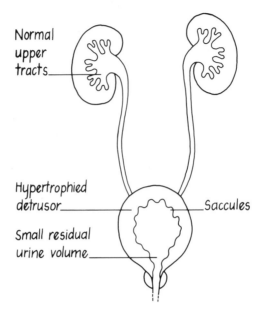

Fig 7.13 Early pathological changes in urethral stricture

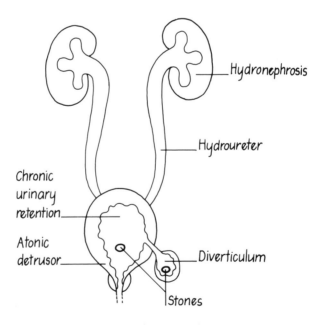

Fig 7.14 Late pathological changes in urethral stricture

as they pass through the thickened bladder wall, and some patients may suffer from vesicoureteric reflux. If untreated the condition may lead to increasing upper tract dilation (obstructive uropathy) and a gradual deterioration of renal function.

After the age of 40 most men suffer from enlargement of the prostate, but only one in ten will have obstruction as a result of it (Blandy, 1992). The degree of obstruction is not always necessarily related to the size of the prostate, and the type and degree of nodular hyperplasia seems to vary from one race to another. Men of Celtic ancestry are thought to have larger glands than Anglo-Saxons, who in turn have larger ones than Mediterranean men (Blandy, 1992). No race is entirely immune, however.

Outflow obstruction may also be a result of a urethral stricture. The patient presents with a poor urinary stream, and may develop the same symptoms caused by detrusor hypertrophy (i.e. poor stream, hesitancy, frequency, nocturia, dribbling incontinence). Urine is trapped in the urethra upstream of the stricture and dribbles away after the patient thinks he has finished voiding. Strictures can occur at any time.

Aetiology of Urethral Strictures

Urethral strictures may be congential or acquired:

1. *Congenital*
   Meatal stenosis
   Bulbar stricture

2. *Acquired*
   (a) Traumatic
       perineal trauma
       ruptured urethra from pelvic injury
       urethral instrumentation
   (b) Infective
       gonococcal
       non-specific urethritis
       tuberculosis
   (c) Inflammatory
       balanitis
       chemical urethritis (e.g. from certain catheter materials)
   (d) Neoplastic
       squamous carcinoma
       transitional cell carcinoma
       adenocarcinoma

The late complications of urethral stricture are shown in Figure 7.15.

Whether the outflow obstruction is caused by the prostate or stricture in the urethra, bladder and renal function can only be conserved by removing the cause.

The prostate can be resected and strictures dilated or divided (using optical urethrostomy). In extreme cases a urethroplasty may be indicated. These procedures are covered elsewhere in this book.

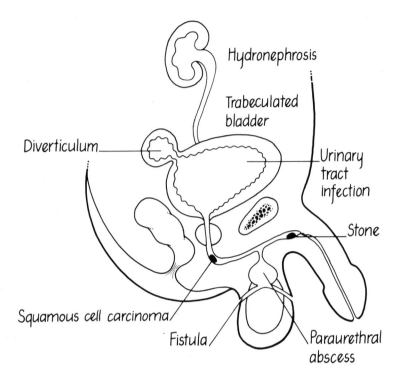

Fig 7.15   Possible complications of prolonged urethral stricture

INCONTINENCE SECONDARY TO FISTULAE OR CONGENITAL ABNORMALITIES

Fistulae may be congenital or acquired. A fistula is an abnormal communication between two epithelial surfaces, or to the exterior. Any part of the urinary tract may be affected. Acquired fistulae may result from:

- Trauma
- Infection
- Tumours
- Surgery
- Radiotherapy

A vaginal fistula is usually the result of pelvic surgery (e.g. hysterectomy). This is the most common cause in the Western world. In developing countries these often form as a complication of obstructed labour. The prolonged pressure of the baby's head against the symphysis involving much of the back of the bladder, lower ends of the ureters and sometimes the external sphincter, causes tissue necrosis and the resulting sloughing leaves a fistula. The repair is done surgically. If the fistula is small, a vaginal repair may be adequate, but if large, then the repair may have to be via a midline incision in the bladder. The bladder is opened down to the fistula and posteriorly, the fistula is excised, and the vagina and bladder closed. A plug of greater omentum is made, and it is mobilised and brought down between bladder and vagina, sealing the vaginal vault.

If the fistula is large it may be seen on speculum examination. A tampon or gauze pack may be placed into the vagina and methylene blue dye instilled into the bladder. If the tampon turns blue this indicates that the fistula is from the bladder. If a ureterovaginal fistula is suspected then an intravenous urogram (IVU) can show the side and level of ureteric injury. Ureters can be damaged during hysterectomy, by being cut, crushed or accidentally caught up in a ligature. Urine escapes through the vault of the vagina, but may not appear for 4–5 days after the procedure. By testing this fluid for its urea content, the fact that it is urine can be confirmed. The ureter may be reimplanted into the bladder, or a flap of tubed bladder used to make up any lost ureteric length (Boari flap); the ureter may also be joined to the unaffected ureter (transureteroureterostomy).

Repair of vaginal fistulae may be done early after the initial procedure, though some units prefer a delay of up to 3 months so that the tissues are not oedematous. Extremely large fistulae may not be successfully closed at times, and a urinary diversion (continent or otherwise) may be the only option. Such a delay in offering treatment only prolongs the misery suffered by these individuals. The patient is constantly wet and has to wear large pads to cope with this sudden incontinence. The patient's quality of life is poor and she may become isolated and depressed. Such patients should be approached with understanding and sympathy and reassured as to the success of the operation proposed to repair the damage. The possibility of failure and the alternative of having a stoma formed should also be discussed, however, to prepare them should the procedure not succeed.

Another type of fistula which is occasionally seen as a complication of prostatectomy is a rectoprostatic fistula. This may be seen especially after an open operation for invasive carcinoma of the prostate, and after severe pelvic fracture injuries with rupture of the membranous urethra and laceration of the rectal wall. Many of these fistulae heal after a period of suprapubic catheterisation of the bladder, and diversion of the faecal stream by temporary colostomy. Complex injuries may also involve urethral reconstruction.

CONGENITAL BLADDER ANOMALIES

Bladder exstrophy is twice as common in males than females and occurs in one in 10 000–40 000 live births. This is only part of a range of defects in which there is failure of fusion of the lower abdomen, genitalia and pelvic bones. The result of this can be defects which range from isolated epispadias to complex anomalies involving the bladder and intestine.

There are other congenital defects which may result in incontinence for the patient. However, many are dealt with immediately after birth with the aim of making the patient continent initially, with reconstructive surgery used as the child grows, to enhance body image and improve quality of life.

References

Blandy JP (1992) *Lecture Notes on Urology*, 4th edn. Oxford: Blackwell Scientific Publications.

Bullock, N, Sibley G and Whitaker R (1989) *Essential Urology*. Edinburgh: Churchill Livingstone.

Norton C (1986) *Nursing for Incontinence*. Beaconsfield: Beaconsfield Publishers Ltd.

Rosenbaum TP, Shaw PJR, Rose GA and Lloyd W (1989) Cranberry juice and mucus production in enterouroplasty. (Unpublished work.) Presented to the British Association of Urological Surgeons, June 1989.

Rosenbaum TP, Shaw PJR and Worth PH (1990) Trans-trigonal phenol failed the test of time. *British Journal of Urology* **66**(2): 164–169.

Sökeland J (1989) *Urology: A Pocket Reference Theime Flexibook*, 2nd edn. Stuttgart: George Theime Verlag.

8

Prostatic Problems

For anatomy and physiology of the prostate gland please refer to Chapter 1.

PROSTATITIS

Definition

Prostatitis is inflammation of the prostate gland and can be acute or chronic. It can result in the formation of abscesses or urethral strictures.

Causes

Prostatitis may occur if the patient has a history of:

- Sexually transmitted disease
- Tuberculosis
- Urinary tract infection
- Instrumentation (e.g. following cystoscopy)

The affecting organism can reach the prostate gland via the blood stream, rectum or pelvic lymphatics.

Signs and Symptoms

The patient usually presents with a history of perineal pain which radiates to the thighs and penis. The patient generally feels unwell, feverish with dysuria and frequency which may result in retention of urine. Haemospermia (blood in sperm) may occur with pain on ejaculation, which affects sexual function.

Investigations

A rectal examination will show a very tender prostate gland which may be enlarged and hot to the touch. The prostate should not be massaged too long because this can cause septicaemia.

A midstream specimen of urine may identify the causative organism.

Treatment and Nursing Care

Treatment is based on finding the causative organism and treating the symptoms.

Problems

Pain in Perineal Area

The patient should be given regular analgesics and their effect should be monitored. The patient may appreciate a soft cushion to sit on and a warm bath to relieve the pain. The patient is encouraged to rest.

Infection causing General Malaise and High Temperature

If the causative organism can be found the appropriate antibiotic should be given as prescribed. This may be for several weeks. Temperature should be recorded 4-hourly and antipyretics given as required. Fluid intake is encouraged. If an abscess is present this might be drained.

Difficulty passing Urine

To relieve this problem a urethral catheter might be inserted, until the inflammation subsides.

Embarrassment with Condition and Inability to Perform Sexually

The patient will need privacy and time to talk and express his concerns. He will require a full explanation of his condition and treatment.

If the prostatitis continues to recur or becomes chronic a transurethral resection of the prostate can be performed or in extreme cases a total prostatectomy (described later in this chapter).

BENIGN PROSTATIC HYPERTROPHY

Definition

Benign prostatic hypertrophy is the benign enlargement of the prostate gland. This occurs in all men over 40 years of age and one in ten of these men suffer with urinary outflow obstruction due to the enlargement.

Causes

The cause is unknown, but it is thought to be due to testicular sex hormone changes as the male ages. Some call it the 'male menopause'. An adenoma (benign tumour), which may develop and cause enlargement of the prostate gland, may be implicated.

Signs and Symptoms

The patient may present with various signs and symptoms, the severity depending on how long the prostate gland has been enlarged.

Common signs and symptoms of prostatic outflow obstruction are:

1. *Frequency of micturition* – more than 10–12 times daily
2. *Nocturia* – the patient wakes up in the night because he wants to void
3. *Hesitancy* – the patient has a delay before he is able to void
4. *Poor urinary stream* – the patient may need to strain in order to void
5. *Urinary tract infection* – due to incomplete bladder emptying
6. *Dysuria* – pain on micturition due to infection
7. *Dribbling incontinence* – due to incomplete bladder emptying
8. *Chronic retention of urine with overflow*
9. *Acute retention of urine*

The patient may present with renal failure or impairment, due to long-term prostatic outflow obstruction. This is caused by the enlarged prostate gland inhibiting the bladder from emptying properly. The bladder compensates by enlarging and thickening. The bladder muscle becomes stretched and ineffective and this results in an atonic bladder. The bladder is therefore unable to contract properly and becomes distended (bladder diverticulae may develop). This in time causes pressure on the ureters and possible ureteric reflux occurs which causes back pressure on the kidneys. This may result in renal failure.

Investigations

1. *A history* of voiding problems is taken in detail
2. *Abdominal examination* may show a distended bladder
3. *A rectal examination* will enable the doctor to feel the prostate gland and detect if it is enlarged
4. *A midstream urine specimen* will detect any infection, which can be treated
5. *Blood samples* are taken to assess renal function, e.g. urea and electrolytes, full blood count
6. *A flow rate* is performed in order to determine the urinary stream
7. *Urodynamics* may be performed to assess the bladder function
8. *An intravenous urogram* is performed to show any damage to the urinary tract from long-term obstruction (ultrasound may also be used for this)

Treatment

Acute Retention of Urine

If the patient presents with acute retention of urine it will probably be due to chronic retention of urine which has not been treated. The patient will be in acute pain and have a very strong desire to void. He should be seen as quickly as possible and have a catheter inserted. A urethral catheter is tried first. If the prostatic obstruction prevents this procedure, a suprapubic catheter is inserted. The patient will require a

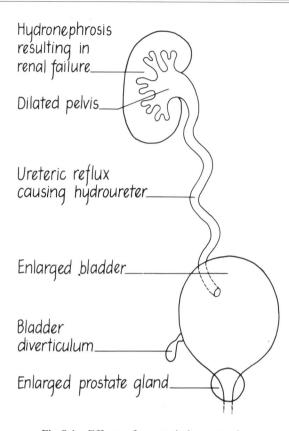

Hydronephrosis resulting in renal failure

Dilated pelvis

Ureteric reflux causing hydroureter

Enlarged bladder

Bladder diverticulum

Enlarged prostate gland

Fig 8.1 Effects of prostatic hypertrophy

lot of support and explanation. Relief from the symptoms is almost immediate once a catheter has been inserted.

There is much confusion as to whether the catheter should be clamped after a certain amount has drained from the bladder. This is done in order to prevent a large diuresis (which could make the patient go into shock) due to the pressure being suddenly released from the kidney. In our experience, clamping is of little use and just a small amount of drainage from the kidney will result in a large diuresis if it is going to occur.

One of the important nursing actions here is to ensure the patient has an input which is equal to the output. This is usually achieved by oral intake but intravenous fluids may be necessary. An accurate fluid balance chart is essential.

Haematuria with clots is quite common after this procedure and bladder washouts may need to be performed or bladder irrigation commenced. If blood loss is a problem the patient's pulse and blood pressure should be carefully monitored and symptoms of shock observed for and reported promptly. The bleeding should subside over 2–3 days. Once everything has settled down further treatment can be decided.

The majority of patients present with voiding problems rather than retention of urine and are admitted routinely for treatment.

TRANSURETHRAL RESECTION OF THE PROSTATE GLAND (TURP)

This involves the passage of a resectoscope via the urethra and a loop for cutting and diathermy is inserted. This instrument cuts slivers of the gland away and diathermy is used to control the bleeding. The surgeon has to be very careful not to damage the external sphincter at the base of the prostate gland because this could result in incontinence.

The bladder neck is resected and consequently retrograde ejaculation occurs. This is when the male ejaculates and the semen goes into the bladder rather than out through the urethra. When the bladder neck is intact and the male ejaculates the bladder neck closes and therefore enables the semen to travel down the urethra. If the bladder neck is damaged then this does not occur and semen goes into the bladder and is passed out during voiding. It is very important to explain this to the male because fertility will be a problem but this should not be used as a form of contraception.

It is also important that the surgeon does not damage the verumontanum. This is a small projection on the posterior wall of the prostate gland and contains the ejaculatory ducts (*see* Fig 8.2).

The whole of the prostate gland is not removed due to the possibility of damaging the prostatic capsule, causing extravasation of urine and also the possibility of damaging the external sphincter, causing incontinence.

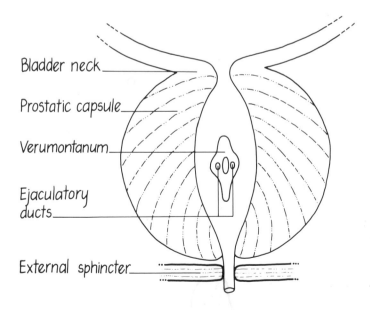

Fig 8.2   Prostate gland

Specific Preoperative Nursing Care

Explanation of Patient Care during Admission

Full explanation of pre- and postoperative care should be given to the patient. Many males are not aware that they have a prostate gland until it causes problems and then they do not understand why it is causing problems. Time should be spent explaining where the prostate gland is and why it is causing a problem. Draw a diagram of the urinary tract and show where the prostate gland is. It is sometimes easier to compare the prostate to a 'doughnut', the hole in the middle representing the urethra. As the prostate gland enlarges it compresses on the urethra and causes obstruction to the outflow of urine.

Other Preoperative Care

● A chest X-ray is performed if the patient has respiratory or cardiac problems.
● Blood specimens are taken for urea and electrolytes and full blood count
● Cross match 2 units of blood
● ECG
● Flow rate
● Antiembolic stockings
● Midstream specimen of urine

Specific Postoperative Care

The patient returns to the ward with an intravenous infusion, urethral catheter and bladder irrigation.

Bleeding from the Prostate Gland following Surgery

The prostate gland is highly vascular and even though diathermy is used during the surgical procedure bleeding and haemorrhage can still be a problem which needs to be carefully monitored.

Blood pressure and pulse are recorded every 15–60 min until stable. A sudden drop in blood pressure and rise in pulse with the patient becoming cold and clammy indicates the patient is hypovolaemic, due to haemorrhage, and the doctor should be contacted immediately. The intravenous infusion may be speeded up or a blood transfusion or plasma expander (e.g. Gelofusine) may be prescribed. The urethral catheter has a bladder irrigation attached and normal saline is used to irrigate the bladder. If the output remains heavily blood-stained then the doctor should be informed. Traction may be applied to the catheter, resulting in the balloon on the catheter being pulled down into the bleeding prostatic area, hopefully stopping the bleeding. The traction should only be applied for 20–30 minutes at a time and then released, even if bleeding continues. If the traction is left longer, necrosis of the area around the catheter balloon will occur. Traction can be applied by tying a piece of gauze around the catheter at the end of the penis and pulling the catheter down or by tying a weight to the end of the catheter and hanging it over the end of the bed. This can be achieved by tying a bandage to the catheter and attaching a 500 ml bag of i.v. fluid to the other end of the bandage (the bag should hang free and not on the floor). If the traction is not effective then the patient may need to go back to theatre for further diathermy.

When bleeding is heavy the irrigation should run fast and this will help to prevent clots forming and blocking the catheter. If the catheter does block the patient usually complains that he wants to void and he will have a distended bladder. If this does occur the bladder irrigation should be turned off to prevent further bladder distension and discomfort. Milking the catheter bag tubing gently may clear any clots. However, a bladder washout may be necessary, but breaking the closed system should be a last resort and performed aseptically to prevent any infection. If a bladder washout is not effective the catheter balloon can be deflated and the catheter gently twisted round. It is important that the catheter is not moved in or out of the urethra because this can cause urethral trauma and introduce infection; also the balloon should be reinflated after this procedure. If following these procedures the catheter is still not draining, it should be changed by the doctor.

Some surgeons also prescribe a drug to help stop the bleeding. An example is tranexamic acid which prevents fibrinolysis (the physiological mechanism that dissolves clots); therefore clotting should occur.

As the urine becomes less blood-stained the bladder irrigation is slowed down and usually after 24 hours the urine is pink in colour and irrigation is discontinued. When the urine is clear or almost clear the urethral catheter is removed. This usually occurs 2–4 days postoperatively.

A full blood count is obtained 24–48 hours postoperatively to detect anaemia.

Maintenance of Hydration and Monitoring Output

The patient comes back to the ward with an intravenous infusion to ensure that he does not become dehydrated and has a good urine output. This is maintained for about 24 hours or until the patient is able to drink without nausea or vomiting. If it is not medically dangerous the patient is encouraged to drink 3 litres of fluid daily to achieve a high urine output and consequently reduce the amount of haematuria. The amount of irrigation has to be carefully monitored and it should be ensured that the total output exceeds the irrigation input. If the irrigation is being absorbed into the blood stream, due to extravasation, TUR syndrome may occur. This is not a common complication but is an emergency situation if it does occur. Symptoms usually start to become apparent soon after surgery. The irrigation fluid is absorbed into the blood stream and causes dilution of the blood and circulatory overload. The patient becomes confused and disorientated. He may fit, due to a low plasma sodium, become comatose and have a cardiac arrest. The doctor should be informed immediately of any significant change in the patient's condition and blood taken to check sodium and potassium levels which, in TUR syndrome, will be low. An ECG should be recorded, irrigation stopped and i.v. fluids reduced. The patient may be transferred to the intensive care unit. Water should never be used as an irrigation fluid because, due to osmosis, it will be readily absorbed from the bladder and prostate area and cause TUR syndrome. Normal saline as an irrigation fluid reduces this risk, because it is isotonic and therefore not easily absorbed. Absorption principally occurs in theatre, where irrigation solution, (devoid of sodium or potassium) is forced under pressure into the prostatic veins.

3. Infection due to Surgery and Indwelling Catheter

Temperature is recorded 4-hourly and any elevation is reported to the doctor. If the patient is known to have a urinary tract infection, antibiotics are given with the premedication or in theatre and continued postoperatively. However, if symptoms occur postoperatively, a catheter specimen of urine is sent for culture and sensitivity and a broad-spectrum antibiotic is prescribed.

To prevent infection the catheter insertion site is kept clean and dry using soap and water. It is better if the patient is able to clean this area himself.

A closed system should be maintained with the catheter and irrigation and if it should be broken an aseptic technique should be used, wearing sterile gloves.

4. Pain due to Catheter

Pain, due to endoscopic, prostatic surgery, is unusual. However, patients may complain either of bladder spasm, or penile pain, both of which are caused by the large, urethral, irrigation catheter inserted postoperatively, and are not a result of the surgery.

Bladder spasm (manifesting as acute, spasmodic, lower abdominal pain, which is often positional in nature) is caused by trigonal irritation, from the large 30–50 ml balloon, which secures the 3 way irrigation catheter in position. Securing the catheter to the leg to prevent 'pulling' will aid comfort and also reduce downward movement of the catheter. This may then reduce irritation of the trigone and thus spasm. However, if the spasms are very troublesome, then antispasmodics (e.g. an anti-cholinergic agent such as Pro-Banthine) may need to be prescribed. Usually, this problem is only reduced when the catheter is removed.

Penile pain (usually at the tip of the patient's penis) is also catheter related and reflects the large diameter of the irrigation catheter. This problem is most effectively treated with lignocaine gel, applied locally to the urethral surface.

5. Constipation due to Restricted Mobility and Fear of Opening Bowels

The patient is usually up and mobile the day following his operation. However, constipation can still be a problem because the patient is afraid to strain with a catheter in situ. Therefore a high fibre diet is encouraged and if the patient expresses difficulty an oral aperient or suppositories are prescribed.

6. Following Removal of Catheter

Following catheter removal the patient is at risk from:

- Retention of urine
- Frequency of micturition
- Incontinence

Occasionally when the catheter is removed the patient is unable to void and will develop retention of urine. If the patient is unable to void he is asked to have a warm bath to try and help him relax. The patient is usually left until he has a strong desire to void and has drank at least a litre of fluid before another catheter is inserted. Once the catheter has been reinserted it is left in situ for between 2 days and 6 weeks and voiding without catheter is tried again. If the patient continues to go into retention of urine further surgery may be necessary.

Most patients suffer with frequency and urgency once the catheter has been removed. This should be explained to the patient. Initially the volumes may be 50–75 ml each void but this does improve over a few days and the patient is encouraged to try and 'hold on' between voiding.

Dribbling incontinence can be a problem. If this does occur the patient is advised to perform pelvic floor exercises. The situation usually improves over a period of days and this is explained to the patient. While the problem is resolving the patient is given incontinence pads which are changed as required. A supply may need to be given on discharge home.

A fluid chart is maintained and each voided volume is recorded. The patient, if able, is taught how to complete his output chart himself. Fluid intake of 2–3 litres is encouraged but the patient is told to cut down on his intake in the evening to prevent nocturia.

A flow rate is recorded before discharge.

Advice on Discharge

An out-patients appointment is made for 6 weeks postoperatively, when a further flow rate will be performed.

The patient is advised to rest during this time and not to perform any heavy lifting. If the patient works this can be resumed after about 4 weeks.

After about 2 weeks an episode of bleeding in the urine is possible due to the 'scabs falling off' in the healing prostate. This is explained to the patient who is advised to increase his oral intake during this period, and if it does not subside to contact his GP.

The patient is told to see his GP if he gets any burning on micturition, or fever. This indicates infection.

The patient is advised to refrain from sexual intercourse for 2 weeks and sexual sensation should not be affected.

Complications of TURP

1. One per cent of patients who have had a prostatectomy suffer with *long-term incontinence* and may require further surgery.

2. *Urethral strictures* may occur due to damage to the urethra from instrumentation during surgery.

3. Impotence, following TURP, has a reported incidence of between 4 and 30 per cent (Tanagho and McAninch, 1992). This wide variation of figures may reflect a reluctance on the part of patients to admit that the problem exists.

4. Postoperative haemorrhage is seen in some 4 per cent of patients. Secondary haemorrhage can occur, which may require the patient to be readmitted to hospital.

5. The overall mortality of TURP is less than 1 per cent, and usually the result of cardiovascular and/or respiratory complications.

The long-term follow-up of patients after TURP reveals the resolution of voiding symptoms in some 80–90 per cent at one year, though this decreases to 60–75 per cent by 5 years. Some 5 per cent of patients will require a repeat TURP within 5 years of their original operation (Tanagho and McAninch, 1992).

Interestingly, a recent study by Roos et al (1989), which compared the mortality rates following both TURP and open prostatectomy, found a higher incidence of death from myocardial infarction at both 3 months, and then later on, in patients who had undergone TURP.

This information is currently being investigated, as it would appear to undermine the usual assumptions regarding the safety of TURP, when compared with an open procedure.

OTHER FORMS OF PROSTATECTOMY

If the prostate gland is over 60g a TURP is not performed because the operation would take much longer than other methods of prostatectomy. One of the following operations may be performed:

Retropubic Prostatectomy

A transverse skin incision is made, the prostatic capsule cut and the gland removed using the finger. The prostatic capsule is sutured and the wound closed.

Transvesical Prostatectomy

A transverse skin incision is made and the bladder is opened. The prostate gland is removed using the finger through the bladder. The bladder is sutured and the wound closed.

Perineal Prostatectomy

This procedure is very rare. An incision is made through the perineum to expose the prostate gland. The capsule is opened and gland removed.

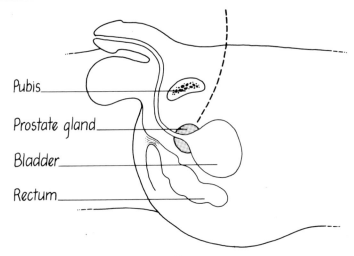

Fig 8.3 Retropubic prostatectomy

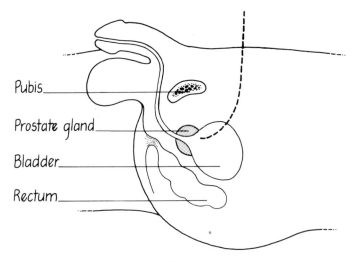

Fig 8.4 Transvesical prostatectomy

Nursing Care

The nursing care required for these methods of prostatectomy is the same as for a TURP plus the following.

Pain due to Abdominal Wound reducing Mobility

Regular controlled analgesia should be given as required and the patient mobilized with help for the first 2–3 days postoperatively.

Care of Abdominal Wound and Wound Drains

The wound is redressed as required and observed for signs of redness, oozing and soreness. Sutures are removed as directed by the doctor after 7–10 days. A wound drain is left in situ and drainage monitored. The drain is removed as directed by the doctor.

With all the types of prostatectomy mentioned there is a chance of regrowth of the prostate gland and further prostatectomy may be required in the future.

ALTERNATIVES TO A PROSTATECTOMY

Patients may present with an enlarged prostate gland causing outflow obstruction but are not fit for an anaesthetic or they do not want to have a prostatectomy and risk retrograde ejaculation or impotence. Therefore alternative treatment is necessary to combat the obstruction.

Balloon Dilatation of the Prostate Gland (McLoughlin and Williams 1990)

A balloon is inserted transurethrally and positioned in the prostatic urethra. The balloon is expanded (usually to 35 mm) for periods of 10–15 minutes.

This procedure can be performed using intravenous sedation and analgesia. Slight bleeding can occur and a urethral catheter may be left in situ for 24 hours. At present results are variable. A study by Gill et al (1989) showed that less than 50 per cent of patients had symptomatic improvement. Perez-Marrero et al (1990) showed 73 per cent had improvement. From the author's own experience the former figure seems more realistic.

At present the improvement in symptoms is short term; therefore it is usually used for younger patients who are concerned about post-prostatectomy retrograde ejaculation or loss of potency who in later life will go ahead with a prostatectomy.

Prostatic Stents (Chappell et al, 1990; McLoughlin and Williams, 1990)

There are two types of stent – macroporous tubular mesh and prostatic spirals.

Macroporous Tubular Mesh

This stent is made of stainless steel woven into a tubular mesh. It is inserted transurethrally into the prostatic urethra using a local anaesthetic. Over a period of 6–8 months epithelium forms around the stent and holds it in place. It can be removed within the first 4–6 weeks if necessary; however, after this time the stent is permanent.

This stent is usually used for patients who are unfit for an anaesthetic and have a limited life expectancy.

Prostatic Spirals

The spiral consists of a tightly coiled metallic spring which lodges in the prostatic urethra. It has a tail which sits outside the external sphincter and can be grasped if it has to be removed. Epithelium does not form around the spiral and it is narrower than the macroporous mesh. It is positioned using a cystoscopy and transrectal ultrasound, using a local anaesthetic.

This spiral, because it can be removed, may be suited for temporary relief of obstruction whilst waiting for a prostatectomy.

With both types of stent the patient is usually able to void following its insertion. If difficulty in micturition occurs a urethral catheter is not inserted due to the risk of displacing the stent. Therefore a suprapubic catheter is inserted. Antibiotic cover is given to minimise the risk of infection. Problems of frequency and urgency following the stent insertion have been reported and these are treated with anticholinergic drugs. The stent can also become displaced and protrude or move into the bladder, necessitating its replacement or removal. See Fig 8.5.

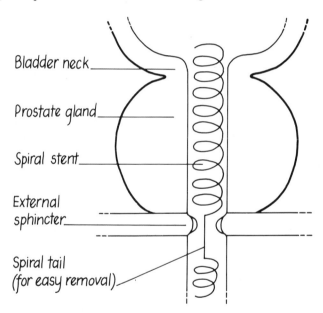

Fig 8.5 Prostatic spiral

Microwave Hyperthermia (Strohmaier et al, 1990; Astrahan et al, 1991)

This involves the prostate gland being heated to a temperature of 42–43°C. The treatment consists of heating the prostate gland for a period of 1 hour, one or two times weekly for 8–10 sessions. The treatment is given as an out-patient and only requires local anaesthetic for insertion of the urethral equipment.

The actual procedure involves a machine which consists of a microwave generator, a heat applicator – which can be either a transurethral applicator or a transrectal applicator (this applicator also has a cooling system to protect the rectal wall from heat damage) – and two temperature monitors – one for the urethra and the other for the rectum.

This method of treatment is still being studied and results at present are variable. The treatment appears to be palliative rather than curative and prostatectomy still has to be performed following treatment.

Laser Treatment

Laser treatment involves the insertion of a laser fibre via the urethra and a laser beam is used at close range in the prostate gland to burn it away.

Medical Treatment (Christmas and Kirby, 1991)

Alpha-1 Adrenoceptor Blockers

The smooth muscle of the prostate gland contains alpha-adrenoceptors and it has been discovered that by blocking these receptors the tone in the prostatic urethra decreases and hence the urinary flow rate improves. Examples of drugs that block alpha-adrenoceptors are prazosin, indoramin and phenoxybenzamine. Side-effects of these drugs include dizziness, palpitations and retrograde ejaculation.

Research is in progress to find an alpha-adrenoceptor that is specific to the prostate gland.

Hormonal

Oestrogen therapy (e.g. stilboestrol) and anti-androgen agents (e.g. cyproterone acetate) are able to reduce the size of the prostate gland but they do have side-effects which are not acceptable. Oestrogens cause sexual dysfunction and gynaecomastia, anti-androgens can cause loss of libido, impotence and hot flushes.

Research is being undertaken to produce an enzyme inhibitor to reduce the amount of dihydrotestosterone, which is essential for normal growth of the prostate gland and is metabolized from testosterone. By stopping the metabolism of testosterone the growth of the prostate will be reduced, thereby reducing outflow obstruction. The normal enzyme is known as finasteride.

This treatment, along with other alternatives to a prostatectomy stated here, are still being researched and are not available as treatment in all urology departments at the time of writing this chapter.

An excellent summary is provided by Christmas and Kirby (1992) and Tanagho and McAninch (1992).

CARCINOMA OF THE PROSTATE GLAND

Carcinoma of the prostate gland is the third most common cancer in males, representing 16 per cent of all malignancies in the adult male. The tumour often arises in the posterior prostatic lobe and is hormone related, depending upon androgens to retain its integrity. The tumour also causes an increase in the secretion of acid phosphatase and prostatic-specific antigen – both of these are reflected in blood serum levels and may indicate a prostatic tumour.

There are no known direct aetiological factors, but it becomes more common with increasing age, and by the time most men reach 90 years of age foci of carcinoma can be found in nearly all prostate glands.

Because of its frequency and the fact that early diagnosis can be made in most cases by a rectal examination, all men should be advised to have an annual check-up after the age of 40. Nurses are advised to include this advice whenever it is relevant in their health teaching.

Pathology

The majority of prostate cancers are adenocarcinomas. Sarcomas occur rarely in the prostate. The prostatic ducts are lined with transitional epithelium and can, therefore, be involved in urothelial cancer. The commonest prostatic cancer is a columnar adenocarcinoma with distortion of normal architecture. Several schemes for assessing differentiation exist and correlate reasonably well with prognosis.

Staging

Although the criteria for staging is well recognised, in practice staging is difficult and therefore sometimes inaccurate.

Carcinoma of the prostate is classified into four stages. These stages are based on the results of rectal examination, serum acid phosphatase and prostatic-specific antigen levels, X-rays of the skeleton and metastases.

Stage I (T0–T1)

Carcinoma in situ is often called latent or focal. Usually there are no symptoms.

Stage II (T2)

The nodule may be palpated on rectal examination.

Stage III (T3)

The growth has spread to the seminal vesicles, the base of the bladder and outside the prostatic capsule, but no distant metastases are present.

Stage IV (T4)

Previously the thick prostatic capsule has kept the lesion localized and prevented spread into the abdominal cavity, but now the blood and lymphatics have carried the disease to distant sites. The bones of the pelvis are most frequently affected. The spread to the bones and liver may result in severe anaemia accompanied by other symptoms of a terminal disease.

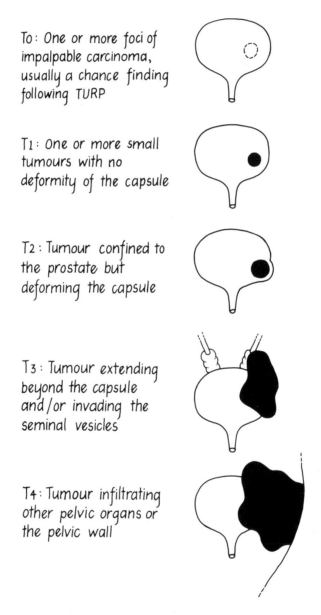

To: One or more foci of impalpable carcinoma, usually a chance finding following TURP

T1: One or more small tumours with no deformity of the capsule

T2: Tumour confined to the prostate but deforming the capsule

T3: Tumour extending beyond the capsule and/or invading the seminal vesicles

T4: Tumour infiltrating other pelvic organs or the pelvic wall

Fig 8.6   Staging of prostatic carcinoma

Presentation

Local Disease

Ninety per cent of carcinomas arise in the peripheral zone of the prostate, and therefore small tumours may not interfere with voiding. As they enlarge, they obstruct the outflow from the bladder, causing poor stream, frequency and nocturia. Some cancers may grow quite large without causing urinary obstruction, and therefore remain undetected until the prognosis is poor. If the tumour extends upwards it may irritate the trigone and cause bladder irritation. A few extend posteriorly and cause tenesmus (painful straining to empty bowel without effect), or even rectal obstruction. Many men present with bladder outflow obstruction caused by benign prostatic hypertrophy and are incidentally found to have carcinoma as well.

Remote Disease

Cancer of the prostate metastasises early to pelvic lymph nodes and bone. About 15 per cent of T1 tumours, 30 per cent of T2 tumours and 60 per cent of T3 tumours have lymph node metastases at presentation (Bullock et al, 1989). Half of those with nodal metastases have bone metastases. Patients may present with bone pain, pathological fractures or even anaemia.

Prognosis

It is very difficult to give a prognosis for an individual patient, as the natural history is so uncertain. Patients with one or two foci of carcinoma, in an otherwise benign gland, and those with small cancers without metastases, have the same life expectancy. The prognosis becomes progressively poorer with increasing stage and grade. For example, the overall survival of T2 cases is about 50 per cent at 5 years. The age of the patient at presentation is irrelevant.

Treatment of carcinoma of the prostate and implications for nursing care are considered in the following section.

Investigations

Before describing the specific investigations into carcinoma of the prostate in detail, it should be stressed that not only can some of the tests prove to be physically uncomfortable and also to generate a high level of anxiety, but some of the investigations, due to their invasive nature, can also be extremely embarrassing for the patient. Therefore, apart from preparing the patient, both physically and psychologically, for these tests, the nurse should also ensure that his privacy and dignity is maintained to a high standard at all times.

Rectal Examination

While a rectal examination of the prostate gland can not prove conclusively the presence of a carcinoma, it is certainly an extremely good indicator. This is because a small tumour will feel hard, like a dried pea on the prostate surface, while larger infiltration into the prostatic capsule will make the gland feel generally 'hard' and 'knobbly'. This compares with a healthy prostate gland which should feel smooth and slightly soft, when palpated rectally.

A rectal examination is one of the first investigations performed, so therefore if a patient suffering from outflow obstruction seeks help promptly from his general practitioner, the latter will undoubtedly perform a rectal examination, and if suspicious, will then order further tests to be done.

Blood Tests

As previously mentioned in this chapter, the prostate gland, under hormonal control, secretes a level of specific antigens (PSA); in a healthy male, this range is between 0 and 4 μg/l. – this level of antigen secretion will be raised, as well-differentiated carcinoma cells have the same enzyme properties as healthy prostatic cells. Therefore if a rise in the PSA occurs, this is due to a growth in the prostate size due to the presence of carcinoma.

Alkaline phosphatase, normal range 80–280 IU/l, and acid phosphatase, normal range <4 IU/l, are also chemicals detected in the blood and are raised if carcinoma is present in the prostate and metastases have occurred.

All such diagnostic indices are rendered unreliable if the patient has undergone a previous, recent, rectal examination of the prostate.

Transrectal Ultrasound

This is an investigation which is occasionally carried out during a TURP, but can also be performed independently in the radiology department. A small ultrasonic probe is inserted into the patient's rectum, and its head rotates to allow for an optimum assessment. The ultrasound will be able to show prostatic growth and the density of the latter, as a malignant growth, will appear darker on an ultrasound monitor. Thus the actual staging of the tumour can be diagnosed using a transrectal ultrasound as the shape, size and infiltration of the carcinoma will be seen. Antibiotic cover may be given prior to this procedure (e.g. gentamicin 80 mg intramuscularly).

This test can be extremely uncomfortable for the patient, whose dignity must obviously be preserved at all times.

Prostatic Biopsy

Obtaining a prostatic biopsy for histology analysis is an extremely convincing test to perform. If a surgeon is suspicious regarding the possibility of a patient having a carcinoma of the prostate during a TURP, a biopsy can be sent to the laboratory for assessment. Otherwise a biopsy can be obtained either transperineally or transrectally. This can be performed in theatre, on the ward or in the radiology department. Following this procedure the patient should be observed for signs of rectal bleeding.

CT Scan

This investigation can be used in conjunction with the transrectal ultrasound to provide an accurate result regarding the staging of the tumour.

Skeletal Survey/Bone Scan

One of the prime metastatic targets for this tumour is the bones. The symptoms that bony metastases cause range from mild backache to an inability to walk, as a tumour pressing on the spinal cord can weaken the legs. The presence of bony metastases can be detected by the use of two investigations:

1. *A plain X-ray* of the abdominal area will illustrate the presence of metastases, shown as osteosclerotic deposits.

2. *Isotopic bone scan.* This is a much more detailed, accurate and easily identifiable investigation than a plain X-ray. An isotopic agent is injected intravenously and 3–4 hours later films are taken. As a tumour receives a blood supply, if there is metastatic bone involvement, then there will be increased blood flow to these areas.

Pelvic Lymphadenectomy

The prostate gland has a large lymphatic supply; therefore, in the presence of prostatic carcinoma, the possibility of nodal metastases around the pelvis lymph area is high. Nodal staging can be achieved by examination of the nodules after a pelvic lymphadenectomy. The latter is usually performed in conjunction with a radical prostatectomy. It is not performed as a separate entity, as the patient's future treatment will depend on where the tumour has metastasised to, beyond the pelvic lymph area (i.e. the spine, chest, liver), as opposed to diagnosing treatment on the pelvic lymph node analysis alone.

Chest X-Ray

This is done if metastases are suspected, as occasionally lung involvement takes place, which can be detected on a plain chest X-ray.

Liver Function Tests

Another site for metastatic spread is the liver, so liver function tests can be performed to establish whether tumour infiltration has taken place. This is detected by a blood test.

Treatment

Treatment for carcinoma of the prostate depends largely on the stage of the tumour when it is diagnosed. As previously mentioned this particular cancer is usually proven to be present following biopsy analysis taken during a TURP. Quite often, if the tumour is small enough and a resection has been done, further treatment will not routinely take place unless the patient shows signs in the future of further outflow obstruction, or if, during a routine follow-up appointment, he shows symptoms of further tumour development (i.e. raised PSA).

The rationale behind this is that carcinoma of the prostate does in fact have a good prognosis if detected early enough, if the tumours are well differentiated and confined to the prostate, and it would ultimately be unnecessary to submit patients to further surgery or treatment when it was not definitely required. Obviously a patient who has been diagnosed as having a carcinoma of the prostate will be seen in the out-patients department on a regular basis to ensure that no further problems occur.

However, not all prostatic tumours are detected at an early stage, and therefore treatment is inevitable. The following are the alternatives available.

TURP

If cancer of the prostate has been diagnosed by blood tests and ultrasound and the latter shows that the tumour is within the prostatic capsule then a straightforward TURP is performed (as described earlier in this chapter). After discharge the patient will be monitored to ensure that no tumour regrowth occurs.

Radiotherapy

Radiotherapy can be given both to the prostate itself and to areas of metastatic involvement. Radiotherapy to the gland itself can take place prior to surgery, such as radical prostatectomy, to limit the chance of tumour spread, and thus shrinking it to as small a size as possible preoperatively.

This treatment can also be implemented without a patient having to undergo surgery. It may be that radiotherapy will shrink the gland and prevent metastatic involvement. Treatment can be undertaken using the linear accelerator, or by using a more recent technique of actually inserting radioactive iodine implants into the gland to cause tumour regression.

Radiotherapy can also be used as a palliative treatment. As mentioned previously bony metastases are common and can cause the patient a great deal of pain and discomfort. A course of radiotherapy can relieve the pain and ensures the bones can heal. (Usually only a short course of radiotherapy is required.)

Hormone Treatment

Before discussing hormone therapy let us briefly re-examine the androgen activity of the male.

The anterior pituitary gland secretes two gonadotrophic hormones: follicle stimulating hormone (FSH) and luteinising hormone (LH). The FSH acts to initiate spermatogenesis, whilst the LH serves to both develop mature sperm and also bring about the secretion of testosterone. The latter is the main androgen in the male and has a vast effect on the body. It ultimately controls the growth and development of the male sex organs, ensures maturation of sperm and is responsible for the development of the male secondary sex characteristics.

The prostate gland and any carcinoma present can develop according to androgen secretion. Hypothetically, if testosterone is given to a patient, it can stimulate prostatic growth, and if a tumour was present this too would be encouraged to develop. Conversely if the androgen supply is stopped, any metastatic spread from the prostate can usually be prevented or severely reduced (by approximately 70–80 per cent).

Hormone manipulation is usually started in patients when metastases are symptomatic. The aim is to prevent testosterone production and there are two main ways to achieve this.

First, as oestrogens inhibit the production of gonadotrophin releasing hormone (which in turn initiates the whole cycle of androgen production), if these are administered the androgen secretion will stop. Commonly used anti-androgen therapy at present are cyproterone acetate, stilboestrol and goserelin (Zoladex). These drugs do have a number of side-effects, including risk of fluid overload due to sodium retention, cardiovascular involvement, liver disease, gynaecomastia, changes in hair pattern and loss of libido.

A small number of androgens are produced in the adrenal glands and an adrenalectomy may be performed (very rarely), or medication given to inhibit adrenal hormone output.

The other hormonal alternative involves surgery where a bilateral subcapsular orchidectomy is performed, which stops all androgen secretion from the testes. This treatment usually puts an abrupt end to pain caused by metastases. It should be remembered and respected that despite the advantage of a subcapsular orchidectomy, it is a change in body image for the patient, and his psychological feeling towards this surgery should be explored. It is a myth that the patient will develop a high pitched voice and this should be explained.

Chemotherapy

This is not a viable treatment at present. Currently there are certain drugs on trial for use in cases of prostatic cancer, but their effectiveness has not yet been assessed, and certainly chemotherapy is not considered as a treatment of choice, even after other alternatives have been exhausted.

Radical Prostatectomy

As the name suggests this is the removal of the whole of the prostate gland including the capsule. A retropubic approach is taken and the urethral endings are anastomosed together.

This operation is often performed with a pelvic lymphadenectomy and ultimately, if the appropriate preoperative tests have been carried out, it would be hoped that the tumour would be removed completely.

Specific Preoperative Care

Psychological Care

The patient should be admitted to hospital at least 2–3 days preoperatively. Psychologically this operation can be extremely daunting for a patient; not only is he about to undergo a procedure which has numerous possible complications (impotence, retrograde ejaculation and incontinence, to name but three), but he will also be aware that he has 'cancer', which is distressing enough anyway. Therefore the patient and his family will need a lot of psychological support. The patient should be given the time and opportunity to discuss any specific fears or anxieties that he may have. The viability of the tumour being removed by surgical intervention can obviously be discussed with the patient by the nursing or medical staff, but the patient may wish to discuss the possibility of impotence or infertility with a sexual counsellor if one is available to the hospital.

Physical Care

1. *Bowel preparation* This is needed due to the possibility of bowel mobilisation during surgery.

Usually the regimen is as follows:

- 3 days preoperatively – low fibre diet
- 2 days preoperatively – free fluids and oral aperient (i.e. Picolax)
- 1 day preoperatively – clear fluids and enema if aperient did not work

2. *ECG* This is required to exclude any cardiac abnormalities as the patient will be anaesthetised for approximately 3 hours and probably suffer a significant blood loss.

3. *Blood assay* The patient will almost certainly have a blood transfusion either during or after surgery, so blood will need to be cross-matched preoperatively. Also the patient's full blood count, urea and electrolytes should be screened to eliminate any abnormalities.

4. *Antiembolism stockings* All patients should have a pair as they will ultimately be immobile for some time postoperatively. If the patient has a history of deep vein thrombosis he should be heparinised too.

5. *Shave* This should be performed in theatre from midthorax down to the scrotal area.

Specific Postoperative Care

Postoperatively the patient will return to the ward with both urethral and suprapubic catheters, a wound drain, an intravenous infusion (which may be blood), an analgesic pump (usually Omnopon) and possibly a central line.

The patient should have no difficulty breathing although the administration of Omnopon (especially intravenously) may lower the patient's respiratory rate, so this should therefore be carefully monitored.

The patient's blood pressure may be lowered in the first 12 hours postoperatively. This may be due either to the Omnopon or opioid pump or to blood loss in theatre (or both). Central venous pressure may be monitored along with the normal blood pressure for the first 24 hours. Blood (or a blood substitute) may have to be given on the ward. The catheters and wound drain should be observed to ensure that there is no significant blood loss.

Pain is usually well controlled using an Omnopon pump. During the days postoperatively the pump can be reduced in the amount administered and possibly rectal analgesia given (e.g. Voltarol).

Urine output must be carefully monitored; the patient may have a bladder irrigation in progress via one catheter and exit via the other. This is discontinued after 24-48 hours. The catheters remain in situ for a further 12 days. This is because the urethral catheter is acting as a splint to aid anastomatic healing. A urethrogram is performed 14 days following surgery and if all has healed well the urethral catheter is removed and the suprapubic catheter is clamped to enable the patient to void normally. If voiding is satisfactory and the bladder is being emptied properly the suprapubic catheter is removed.

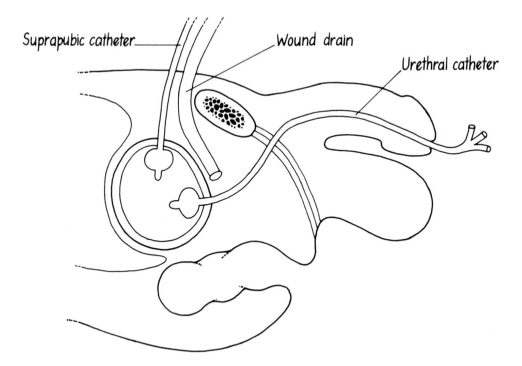

Fig 8.7   Positioning of drainage apparatus post-radical prostatectomy

Complications

The majority of complications of this operation are the same as for a TURP. However, the incidence is much higher (e.g. retrograde ejaculation, incontinence due to sphincter damage). Impotence is almost certain.

Nerve sparing operations are now available to try and reduce such complications (Tanagho and McAninch, 1992), Kirby (1991).

Other complications are:

1. *Chest infection and deep vein thrombosis* due to restricted mobility postoperatively

2. *Infection* due to abdominal wound, drains and catheters

3. *Stricture formation* at the anastomotic site resulting in retention of urine

Following discharge the patient is seen regularly in the out-patients department and if progress is good further surgery may be offered to treat any incontinence or impotence.

References

Astrahan MA, Ameye F, Dyen R (1991) Interstitial temperature measurements during transurethral microwave hyperthermia. *Journal of Urology* **145**: 304–308.
Bullock N, Sibley G and Whitaker R (1989) *Essential Urology*. Edinburgh: Churchill Livingstone.
Chappell CR, Milroy JG and Rickards D (1990) Permanently implanted urethral stent for prostatic obstruction in the unfit patient. *British Journal of Urology* **66**: 58–65.
Christmas TJ and Kirby RS (1991) Conservative treatment for benign prostatic hyperplasia. *Hospital Update* **17**: 635–641.
Gill KP, Machen LS, Allison DJ and Williams G (1989) Bladder outflow tract obstruction and urinary retention from prostatic hypertrophy treated by balloon dilatation. *British Journal of Urology* **64**: 618–622.
Kirby RS (1991) Nerve-sparing radical retro-pubic prostatectomy for localised cancer of the prostate. In: Hendry WF (ed.) *Recent Advances in Urology/Andrology*. Edinburgh: Churchill Livingstone.
McLoughlin J and Williams G (1990) Prostatic stents and balloon dilatation. *British Journal of Hospital Medicine* **43**: 422–426.
Perez-Marrero RA, Lee LM, Emerson L and Goldberg SL (1990) Endoscopic balloon dilation of the prostate: early experience. *Journal of Urology* **144**(1): 83–87.
Roos NP, Wennberg JE, Malenka DJ (1989) Mortality and reoperation after open transurethral resection of the prostate for benign prostatic hyperplasia. *New England Journal of Medicine* **320**: 1120–1124.
Strohmaier WL, Bichler KH, Fluchter SH (1990) Local microwave hyperthermia of benign prostatic hyperplasia. *Journal of Urology* **144**: 913–917.
Tanagho EA and McAninch JW (eds) (1992) *Smith's General Urology*, 12th edn. London: Prentice Hall International.

9
Penile Disorders

The penis consists of

- A root
- A body
- A glans

The root involves three masses of erectile tissue called the bulb and left and right crura which lie within the perineum. The bulb may be felt on deep palpation in the midline of the perineum, posterior to the scrotum. It is transversed by the urethra and forms the corpus spongiosum. The two crura converge anteriorly and come to lie side by side in the dorsal part of the body of the penis, forming the corpora cavernosa. The corpora are contained within a fibrous sheath – Buck's fascia.

The body is suspended from the symphysis pubis by a suspensory ligament and surrounds the urethra.

The glans is situated at the extremity of the body of the penis. At the tip of the glans is the external urethral meatus. Just above, the skin is folded upon itself and forms a movable double layer, i.e. the foreskin or prepuce. It is connected to the glans just below the urethral orifice by a fold called the frenulum.

MALE PELVIS

Blood Supply

Arterial

The right and left internal pudendal arteries divide into superficial and deep arteries of the penis which arise from the internal iliac artery.

The deep artery supplies separate branches to the spongiosum, urethra and corpora cavernosae. Arterioles connect the spongiosum and dorsal vessels.

Venous

The veins form two main channels – superficial and deep. The superficial dorsal vein passes beneath the skin to the pubis and there divides into branches which empty

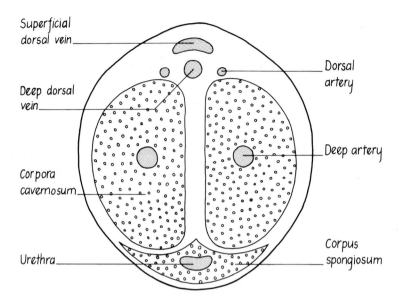

Fig 9.1   Cross-section of the penis

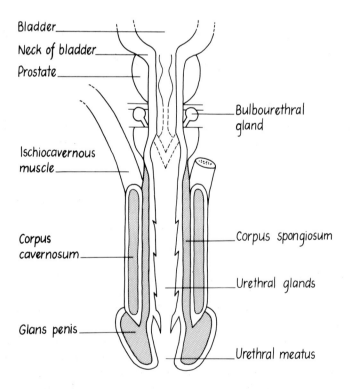

Fig 9.2   Longitudinal section through the penis

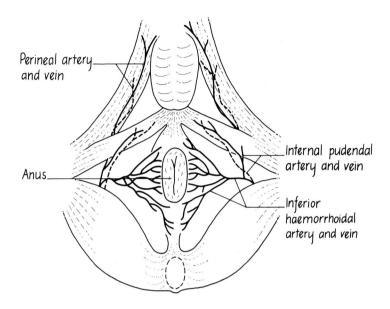

Fig 9.3   Blood supply of male perineum

into the saphenous system or directly into the femoral veins. The deep dorsal vein follows a similar course but additionally drains via the prostatic plexus. This network of dorsal veins drains the peripheral blood from the penis during detumescence.

Lymphatic Drainage

The skin of the penis is drained into the medial group of superficial inguinal nodes. The deep structures of the penis are drained into the internal iliac nodes.

Nerve Supply

The penis is supplied by autonomic and somatic (voluntary) nerves:

1.   *Internal pudendal nerve* — cerebrospinal system.

2.   *Hypogastric plexus* to the erectile tissue — autonomic system.

The principal nerve supply to the penis is the pudendal nerve. This was once known as the nervi erigentes — the nerves of erection. The word pudendal originates from the Latin 'pudeo' — 'I am ashamed!'. In polite society the genitalia were once called the pudenda.

The pudendal nerve arises from S2:3:4 of the sacral region of the spinal cord, supplying the musculature of the levator ani and the pubococcygeus and the muscles of the penis, the ischiocavernosus and the bulbospongiosus. The nerves supplying the blood vessels to the genitalia and involved in the neural control of vasocongestion derive from the sympathetic and parasympathetic systems.

Erection and Ejaculation

The penis consists of three cylindrical bodies of erectile tissue. These are the two corpora cavernosa and the corpus spongiosum. The corpora cavernosa consist of a network of fibrous tissue which becomes filled with blood during erection of the penis. The two corpora cavernosae lie next to each other and have a deep central artery – a branch of the internal pudendal artery. The corpora separate posteriorly to form the two crura which are attached to the ischiopubic rami of the pelvis. The crura are covered by the ischiocavernous muscle, which provides the penis with a secure attachment to the pelvis. The corpus spongiosum is expanded to form the glans penis anteriorly and the bulb of the penis posteriorly. The bulb is covered by the bulbospongiosus muscle which has many fibres closely associated with the corpus spongiosum which surrounds the urethra. The muscle has an important role in propelling semen along the urethra during ejaculation. The 'bulbospongiosus reflex' is elicited by stimulation of the glans penis and this results in reflex contraction of the bulbospongiosus muscle. The reflex requires the integrity of the sensory and motor branches of the pudendal nerves and of the segments S2:3:4 of the spinal cord.

Sexual Response Cycle

Erection in the male is gradually built up as a consequence of various sexual stimuli. Four phases have been identified which rather than being distinct tend to overlap each other.

The excitement phase is initiated by whatever the individual finds sexually stimulating, thus resulting in the bombardment of the central nervous system by afferent stimuli. Efferent nervous impulses pass down the spinal cord to the parasympathetic outflow in the second, third and fourth sacral segments. If the stimuli are interrupted for any reason the cycle may stop here or become extended.

If stimulation continues, sexual tension increases, entering the plateau phase. During this phase the efferent nerve impulses pass into the tissue at the root of the penis. Vasodilation of the arteries now occurs, producing a great increase in the blood flow through the blood spaces of the erectile tissue.

The third phase – the climactic or orgasmic phase – involves a completely involuntary response. The corpora cavernosae and corpus spongiosum become engorged with blood and expand while compressing the vessels of venous drainage against the surrounding tissue, thus retaining the blood, causing rigidity and an increase in both length and diameter of the penis. Secretions from the bulbourethral glands moisten the glans penis and continued friction results in increased nervous impulses along the sympathetic nerve fibres to the smooth muscle of the duct of the epididymis, vas deferens, the seminal vesicles and the prostate. On contraction of the smooth muscle the spermatozoa are discharged into the prostatic urethra along with seminal fluid. Ejaculation from the penile urethra occurs as a result of rhythmic contractions of the bulbospongiosus muscles which compress the urethra. During this phase the sphincter of the bladder contracts to prevent reflux of sperm into the bladder.

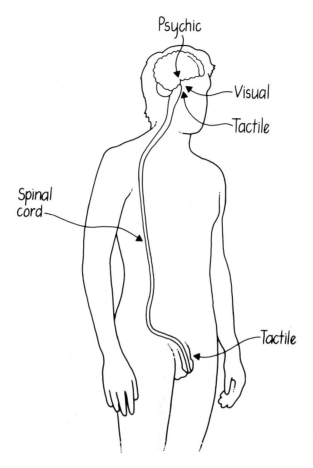

Fig 9.4   Neural mechanisms for erection

The fourth or final phase, resolution, is characterised by decreased sexual tension as the individual returns to an unstimulated state. The arteries supplying the erectile tissue undergo vasoconstriction and the penis returns to its flaccid state.

PENILE CONDITIONS AND SURGERY

Phimosis

Phimosis is the inability to retract the foreskin back over the glans. This can result in a pinhole meatus, thus impeding flow of urine, and can cause urinary retention, meatal infection and symptoms of lower urinary tract obstruction.

Paraphimosis

This is swelling of a retracted foreskin behind the glans penis. This condition may arise after sexual intercourse, masturbation or surgical instrumentation of the penis (e.g. cystoscopy or transurethral resection). It is therefore very important to check that the patient's foreskin has been pulled forward following instrumentation. If unresolved the compression of the glans may become so severe that gangrene of the glans may ensue.

Treatment

This condition can be treated conservatively in the early stages. Application of an anaesthetic gel (e.g. lignocaine) and gentle, firm compression may be sufficient to restore the position of the foreskin. If this is unsuccessful it may be necessary for the surgeon to perform a dorsal slit under general anaesthetic. Both phimosis and paraphimosis may need to be treated surgically by formal circumcision.

Circumcision

This procedure is also commonly performed within certain religious communities and it can be stated that neonatal circumcision does protect against the chance of certain types of penile carcinoma.

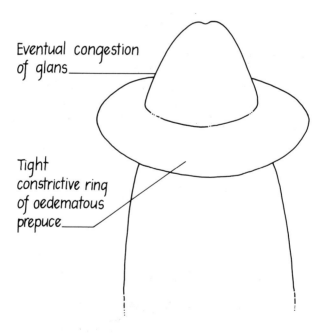

Eventual congestion of glans

Tight constrictive ring of oedematous prepuce

Fig 9.5 Paraphimosis

Procedure

A dorsal slit is made and the foreskin excised to the base of the glans. The individual bleeding vessels are ligated and interrupted catgut sutures circumscribe the base of the glans.

Complications and nursing care are shown in Table 9.1.

Table 9.1 Complications of circumcision and specific nursing care

Problem	Action
Bleeding – close proximity of dorsal vein and frenular arteries	Regular observation Light paraffin dressing Inform medical staff immediately of any excessive bleeding and possible return to theatre
Pain – particularly post-operatively if patient has erections	Regular analgesia Surgeons may prescribe diazepam to reduce erections Application of anaesthetic gel
Oedema	Supportive pants and pad with penis in upright position

Balanitis

Balanitis (inflammation of foreskin and penis) is often a result of poor hygiene. A resulting infection can produce itching and burning.

The foreskin and glans penis can be exposed to a number of potential infections. In the presence of any additional problems of maintaining hygiene (e.g. phimosis), the underlying infection may produce oedema, exudate, erythema and scarring.

Sources of Infection

Sources of infection include:

1. *Poor hygiene*

2. *Urethral discharge of bacterial origin*

3. *Certain skin diseases*, e.g. psoriasis, lichen planus, leucoplakia

4. *Vulvovaginitis* – cross-infection from an infected partner

5. *Underlying illness*, e.g. diabetes, resulting in secondary infection

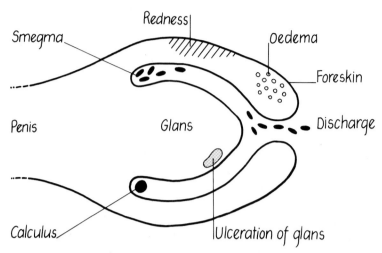

Fig 9.6   Inflammation of the foreskin and penis (balanitis)

Treatment

The main aim of any treatment will be to eradicate any infection present and to maintain careful hygiene. Local washing and careful drying are extremely important. The use of systemic antibiotics may be necessary, accompanied by the use of localised antibiotic cream or lotion. Circumcision may be considered if there is no improvement due to tightness of the foreskin.

Priapism

Priapism (painful persistent penile erection) is accompanied by venous congestion of the penile cavernous structures. The prolonged erection is not accompanied by sexual desire or excitement.

Possible Causes

Possible causes of priapism include:

1. *Vascular-venous thrombosis* in the vessels that drain the penis in certain blood disorders (e.g. sickle cell anaemia, leukaemia)

2. *Obstructive tumours* around the base of the penis, bladder, prostate or rectum

3. *Spinal cord injuries*

4. *Idiopathic* – often no definite cause can be found, but there may be a history of prolonged vigorous sexual intercourse

5. *Drugs*, often in overdose – anticoagulants, phenothiazines, marijuana, antihistamines

6. *Post-papaverine injection* – drug used to produce erection when injected into the base of penis. Erection should subside naturally but occasionally does not.

Treatment

This condition should be recognised as a urological emergency. Initially the erection may be resolved by sedation with, for example, Valium.

Sedation with intravenous procyclidine hydrochloride (Kemadrin) may produce a dry mouth, dizziness and blurred vision after administration and the patient should be reassured that this will resolve. Aspiration of the corpora with a butterfly needle and syringe and flushing with heparinised saline may thin and relieve the pressure of the thick viscous blood. Metaraminol (Aramine) or phenylephrine hydrochloride (drugs used in the treatment of acute hypotension) can be injected intracorporally into the penis.

Specific nursing care of priapism is shown in Table 9.2.

If medical management is unsuccessful it will be necessary for the surgeon to bypass the blocked channel by means of a shunt. This can be created by three routes:

- Glans/cavernosus
- Spongiosus/cavernosus
- Corporosaphenous

By providing this escape route for the blood, the erection will then subside. The effect of performing shunts is often a damaged erectile system and permanent impotence.

Table 9.2 Nursing care for priapism

Problem	Action
Potential sudden severe hypertension	Frequent monitoring of the patient's blood pressure within the first hour is essential
Psychological effects of:	
Embarrassment	Provide privacy
Worry about impotence	Keep patient informed before each treatment is commenced
Pain and discomfort	Provide reassurance. Analgesia as required (studies have shown that giving information reduces anxiety and pain due to drug treatment)
Potential bruising and bleeding around injected site	Provide scrotal support/pants and a soft sterile pad. The penis should be supported upwards to prevent further oedema

Peyronie's Disease

This disease is characterised by the formation of plaques of fibrous tissue in the sheath of the corpora cavernosa, which are adherent to the overlying Buck's fascia. The plaques prevent the penis from distending fully on erection, producing varying degrees of curvature. Although the aetiology is unknown, the tissue is similar in its histology to that found in Dupuytren's contracture and retroperitoneal fibrosis. This is a benign condition.

Clinical Examination

Papaverine injected into the corpus cavernosum will produce an erection and the degree of curvature can be assessed. During erection the area of fibrous tissue fails to distend. Varying degrees of bend are produced according to the site and overall area of scarring. On questioning, the patient may report that there is a tendency for his erection to be painful and penetration may be difficult or even impossible, especially if there is complete failure of erection distal to the plaques.

Surgical Treatment

The most successful surgical treatment for this condition is known as a Nesbit's procedure. During the operation, the surgeon makes an incision in the area of Buck's fascia opposite that of the plaque. The tissue is then reefed and sutured. Often the

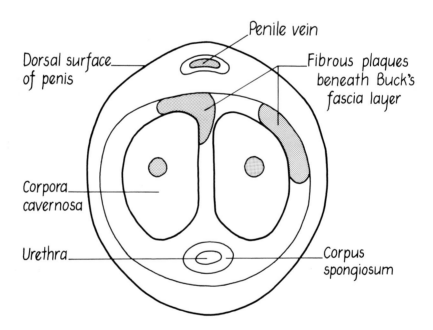

Fig 9.7 Peyronie's disease

patient is circumcised at the same time. The medical staff will advise the patient that a certain amount of shortening will occur. This may cause anxiety and counselling may be required by both medical and nursing staff. Problems and nursing care after correction are listed in Table 9.3.

Table 9.3   Nursing care following correction of Peyronie's disease

Problem	Action
Potential pain and discomfort	Light supportive dressing. Analgesia offered (usually mild to moderate medication is sufficient)
Potential haemorrhage	Frequent checking of sutured areas. Inform medical staff promptly as patient may require further suturing if bleeding is excessive

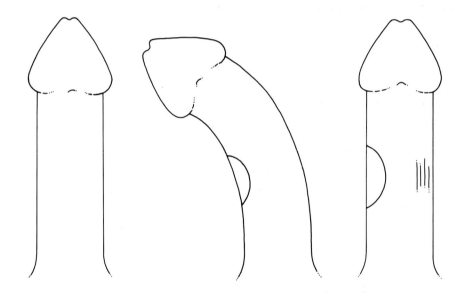

Fig 9.8   Peyronie's disease: curvature and correction

Venous Leaks

In the event of a venous leak there will be failure of the erectile bodies to fill with blood and therefore inability to form an erection.

Causes

Causes are congenital or acquired:

1. *Congenital* The patient may always have been unable to achieve erection because of congenital leakage within the venous system of the spongiosus or glans. Abnormal veins may also be present.

2. *Acquired* Venous leaks can be acquired post-surgery (e.g. priapism or urethral surgery), as a result of atheroma or after fracture of the pelvis.

Diagnosis

Detailed history will establish the onset of impotence. An injection of papaverine, a drug which causes the penile arteries to relax, will produce an erection providing the blood supply is not obstructed or leakage present. Impairment of the arterial blood supply may be shown by Doppler studies of the penile blood flow. The site and extent of the leakage can be more specifically identified under X-ray conditions using pelvic angiography or cavernosogram.

Venous Leak Repair

This operation will vary in severity depending on the site and extent of the leak. Specific nursing care is shown in Table 9.4.

Table 9.4 Specific nursing care for venous leak repair

Problem	Action
Embarrassment and anxiety about success of operation	Obtain information from surgeon for patient as to severity of operation and success rate. This is essential as the operation may be fairly minor or patient may return to ward with intravenous infusion, wound drains and large wound incision
	Reduce embarrassment by providing privacy for patient as far as possible

Impotence

Impotence is the inability to sustain an erection to allow sexual intercourse.

Causes of Impotence

1. *Vascular* (e.g. diabetes, atherosclerosis)

2. *Neurological* (e.g. CVA, head injury, diabetes, post-pelvic fracture, surgery)

3. *Endocrine* (e.g. pituitary dysfunction, hypothyroidism)

4. *Congenital* (e.g. extrophy, epispadias, hypospadias)

5. *Acquired* (e.g. Peyronie's disease, carcinoma of penis)

6. *Drugs* (e.g. antihypertensives, anticonvulsants, alcohol)

Clinical Diagnosis

The medical staff will take a detailed history of the onset of impotence. Various questions will be asked:

1. *Early morning erections* – presence suggests psychogenic origin to the impotence.

2. *Gradual or sudden onset* – gradual, usually organic; sudden, psychogenic (unless known injury)

3. *Life-style* – smoking can cause atheroma in the arteries of the penis. Drinking habits are also relevant

4. *History of any pelvic injury*

5. *Drug history*

Blood may be taken to establish hormonal levels. Examination of the patient will include observation of facial hair, development and pitch of voice; neurological and vascular examination of sacral sensation and peripheral pulses.

Investigations

The following investigations are performed:

1. *Urine* will be tested for glucose

2. *Doppler ultrasound flowmeter* – assesses blood flow in penis

3. *Papaverine injection*

4. *Cavernosogram* – X-ray to establish venous drainage

5. *Nocturnal penile tumescence studies* – this test requires an overnight stay in hospital. Gauges are attached to the penis. These record changes in penile length and circumference. Erections occur naturally several times during the night, especially during periods of deep sleep (during periods of rapid eye movement). Results are computerised. Graphs showing no movement suggest impotence of neurogenic origin whilst graph activity shows impotence of psychogenic nature.

Treatment

Once investigations establish the cause of impotence, potential treatment can be discussed with the patient. If nocturnal tumescence studies show night-time erections, the patient can be referred to a psychosexual counsellor. If surgery is not advisable or desired, the patient can be taught to inject himself with papaverine to initiate erection.

Prosthetic implants

This operation involves the insertion of materials into the corpora cavernosa. There are three basic types of penile implants:

1. *Rigid rods* – these are less commonly used nowadays.

2. *Flexible rod implants* – these produce a permanently erect penis which can be bent to accommodate intercourse and be flexible enough to be moved into a position of concealment afterwards.

3. *Inflatable implants* – these consist of two penile cylinders, a pump and a reservoir. Each part is interconnected by tubing. The pump is situated within the scrotum and if squeezed by hand several times the fluid fills the cylinders and an erection develops. The erection can be maintained as long as the patient desires and once the release bar on the pump is activated the fluid in the cylinders returns to the reservoir where it is stored again and the penis returns to its normal relaxed position.

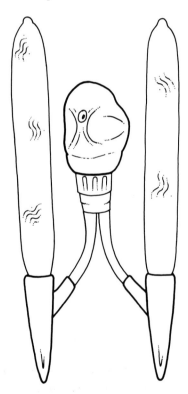

Fig 9.9 Inflatable penile prostheses

Preoperative Preparation

As one of the most common complications following penile prosthesis is infection, work begins preoperatively to minimise this problem.

Table 9.5   Penile prosthesis — *Specific nursing care*

Problem	Action
Potential risk of postoperative infection	The patient will be required to have preoperative Betadine or Hibiscrub baths
	Naseptin cream is inserted into each nostril on preoperative day (one of the most common bacteria isolated from rejected prostheses, *Staphylococcus aureus*, is often found in the nose)
	Shaves are carried out in theatre
	Intravenous antibiotics are given at induction
Potential psychological trauma of altered body image, low self-esteem and loss of feelings of masculinity	Ensure patient is given enough time to express his fears and worries and given support
	Provide pre- and postoperative information.
	Show prosthesis to patient if required
	Involve session with psychosexual counsellor if required
	Ensure privacy as far as possible

During Surgery

The implants are measured and cut to the correct size in theatre before insertion into the corpora cavernosa. Prophylactic antibiotics are now commonly used (e.g. gentamicin) and injected locally into the area of insertion.

Postoperative Care

Postoperative care is shown in Table 9.6

On Discharge

Patients are advised to return to their surgeon immediately if they have any problems after discharge.

Depending on the surgeon, the patient will be advised either to attempt intercourse 1 week before returning to the out-patients department or to abstain until he is seen in clinic 6 weeks after discharge.

Table 9.6   Specific nursing care for penile prosthesis

Problem	Action
Potentially swollen and bruised penis	Elevate penis with scrotal support or pants and pad
	Regular analgesia should be offered
	Encourage rest
Potential inability to pass urine	Support patient standing at the side of the bed if unable to pass urine while lying flat
	Ensure adequate hydration
	Inform surgeon if patient unable to void (may require catheterisation)
Potential infection and/or rejection	Prophylactic antibiotics are given for 48 hours postoperatively
	Wound examined regularly for breakdown or dehiscence
	Temperature and pulse recorded 4-hourly.

10

Urological Cancer

'Cancer' is a generic term, encompassing a variety of different illnesses which individually affect a wide range of organ systems and tissues.

However, common to all cancers is a deregulation of the normal processes of growth and differentiation, such that uncontrolled cellular proliferation is seen. Such proliferation occurs because cancer cells no longer respond to normal mechanisms of growth control and the uncoordinated growth pattern which results can then lead to invasion of surrounding tissues and/or subsequent haematological or lymphatic spread.

It is this characteristic pattern of invasion and spread that accounts for the morbidity and mortality of cancer. In any discussion of cancer-related illness, one needs first to distinguish between the descriptive terms malignant and benign, which refer to different types of growth control deregulation.

A summary of the differences between these two types of growth are shown in Table 10.1.

Table 10.1 Malignant and benign growth: characteristics

Malignant	Benign
Do not remain encapsulated	Remain encapsulated
Grow in an invasive manner	Do not grow invasively
Metastasize	Do not metastasize
Are life threatening	Generally, non-life threatening
Tend to be less well differentiated	Generally well differentiated
Usually grow faster than benign tumours	

There are other cancer-related terms in common usage which may result in confusion. To try to avoid ambiguity, the key terms used in this chapter are listed in Table 10.2 along with their definitions.

Cancer is an increasingly common disease within industrialised populations, and this may reflect the combination of an environmental aetiology alongside possible genetic predispositions for certain types of cancer. Table 10.3 illustrates the incidence of some specific types of cancer, and includes some of the more common urological cancers for comparison.

Table 10.2   Some key terms used within the context of cancer

Term	Contextual Meaning
Tumour	A distinct region of growth deregulation, resulting in a dividing colony of cells of varying size, which may display either malignant or benign characteristics
Differentiation	The process whereby dividing cells maintain a degree of morphological and biochemical similarity to their parental cell type. Loss of differentiation is a characteristic of cancer cells, which may be highly undifferentiated and thus very different from their cell or tissue of origin. Loosely, the higher the degree of undifferentiated character, the poorer the prognosis
Malignant	A pattern of tumour growth characterised by uncontrolled cellular division, invasion of surrounding tissues and usually metastatic spread, if untreated
Benign	A pattern of tumour growth characterised by uncontrolled cellular division, but which remains localised, without invasion of surrounding tissues or metastases
Cancer	A generic term used to describe any malignant tumour
Carcinoma	A malignant tumour of epithelial tissue

Table 10.3   Incidence of some common forms of cancer

Primary site	Site of occurrence in England and Wales (%)
Males	
Lung	9.15
Colon	1.89
Pancreas	0.94
Stomach	2.23
Bladder	1.99
Prostate	2.17
Females	
Breast	5.96
Ovary	1.26
Colon	1.65
Cervix	1.21
Lung	2.42

Adapted from Muir et al, 1987.

Clearly, causative agents for cancer are extremely varied and, in many cases, unknown at this time. Table 10.4 lists some common urological cancers and illustrates possible risk factors for the development of malignant tumour growth in these tissues.

Table 10.4 Possible/established aetiology of urological cancers

Site	Incidence (%)	Overall mortality (%)	Male:female ratio	Established risk factors
Prostate	4.7	4.8	Male only	Black racial group Endogenous hormones High fat intake
Bladder	4.7	3.3	2.1:1.0	Smoking Aromatic amines Certain anticancer drugs Schistosomiasis infection (not in UK)
Kidney	1.6	1.6	1.6:1.0	Smoking Aromatic amines Phenacetin
Testis	0.5	0.1	Male only	White racial group Undescended testis Foetal exposure to endogenous hormones
Penis	0.1	0.1	Male only	Early circumcision is preventative Specific types of papillomavirus Poor penile hygiene may be involved in causation

Overall mortality refers to the number of patients dying per year as a percentage of total deaths from cancer per year, and incidence is expressed as a proportion of all cancers.

The typical pattern of urological cancers, in terms of their location and incidence, is shown in Figure 10.1. The problem with cancers of the urothelium is that they have the potential for rapid spread throughout the urinary tract, because of the uniform nature of the transitional cell epithelium. Therefore, a bladder carcinoma may readily spread in a retrograde direction, to involve the ureter, or via an antegrade route to involve the urethra and penis. Likewise, a renal cancer may well spread in an antegrade direction to involve the ureter and perhaps the bladder. This therefore underlines the importance of early diagnosis and treatment whenever possible.

BLADDER CANCER

Bladder cancer, along with prostatic cancer (see Chapter 8), is by far the most common urological malignancy, accounting for 90 per cent of tumours seen. It is found in approximately 20 per 100 000 of the population and this means that some 8000 new cases of urothelial cancer present within the United Kingdom each year.

World wide, a significant geographical variation in incidence is seen, with bladder cancer common within the industrialised world but less common within developing

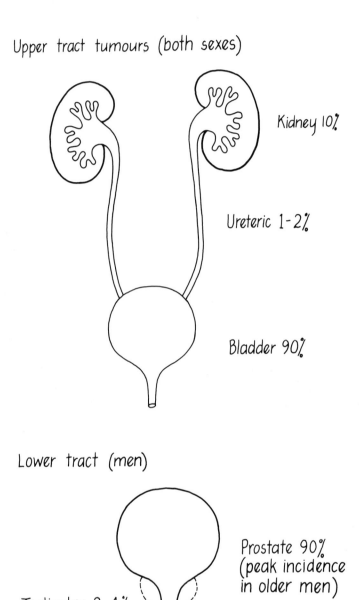

Upper tract tumours (both sexes)

Kidney 10%

Ureteric 1-2%

Bladder 90%

Lower tract (men)

Prostate 90%
(peak incidence
in older men)

Testicular 2-4%
(seen in men
20-40 years)

Urethral and penile 1%

Fig 10.1   Incidence and location of common urological cancers

countries (except those where schistosomiasis is common). In the UK and Europe the peak incidence of bladder cancer occurs at around 65 years of age. In other areas the age of presentation is lower, because of the nature of the chronic inflammation and irritation caused to the bladder mucosa by schistosomiasis infection.

Histology

Histology refers to the type and morphology of cells which make up an organ or tissue and, histologically, certain types of urethelial tumours can be identified. These are:

1. *Benign* – papilloma; fibroepithelial polyp.

2. *Malignant* – transitional cell carcinoma (90 per cent); squamous cell carcinoma (5–8 per cent); adenocarcinoma (1–2 per cent); sarcoma (<1 per cent); undifferentiated, highly anaplastic cancer.

These basic categories of malignancy may also present within the upper tracts, such as in the kidney or ureter. Sadly, however, the presentation of such upper tract tumours if often later, so that a proportion of them are more advanced at the time of diagnosis and thus the prognosis of these patients may well be less favourable.

Further, a specialised form of cancer, not shown above, but which may present anywhere within the urinary tract is that of carcinoma in situ. Urothelial carcinoma in situ is analogous to carcinoma in situ within other bodily sites (such as the cervix) and is characterised by malignant change within the surface epithelial lining of either the bladder or upper tract mucosal surface. Such carcinoma in situ, within the bladder, however, may occasionally behave in a very aggressive manner with early invasion and metastatic spread and this can present difficult problems in relation to management.

Staging of Bladder Cancer

For enhancement of diagnosis and treatment, in relation to bladder and prostatic cancer, an internationally agreed system of staging is used, thus ensuring that all urological units are working from the same uniform diagnostic criteria. This system is the so-called TNM + G stage, where the initials T, N and M stand respectively for *Tumour*, *Nodes*, and *Metastases* and the G for *Glesson*, which relates to the degree of differentiation of the tumour (this is clearly, therefore, a histological diagnosis).

Figure 10.2 and Table 10.5 illustrate both the use of TNM staging and also how such diagnostic criteria relate to the extent of the presenting disease. The T stage is thus ascertained both by the histological examination of biopsy specimens and also by means of examination under anaesthetic (EUA). Nodal status is also ascertained via EUA and biopsy and metastatic disease assessed largely by bodily screening procedures such as ultrasound or CT scanning.

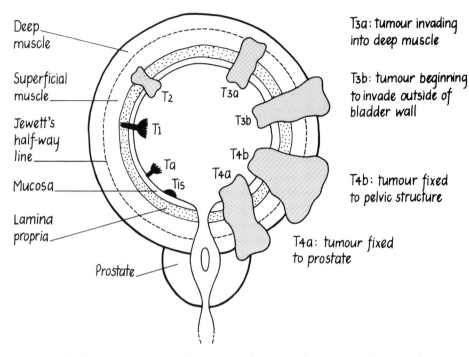

Fig 10.2 Bladder cancer staging. Tis: flat, carcinoma in situ: Ta: papillary, confined to
mucosa. T_1: invasion of lamina propria. T_2 invasion of superficial muscle. T_{3a}:
invasion of deep muscle. T_{3b}: invasion of perivesical tissue. T_{4a} tumour fixed to
prostate. T_{4b}: tumour fixed to other pelvic structures

Table 10.5 Staging of metastasis and lymph nodes in bladder cancer

M_0	No evidence of metastatic disease
M_1	Metastasis present
M_x	Metastatic state unknown
N_0	No nodal involvement
N_1	Single, adjacent node involved, on same side of body as the tumour (i.e. ipsilateral)
N_2	Bilateral nodal involvement or opposite side nodal involvement (contralateral) or multiple regional nodes involved
N_3	Fixed, regional nodes involved (i.e. tumour spreading out of nodes into adjacent structures)
N_4	Juxta, regional nodes involved (i.e. wider metastatic disease)
N_x	Nodal status unknown

Clearly the G stage is a histological diagnosis. It can also be seen that it is actually
very difficult to stage metastatic disease accurately because, even with CT scanning
or NMR, or tumour markers, one can never totally eliminate the presence of
microscopic metastases, which may actually consist of only one or two cells. Thus,

the absence of metastases can probably be assumed if the patient reaches 5 years with no further symptoms.

Presentation of Urothelial Cancer

Patients who have developed a urothelial cancer classically present with one or more episodes of painless haematuria. Bullock et al (1989) report that 20 per cent of such patients are then subsequently found to have a urinary tract tumour. Thus, although a common mode of presentation, painless haematuria is by no means 'proof' of a urothelial tumour.

Also, because of the intrinsic sensitivity of the urine testing sticks used for routine health screening, more patients are now being referred for urological investigation, with microscopic haematuria having been discovered on stick testing. Many of these individuals are younger patients and, in the vast majority of cases, the haematuria is idiopathic and no abnormal lesion or disease process is discovered on subsequent investigation. So-called 'March' haematuria (first seen in soldiers following long route marches) is one such example of idiopathic haematuria.

Bullock et al (1989) further report that approximately 10 per cent of patients with such microscopic haematuria, who are over the age of 45 years, have a urological malignancy as the cause of the bleeding.

A tumour of the bladder urothelium may also be an incidental finding at cystoscopy for other urological problems (e.g. prostatic resection or recurrent urinary tract infection) and such a method of discovery accounts for about 10 per cent of all urothelial tumours (the vast majority of which are bladder cancers).

Other problems caused by urothelial cancers, which may cause a patient to present, are shown in Table 10.6.

Sterile pyuria (i.e. pus cells in the urine, but the specimen does not then grow any causative organism on routine growth media) is a potentially sinister presenting problem, and is generally indicative of either tuberculosis or cancer within the urinary tract. However, sterile pyuria may also result from recurrent established calculi (e.g. stag-horn calculus and/or other infection type stones) because antibiotic agents do not penetrate right into the interior of such stones and thus viable bacteria are always left intact. Also, sterile pyuria may result from partially or ineffectively treated urinary tract infections. Further, the irritant effect of calculi can lead to localised inflammation and scarring within the kidney, as a result of which white cells may again appear within the urine.

As stated above, tuberculous bacilli do not grow on routine growth media and therefore require a more specialised method of laboratory culture, if suspected. Also, such bacilli have a lipid, hydrophobic cell wall, which prevents the penetration of normal acidic staining reagents (hence the term 'acid-fast' bacilli). Thus, a staining method such as the Ziehl–Neelsen procedure is required, which is able to penetrate the lipid cell wall and therefore highlight the presence of such bacilli.

Pus cells may also result from urothelial cancers, because leucocytes are part of the normal immune response which seeks to prevent tumour growth, and thus cause regression/destruction of cancer cells. Such immune cells may be shed from the tumour surface, or from blood vessels which the cancer has eroded, and thus appear in the urine.

It is a useful protocol, therefore, for any patient with sterile pyuria to be assumed to have either tuberculosis or cancer, unless/until proven otherwise.

Table 10.6 Presenting problems which may be caused by malignancy of the urinary tract

---

Painless haematuria (70–90 per cent), which is *overt* or *microscopic* (i.e. found on routine urinalysis)
Cystitis (some 15 per cent of patients present with symptoms of cystitis and of these 40 per cent have urinary tract infection)
Bladder outflow obstruction (due to tumours which are close to the trigone or bladder neck)
Ureteric obstruction (either at the level of the ureteric orifice or higher up), which can then result in renal failure or loin pain
Non-specific symptoms (e.g. weight loss, anaemia, pyrexia of unknown origin)
Established metastatic disease
Perineal or abdominal pain (this may be a late onset sign which correlates with both soft tissue and nervous invasion by tumour cells

---

Patients who present with symptoms of urothelial cancer, in association with abdominal or perineal pain, may well have advanced cancer of the bladder or kidney, the pain suggesting that the tumour has begun to infiltrate and invade surrounding tissues, causing both tissue destruction and nerve compression or damage. Generally such pain is characteristic of more advanced urological tumours (e.g. T_3–T_4 bladder cancers, or prostatic tumours).

The specific management of some common urological cancers has already been discussed in Chapters 8 and 9 and so will not be discussed here. However, a description of the management and nursing care of patients with bladder, kidney and testicular cancers, all of which have not been discussed elsewhere, follows.

Investigation

Urothelial cancer is normally investigated by three principal methods. These are:

- Urinary culture and microscopy
- IVU or ultrasound or CT scanning
- Cystoscopy and examination under anaesthetic

Clearly, if IVU or ultrasound suggests the presence of an upper tract lesion (i.e. within the kidney) then other investigations, such as abdominal CT scanning, are more likely to be employed. If IVU or ultrasound suggests a ureteric or bladder lesion then cystoscopy and EUA is performed, in conjunction with transurethral resection, as this then allows effective staging of such tumours.

Tumour staging requires examination under anaesthetic because the abdominal muscles are then completely relaxed, which allows determination of whether the cancer has invaded through the bladder wall into adjacent structures, which one clearly could not discern by cystoscopy alone.

It must also be stated that a negative urinary cytological examination does not necessarily exclude the presence of urothelial cancer, but a positive result is very useful in terms of establishing a diagnosis.

For carcinoma in situ, urinary cytology is a particularly useful investigation because random biopsy of the bladder mucosa, via cystoscopy, in such patients may not actually display a typically malignant histology. However, malignant cells are often shed into the urine in patients with carcinoma in situ, and these may well be detected via urinary cytology, especially in early morning specimens (EMU), due to their increased bladder dwell time.

Management of Urothelial Cancers

Clearly the exact medical and nursing management of individual patients will vary according to the clinical unit in question. Table 10.7, therefore, provides a summary of common approaches for specific types of urothelial cancer, and each of these will clearly require specific nursing care measures.

Table 10.7 Summary of management strategies for specific urothelial cancers

Location of tumour	Likely management

Kidney	Partial nephrectomy
	Radical nephrectomy
	    + /− radiotherapy
	    + /− systemic chemotherapy
	    + /− localised chemotherapy via nephrostomy

Ureter	Ureterectomy (partial/total)
	Ureteral reconstruction once tumour removed
	    + /− deep X-ray (DXR)
	    + /− systemic chemotherapy

Bladder	
Superficial tumours	Systemic chemotherapy (generally poor response) Intravesical chemotherapy (30–50 per cent response rate) Helmstein balloon distension Cryosurgery/laser surgery Mucosal stripping procedures Immunotherapy

More extensive tumours	Resection of varying depth according to nature of cancer
	    + /− DXR radiotherapy
	    + /− systemic chemotherapy
	    + /− Intravesical chemotherapy
	Cystectomy and conduit-type diversion
	Cystectomy and continent diversion
	Partial cystectomy (though not advocated by all centres because of the risks of tumour dissemination or further tumour growth in remaining segment)

Location of tumour	Likely management
Prostatic tumours (see Chapter 8)	Resection (classical TUR) Cryotherapy Thermotherapy (microwave) Testosterone antagonists or blockers of testosterone synthesis Synthetic oestrogens (generally, have very significant side-effects)

Penile	Partial or total amputation, depending on size of lesion at
	   diagnosis
	   $+/-$ DXR
	   $+/-$ systemic chemotherapy
	 Lymph node dissection if required

Testicular (e.g. seminoma, teratoma)	DXR (especially for seminoma, which is very radiosensitive) Orchidectomy Systemic chemotherapy (sperm save prior to treatment) Monthly tumour markers (e.g. AFP or HCG) to follow response to treatment, for up to 2 years

The majority of management strategies in Table 10.7 and their nursing implications are covered in other chapters, and therefore are not repeated here. However, tumours of the bladder and kidney and also testicular cancers are discussed more fully below.

Management of Bladder Cancer

As can be seen from Figure 10.3, bladder cancers can affect either very little of the overall mucosal surface, or they may be far more widespread (e.g. carcinoma in situ). Also, such urothelial cancers may either already have invaded deeply into the wall of the bladder by the time of presentation (e.g. T_3–T_4) or be far more 'superficial' in nature (e.g. T_a or T_1).

Bladder cancer usually presents with one of three principal appearances. These are:

1. *Papillary* – a 'fronded' appearance, projecting outward from the mucosal surface into the bladder lumen.

2. *Solid* – usually more invasive tumours, remaining within the bladder wall.

3. *Ulcerated/erythema type* – often mistaken for regions of cystitis or cystitis affecting the whole mucosal surface. (Biopsy, at time of cystoscopy, is therefore very important.)

Certain histological types of cancer are also common. Within the UK and Europe by far the most common (approximately 95 per cent) are transitional cell carcinomas, which reflect malignancy of the normal transitional cell lining of the urinary tract. The problem with such tumours is that they may rapidly spread to involve other parts of the urinary tract, and thus cancers originating within the bladder or kidney may undergo either retrograde or antegrade spread, sometimes with alarming rapidity.

Thus it is normal, if removing a kidney for cancer, to remove the associated ureter also (to minimise the risk of recurrence), or, if removing the bladder, also to remove the lower part of the ureter and the urethra.

Non-European Regions

Outside of Europe, other histological types of bladder cancer are more common, and transitional cell carcinoma in such regions is actually rarely seen. Thus, within parts of the African subcontinent, where schistosomiasis infection is endemic, squamous cell carcinoma of the bladder is far more common, as a result of the chronic irritation and inflammation caused to the mucosal lining of the bladder by the schistosomiasis parasite.

Squamous cell bladder cancers are seen within Europe, but far less commonly than transitional cell tumours and not usually associated with parasitic infestation. Squamous cell bladder carcinoma may also present within a poorly draining diverticulum where the constant irritant effect of urine ± infection (caused by urinary stasis within the diverticulum) can induce squamous metaplasia and then cancer.

Thus bladder diverticulae, which do not empty upon voiding, are potentially serious and require treatment. Squamous cell bladder carcinoma is therefore commonly associated with long-standing irritation to or inflammation of the bladder mucosa.

Adenocarcinoma is also seen within the bladder, as one might expect of a secretory (glandular) epithelium, such as that lining the bladder (which is mucus secreting). Most commonly, adenocarcinoma is a result of chronic infection, over a prolonged period, but actually can occur *de novo* anywhere within the bladder lumen, most commonly in the region of the vault from possible urachal remnants (embryological remnants of the bladder). Generally, adeno- and squamous cell carcinomas of the bladder carry a poorer prognosis because they are more dedifferentiated (i.e. less like their tissue of origin) than many transitional cell tumours.

Overall the most common sites for metastatic spread from malignant bladder tumours (and also prostatic cancer, because the lymphatic and venous drainage of the two organs is very similar) are the bony pelvis, upper femurs, rib cage and liver.

Staging and Treatment

An overview of staging and possible management is shown below.

Tumour in situ or Tumour stage 1

1. Intravesical chemotherapy

2. Cryotherapy

3. Laser therapy

4. Helmstein's dilatation

5. BCG treatment

6. Mucosal stripping

Recurrent, invasive tumour in situ may require cystectomy and urinary diversion to prevent advancement of the disease.

Tumour stage 2

1. Transurethral resection
  + /– Radiotherapy
  + /– Systemic chemotherapy
2. Cystectomy may be performed if viable tumour remains within the bladder six months after radiotherapy or if invasive cancer recurs after initially successful treatment.
3. Cystodiathermy is usually employed for superficial recurrences following radiotherapy.

Tumour stage 3

1. Radiotherapy is the mainstream treatment, especially in younger patients. This can then be followed by salvage cystectomy if recurrence occurs or if severe side-effects result (e.g. bladder contracture or fistulae formation, as a result of radiotherapy).
2. Conduit type diversion
3. Continent diversion, with the formation of a neo-bladder.
4. + /– Systemic chemotherapy

Tumour stage 4

This falls within the realm of palliative care. Radiotherapy may be used to help control pain caused by both local tumour spread and also bony metastases. Radiotherapy may also be useful in helping to reduce haematuria, should this be a problem. Intravesical formalin and internal iliac arterial embolisation may also be employed, to reduce blood loss caused by haematuria. Temporary urinary diversion (e.g. ureterostomy) may also be employed.

The major methods employed in the treatment of bladder tumours are shown, and some of these have already been covered in terms of nursing care (e.g. continent diversion, transurethral resection). However, over recent years a number of newer treatments have been developed and these are described below (in association with more established methods) along with the required nursing care of patients receiving them.

Superficial Bladder Tumours

Intravesical chemotherapy

This is generally used for superficial bladder cancers (e.g. T_a or T_1) or for regions of Tis (see Figure 10.2). Usually such patients will be treated as day cases. The principle behind this treatment is to expose the bladder mucosa to a uniform treatment with a chemotherapeutic agent, thus killing as many of the malignant cells as possible, but preventing or minimising damage to the normal mucosa.

Such chemotherapeutic agents directly disrupt the normal cell cycle, either by blocking synthesis of key components required for cellular division (e.g. ribonucleotides) or by disrupting the process of division itself (e.g. by inhibiting microtubule formation). They are instilled via a urinary catheter, which remains in situ for the duration of the treatment.

The patient is asked to lie first supine, then prone, then on either side (laterally), typically for approximately 15 minutes each – giving a total dwell time of 60 minutes. A key problem with such an approach is that the agents used are often very irritant (as one might expect) and therefore not all patients may be able to retain them for the full treatment period. Thus, patients require both support and encouragement during treatment, and perhaps simple diversional measures such as music, reading or conversation with the nurse. Normally, patients are asked to void prior to the instillation of the drug, to reduce the likelihood of dilution and/or voiding during treatment. At the end of the specified time period (usually 1–2 hours in total) the drug is then allowed to drain out, and the catheter removed.

The patient should be warned, prior to voiding, that his/her urine is likely to be coloured, and that this is normal, especially as some of the drugs used are red in colour and give the impression of haematuria for the first or second void. Once the patient has passed urine successfully he/she is then encouraged to drink normally, whilst the voiding pattern is monitored to ensure that a normal pattern for that individual has been restored (e.g. cystitis and frequency are common for the first 24–48 hours after the procedure).

Usually a series of treatments is given over 4–8 weeks (approximately one per week) and the patient is then re-endoscoped at 3 months, to assess the response to treatment. Clearly, instillation of such anticancer drugs (because of their inherent toxicity) requires suitable precautions (e.g. eye protection, and gloves whilst drawing up and administration) on the part of all staff.

Patient responses to such intravesical chemotherapy may vary, but only 50 per cent of patients actually show any response at all. Thus, intravesical chemotherapy is not a particularly successful treatment for superficial bladder tumours.

Laser therapy

The initials LASER stand for Light Amplification by Stimulated Emission of Radiation. In essence, particles within a laser medium are raised to a high energy state by the application of energy from a suitable external power source. These unstable, excited particles then return to their normal resting state via a photon release of light energy (i.e. stimulated emission of radiation). In a laser, such photon release itself is caused by the impact of a separate photon, and thus the process can rapidly generate a chain reaction which effectively amplifies the light to very high energy levels. (For a detailed consideration of laser therapy, within urology, see Etchells, 1988).

Simply, lasers with a frequency range within the infrared region of the visible spectrum are used for incision, vaporisation of tissue and/or coagulation (i.e. thermal mechanisms). In contrast, lasers of lower frequency interact with naturally pigmented tissues or with compounds added to cells (i.e. photosensitisers), inducing cellular disruption and cell death.

Not all lasers are suitable for endoscopic use, however. The CO_2 laser, for example, does not function well urologically, because this wavelength is absorbed by fluid within the bladder.

The most versatile laser for urological use is the Nd:Yag (yttrium aluminium garnet) and this can be used either as an alternative to conventional treatment or as an additional treatment following the electroexcision of tumour, via cautery. The Nd:Yag laser can thus induce bulk tissue necrosis, which allows it to be used for the destruction of bladder cancers. Because of its infrared wavelength (1064 nm) the Nd:Yag beam is invisible to the naked eye: thus it is used with a so-called 'pilot' laser (helium–neon) which provides a red light beam, which can then be aimed on to the target area. Activation of the Nd:Yag beam increases the temperature of tissues within the target area to approximately 60°C, which is more than sufficient to denature most of the intracellular proteins.

Thus, even though the gross architecture of the treated area remains intact, the cells composing it die. The wavelength of the Nd:Yag laser means that such thermal damage to tissues is possible up to a depth of 1 cm and the laser also has the advantage that it can be directed down a fine, flexible, quartz fibre, fed down the channel of a suitable endoscope. Fowler (1991) reports that such laser energy can be transmitted either by specialised 'contact tips' which allow the fibre to penetrate below the tissue surface or the beam can simply be applied to the surface alone. For such 'non-contact' application, the laser is usually held between 0.25 and 0.75 cm away from the tumour surface, and pulses of less than 5 seconds applied to the tumour.

Clearly, laser treatment requires strict precautions to protect the eyes of both operator and patient and thus safety goggles/glasses of appropriate colour (this will vary according to the type and frequency of the laser) are mandatory for both staff and patient. (If anaesthetised, the patient's eyes may be taped closed). Black instrumentation is also needed, to prevent reflection. A comprehensive consideration of such safety methods is given by Etchells (1988).

Patients generally report only minor discomfort following laser treatment of superficial bladder cancers, such as suprapubic burning pain or 'prickling' type pains. Fowler (1991) reports that this type of postoperative pain can be avoided/ lessened by moving the laser beam during treatment so that local heating of adjacent healthy tissues is reduced. Also, installation of 20 ml lignocaine solution (1 or 2 per cent) into the bladder, 20 minutes prior to the procedure, has been used to reduce the sensitivity of the urothelium.

Laser treatment produces very little bleeding, such that postoperative urethral catheterisation is usually unnecessary (unlike endoscopic resection, where post-operative loss may be significant) and thus patients can be treated on a day case basis. Follow-up of such patients would seem to indicate that the rate of tumour recurrence is no more than for other treatments and has the advantage of being suitable for day case use.

However, although lasers reduce the time the patient stays in hospital, they remain extremely expensive. Safety precautions must be used and rigidly enforced to protect both the users and patient from retinal damage. All surfaces which could reflect must be dulled and doors alarmed and locked to prevent unshielded people entering during treatment. According to Fowler (1991), the main danger from the use of the Nd:Yag laser, in treating bladder cancer, is late perforation of the bowel, caused by heating of bowel loops adjacent to the bladder wall. As the wall of the heated bowel then begins to necrose (because the cells die) intestinal enzymes will begin to digest the necrotic tissue, resulting in the possibility of perforation up to 72 hours after laser treatment. Using limited power settings on the laser seems to reduce the incidence of this complication to very low rates.

Thus, the nursing care of patients undergoing laser treatment is minimal, especially if they are receiving their treatment under local anaesthetic. Clearly, adequate preparation and explanation are vital, as is support during the procedure. It also should be ascertained that the patient has voided postoperatively, and that urinary bleeding is not significant. Likewise, monitoring the patient for pain is an important aspect of postoperative care.

Photodynamic Therapy

Photodynamic therapy (PDT) is a major application of laser therapy, relevant to urology. Photodynamic therapy is a method whereby superficial solid cancers, containing a previously injected photosensitiser, are destroyed with a laser beam of suitable frequency. Red (633 nm) is common but green and other colours are also used.

The patient receives an intravenous injection of a photosensitising agent (e.g. a haematoporphyrin derivative or its purified form, dihaematoporphyrin) which is then taken up by both normal and cancerous tissue. Cancer cells, because of their altered metabolism, retain such drugs, whereas they are gradually removed from normal cells and excreted via the kidneys in urine.

Normal cells when exposed to laser energy, suffer a reaction similar to sunburn (just as people with porphyria suffer if they go out in bright sunlight) which normally subsides after a few days and thus cell death is avoided because of the lower concentration of drug within such cells. Cancer cells, however, retain far more of the pigment and therefore are much more susceptible to damage and death. Thus, if a laser is applied to a localised area of bladder tumour, effective cellular destruction should occur with minimal damage to other normal tissues. Patients are prepared for surgery, having received the photosensitising drug beforehand.

In theatre, the patient's eyes are protected and the tumour then treated with the laser under direct visual control. Post-procedure, the patient is observed for pain, urinary output and voiding pattern.

Commonly patients can experience frequency and suprapubic pain, and usually require analgesia. They may also be given prophylactic antibiotic treatment. When discharged the patient is warned to stay away from bright sunlight for 2–3 weeks until such time as the photosensitising compound has been metabolised.

Irritation can be experienced for up to 3 months and tissue fragments (e.g. sloughed off urothelium) or blood can also appear in the urine. Patients may also suffer bladder contracture, though significant contracture would appear to be uncommon. Patients clearly require comprehensive information, in a manner that they can comprehend, especially as this type of treatment remains very new within the UK.

Patients receiving PDT are followed up at 3 months with a check endoscopy and urinary cytology, to assess response to treatment.

Helmstein's Balloon Dilation

Helmstein's balloon dilation is a method of treating superficial bladder cancer which utilises the mechanism of applying pressure, directly to the bladder mucosa, of sufficient magnitude and time to induce mucosal necrosis (thus killing the cancer cells).

Helmstein's dilation uses a balloon (of typical volume 300–500 ml) incorporated into a modified urethral catheter. This is then inserted, with the patient under general or spinal anaesthetic (in the lithotomy position), and water is then pumped into the balloon under pressure. Thus the catheter 'balloon' comes into contact with the whole mucosa of the bladder and, once arterial pressure (i.e. $\geqslant 120$ mmHg) is reached, the balloon is left inflated for approximately 40–60 minutes. Clearly there is a danger of inducing severe necrosis of the bladder wall or rupture or causing permanent muscular/nervous damage to the bladder. Tumours may also recur if all the cancer cells are not removed by the initial treatment.

Postoperatively, patients require the same generalised care as a patient who has undergone general or spinal anaesthesia, and also observation of voiding to ensure that the detrusor muscle is intact and a normal pattern of voiding restored. Patients should also be observed for any sign of perforation, such as pain or urinary retention. Abdominal pain and guarding could indicate an intraperitoneal rupture, and pain in the region of the lower back is suggestive of extraperitoneal bladder rupture, with fluid accumulating within the retroperitoneal space.

Patients are usually re-endoscoped 3 months after treatment, to assess the tumour response, during which biopsies will again be taken from the bladder mucosa. A series of Helmstein dilations may be given.

Bladder Thermotherapy

Thermotherapy of the bladder remains a very new development in the treatment of superficial bladder cancers, and really falls within the realm of an experimental technique offered, at present, only in a small number of centres.

Thermotherapy of the bladder is based upon the same principle as that of prostatic thermotherapy, namely microwave energy applied to localised areas of tissue, via a modified flexible endoscope. (A metal endoscope can not be used because of heating effects.) Such localised thermotherapy is designed to cause extensive damage to intracellular proteins and thus cell death within the specified treatment area. The treatment is usually performed under local anaesthetic, as a day case, but its efficacy remains debatable at this time.

Patients are discharged once they have voided, and should be advised that some haematuria and loss of tissue fragments may occur after the procedure.

Thermotherapy of the bladder mucosa (i.e. to areas of superficial tumour growth) poses the same potential risk as that of laser therapy, regarding the heating of adjacent bowel loops, which could then necrose and subsequently perforate.

Cryosurgery

Cryosurgery is a further 'experimental' procedure at this time, which still awaits comprehensive evaluation and, like thermotherapy, is offered only in a very few centres within the UK.

Cryosurgery utilises a specialised probe, inserted into the bladder under direct vision (via an endoscope), which then has the ability to become extremely cold, very quickly. The probe is applied to areas of localised tumour growth, and the intense cold generated by the probe is then sufficient to kill cells within the immediate vicinity, by destroying the integrity of cellular membranes.

Patients are usually treated as day cases and should be advised that some urinary blood loss and/or loss of tissue fragments may occur during the immediate period following the procedure.

Biological Response Modifiers (BRM)

Biological response modifiers are naturally occurring proteins which form the basis of the genetic treatment known as cancer immunotherapy. Such immunotherapy is based upon the assumption that if the host immune system is able to recognise invading tumour cells as foreign, then they will be targeted and destroyed by immunoactive cells and proteins. Thus, biological response modifiers can either augment *or* both augment *and* direct overall immune function. At present, such treatments remain experimental and regimens are changing constantly.

Three major subdivisions of BRM are recognised. These are:

1. Proteins which restore, enhance or modify mechanisms of immunity (e.g. interferon and interleukin-2)

2. Cells that have direct anticancer activity (e.g. monoclonal antibodies)

3. Proteins which have other biological effects, such as interfering with the ability of cancer cells to survive or metastasise, or undergo malignant transformation (e.g. bacterial agents such as Bacillus Calmette-Guérin).

Two of the above categories have particular relevance to the treatment of superficial bladder cancer, and these are discussed below.

Interferon

It was discovered in 1957 that cells produce a specific substance which helps them defend very effectively against invading pathogens (i.e. viruses). The substance was named interferon because it seemed to 'interfere' with viral replication and also to protect bodily cells from infection.

Interferon was also found, in the early 1960s, to possess antitumour potential. However, it was not possible, until the advances of molecular biology in the early 1980s (e.g. via cloning of genes and then insertion into a suitable vector) to produce enough of the substance for clinical testing. It was then discovered that interferon was not a single protein but in fact an aggregate of proteins, and could be divided into three major subtypes, alpha, beta and gamma.

Interferons belong to the same group of biological response modifiers as do the group of compounds known as interleukins, and this collective grouping are called the lymphokines. The lymphokines (and thus interferon and interleukin) are produced by specific white blood cells, namely the activated T lymphocytes.

Interferon would appear to perform three major functions. These are:

1. *Inhibition of DNA replication in viruses*, once these have invaded cells, and also protection of the infected cell from invasion by other viruses.

2. *Interaction with T lymphocytes*, stimulating the production of other cellular products. Such T-cell products then signal monocytes, natural killer cells and other T lymphocytes to recognise and destroy cancer cells.

3. *Inhibition of the growth and division of cancer cells*. It also stimulates the expression of HLA and tumour-associated antigens onto the surface of cancer cells, making such cells more recognisable to the immune system.

It is not understood exactly how interferon causes specific types of cancer to regress although in some types of tumour (e.g. renal cell carcinoma) its effect seems to be dose related, suggesting direct cytotoxic activity.

Alpha-interferon has been more fully studied than either beta- or gamma-interferon. The maximum tolerated dose is dependent on the route, the administration schedule and its frequency, but generally not more than 30 megaunits/M^2 are given daily and not more than three such doses are given per week.

Intermittent dose schedules seem more effective than daily doses, because the build-up of serum interferon levels can suppress some aspects of immune response. Once given (usually intramuscularly or via slow intravenous infusion) key nursing responsibilities centre upon support of the patient and observing for significant side-effects.

Acute side-effects include fever (up to 40°C), rigors, headache, muscle pain, fatigue, malaise and confusion. Tolerance to side-effects generally occurs with increasing treatment frequency.

Interferon-induced toxicity is common with doses of greater than 1 megaunit/M^2, becoming more severe as the dosage is increased. Such toxicity can also be seen with moderate to high doses of interferon if given for longer than 1 month and can manifest as unacceptable fatigue, anorexia, weight loss, confusion, leucopenia and possible problems with liver enzymes (e.g. transaminase).

Less severe toxic side-effects, which are usually reversible once treatment has stopped, include nausea, vomiting, diarrhoea, hypotension, central nervous system depression, paraesthesia and proteinuria.

Interferon should be used with caution in patients with a history of cardiovascular disease, because acute cardiac failure with arrhythmia and/or ischaemia can occur.

Interleukin-2

Interleukin-2 is more commonly used within the USA but has been trialled within the UK for superficial bladder carcinoma. It can be administered by intravenous bolus injection, continuous i.v. infusion, subcutaneous injection, intrahepatic infusion or by peritoneal infusion. The pattern of dose frequency can vary, from three times a week, a weekly 24-hour infusion, a weekly i.v. bolus or by continuous infusion over 5–6 days (usually by micrograms per kilogram body weight).

Interleukin-2 affects every major bodily system and patients must therefore be relatively well before receiving treatment. As in the case of interferon, side-effects are varied and can include malaise, flu-like symptoms, nausea, skin desquamation, anorexia, peripheral oedema, vasodilation and dramatic hypotension due to 'third spacing' (this reverses rapidly when treatment is stopped). Most symptoms resolve within 96 hours of stopping interleukin-2 treatment.

Both interferon and interleukin-2 may result in the patient becoming drowsy or confused and memory loss may also be seen. Thus the nursing care of patients centres upon observation for and assisting in the alleviation of such side-effects. To date, both interferon and interleukin-2 have been used on a trial basis only, and remain essentially experimental treatments.

Bacillus Calmette-Guérin (BCG) Therapy

The use of BCG to treat cancer in humans was first reported in 1935. Modern usage began in 1969 when Mathe et al (1969) demonstrated the successful use of BCG in the treatment of acute childhood leukaemia. Morales et al (1976) then reported the application of BCG in the management of bladder cancer.

BCG is now recognised as an effective biological agent for the treatment and prevention of recurrence of superficial bladder cancers. BCG therapy is currently used more in North America than in the UK and some reservations have been expressed within the UK regarding the long-term effectiveness and potential complications of intravesical BCG therapy.

Several vaccine strains are available (e.g. Pasteur and Evans: previously Glaxo) and these differ in the number of colony-forming units per ml of solution (e.g. Pasteur 6×10^8 CFU/ml, Evans $1–5 \times 10^9$ CFU/ml).

Mechanism of Action

Numerous mechanisms have been proposed for the effects of BCG upon urothelial tumours. These include sensitisation of lymphoid cells against tumour cell antigens (thus, lymphoid cells are then more likely to attack the cancer), activation of macrophages (which then cause lysis or inhibition of cancer cells) and increased natural killer cell activity.

The production of interleukin-2 has also been reported as a response to BCG treatment in the urine of patients and this may constitute a further mechanism of action.

Other mechanisms centre upon enhanced immunological recognition of cancer cells, similar to the process seen in autoimmune disease. Clearly, however, the exact mode of action is, as yet, not understood.

Patients receiving BCG are those with T_a and T_1 tumours. It is also increasingly being used for Tis (carcinoma in situ), especially in those patients who have not responded to intravesical chemotherapy.

Prior to treatment, all visible papillary-like lesions are removed by transurethral resection or laser, and multiple biopsies are also taken. Urinary cytology also forms an important assessment for gauging response to treatment.

Administration

BCG therapy is started within weeks of endoscopy. Mukherjee et al (1992) suggest a 10-day limit for treatment initiation, because the disrupted urothelium may facilitate localisation of bacterial antigens (i.e. cellular components) to areas of previous tumour growth.

BCG vaccine, freshly prepared, is mixed with between 50 and 200 ml normal saline, and administered intravesically via an 'indwelling' urethral catheter. The BCG suspension is then kept within the bladder for 1–2 hours, with the patient lying alternately supine, prone and laterally to 'coat' the urothelium evenly with suspension.

The bladder is then emptied and the catheter removed. Clearly, the catheter must be inserted and removed with care, to minimise urethral trauma. However, should bleeding ensue, BCG therapy should not be used for at least 48 hours, to avoid bacterial inoculation into blood and the induction of a possible bacteraemia.

Initially, patients were also given BCG intradermally, to try to create plasma antibodies to BCG, so that its effects would then only be exerted within the bladder. (i.e. any organisms absorbed intravenously would therefore be destroyed). However, this practice has been abandoned because no value has been demonstrated from such 'additional' dosage.

Usually, 6-weekly BCG installations are given. Patients then undergo re-endoscopy at 12 weeks, with associated biopsy and urinary cytology, to assess response to BCG therapy. If complete remission has occurred (i.e. no recurrence on biopsy and negative urinary cytology), a monthly maintenance dose can be given, with regular re-endoscopy (i.e. 3–6-monthly). However, BCG treatment within the UK is so recent that no standard protocol has yet been developed. Also, the need for maintenance therapy is not firmly established at this time.

One protocol which has been suggested includes weekly administration for 6 weeks, biweekly twice, 3-monthly for 2 years, 6-monthly for 2 years and then yearly after that. A further protocol simply suggests six weekly installations, then no further treatment. Others suggest six weekly installations, then a further six weekly installations if tumour recurrence occurs.

Nursing Implications

These include support of patients during installation of BCG suspension, effective safe catheterisation and catheter management, and ensuring the patient is able to void after the procedure. Also adequate explanation is clearly vital.

Side-effects/Complications of BCG Therapy

Patients may experience haematuria and dysuria lasting between 2 and 7 days on average. In addition, BCG treatment requires a high frequency of urethral catheterisation; therefore skilled aseptic practice is essential.

Mukherjee et al (1992) report that the effects of BCG seem to be localised to the urothelium, because some patients found to be free of tumour on re-endoscopy also had coexisting metastatic disease (though the number of such patients was very small). Further, Lamm et al (1991) (cited in Mukherjee et al, 1992) has reported serious side-effects from BCG therapy, in a study consisting of 2589 patients. These include fever ($> 39°C$), haematuria, granulomatous prostatitis, joint pain, epididymitis, sepsis, skin rashes, ureteric obstruction and bladder contraction. Clearly, therefore, at this time much remains to be discovered about the exact mechanism of action of BCG and its optimum administration regimen, and nursing staff may need to support patients particularly because of this.

Renal Use

BCG has also now been used in the treatment of some renal cancers, especially those in the pelvicalyceal region, where the BCG suspension is administered via a nephrostomy tube directly into the renal pelvis.

Overall, BCG would appear a very useful alternative to the use of intravesical chemotherapy for the treatment of superficial bladder cancer, though it is clearly still a very new biological agent which remains to be fully evaluated.

Systemic Chemotherapy

Systemic chemotherapeutic agents are sometimes used in the treatment of superficial bladder cancer, but generally their role is more pronounced in patients with more advanced tumours. Commonly administered drugs include cyclosphosphamide and methotrexate. Generally, however, such drugs have a limited role because both bladder and prostatic cancer are usually poorly responsive to systemic agents. Also, such drugs can cause profound side-effects, which clearly require skilled and coordinated nursing and medical management. Systemic chemotherapy may also induce problems with wound healing, should subsequent surgery be required.

Mucosal Stripping

The treatment of mucosal stripping is founded upon the fact that recurrences of superficial bladder tumours usually arise from areas of unstable mucosa known to exist in this disease. Mucosal stripping is a method which aims to remove the entire vesical mucosa, to prevent tumour recurrence.

Method

Under spinal or general anaesthesia, the anterior wall of the bladder is exposed suprapubically. The bladder is secured with sutures, with the peritoneal reflection displaced upwards, and the wall of the bladder incised. The internal surface can then be inspected and the number and nature of tumours confirmed. Ureteric catheters are then inserted into each ureter. A submucosal injection of normal saline solution is then inserted at the incisional margin, such that it forms a small wheal and the entire mucosal membrane is then elevated from the underlying mucosal layer. Thus, a plane of cleavage is developed between the elevated mucosa and the muscularis layer. The mucosal membrane can then be removed as an intact sheet with the muscle layer left beneath. Thus, tumours which have not infiltrated beneath the mucosa will be removed along with the mucosal membrane.

Haemostasis, via electrocoagulation, especially to points of previous tumour growth, is then performed and the bladder closed and the ureteral catheters brought to the surface suprapubically. These are then removed 2–3 days after the operation. Patients also usually have a three-way (urethral) irrigation catheter inserted, as severe haematuria may commonly occur following surgery. Bladder irrigation can then be performed, should this be required.

In many ways, therefore, the nursing care of such patients is similar to that of patients who have undergone transurethral resection of bladder tumours, except that these patients initially also possess ureteric catheters.

The problem with mucosal stripping is that any procedure used to treat urothelial cancer is rarely curative, because of the generalised epithelial involvement and instability of the remaining urothelium, which may then become the site of new tumours. Connolly (1972) found that though the mucosa may have been macroscopically stripped, microscopic islands of epithelium remained. Further, in man, it was even more difficult to remove all the mucosa, due to trabeculation; thus such islands of urothelium were even more likely to remain. These islands of mucosa and unstripped urothelium are sources of epithelial regeneration and, because the entire urothelium is often involved in bladder cancer, mucosal stripping would seem to offer little benefit.

The lining of the internal bladder surface is usually regenerated within 4 weeks of treatment and complete regeneration of the transitional cell epithelium normally occurs within 3 months. Further, mucosal stripping assumes that bladder carcinoma has a low malignancy, which may not always be the case (e.g. Tis can be very invasive). During the stage of mucosal regeneration (normally 3–5 weeks) complications such as continuous bleeding from the 'sore' surface, reabsorption via the stripped bladder wall or circular stricture can develop. Also, the ureterovesical junction presents a particular problem and to prevent ureteral stenosis a rim of mucosa is usually left around the ureteric orifice, which would again seem to undermine the overall procedure.

Stage 2 Bladder Cancers

Stage 2 tumours, by definition, are more invasive, and around 15 per cent of bladder cancers fall into this category. Thus, the management of such patients centres upon methods which penetrate beyond the superficial layers of the bladder mucosa.

The main method of treatment employed is that of endoscopic resection (which also has the advantage of allowing staging to be performed) in association with radiotherapy or chemotherapy. Resection is performed under general or spinal anaesthesia, using diathermy and cautery (i.e. high-frequency electric current, in a suitable liquid medium such as glycine), which is exactly the same method employed for transurethral prostatic resection.

Patients normally return from theatre with a three-way urethral irrigation catheter in situ, which remains for the initial 24–48 hour period, along with isotonic normal saline bladder irrigation if required (i.e. if significant haematuria is present postoperatively, which could cause obstruction from clot formation). The urinary catheter is removed when the urine is a suitable colour (approximately 24 hours postoperatively) and the patient can be discharged once he/she is voiding adequately. Thus, care of such patients, apart from routine postoperative measures, centres upon catheter and/or irrigation management (if either is present) and ensuring a normal voiding pattern is restored once the catheter is removed.

Most units will obtain an MSU specimen once the catheter is removed, to screen for possible urinary infection. However, the use of testing sticks containing leucocyte esterase and nitrite assay pads are sufficiently accurate to render this practice unnecessary.

Patients may also receive radiotherapy and/or intravesical chemotherapy, depending on the nature of the tumour and the degree of differentiation (gained from histology). If a residual mass is palpable in the bladder wall following resection (i.e. on EUA) or if the cancer is poorly differentiated, then radiotherapy and/or cystectomy is usually advised.

Patients with both superficial and T_2 tumours will be re-endoscoped to a suitable regimen for at least 10 years, to ensure no recurrence occurs and also to monitor the effectiveness of treatment given. (Most units advocate that if an individual patient remains free of recurrence for 10 consecutive years, then no further checks are required.) Thus, if a superficial or T_2 tumour is diagnosed and treated the patient is likely to be re-endoscoped 3-monthly for 12 months, 6-monthly for 2 years and then yearly for 10 years, assuming no recurrence is seen. Bullock et al (1989) state that if viable cancer is present in the bladder 6 months after radiotherapy, or if an invasive tumour recurs, then cystectomy is the treatment of choice. However, if the recurrence is superficial following radiotherapy then treatment by cystodiathermy is indicated.

Stage 3 Bladder Cancers

Stage 3 cancers of the bladder are potentially far more serious in terms of threat to the patient's survival and may involve very profound management measures which require intensive nursing care. By definition, such tumours have already invaded deeply into the muscular wall of the bladder and will spread outside the bladder if left untreated. Also, as for all stages of bladder cancer, metastatic disease may already be present at the time of presentation, and the more likely is this process as the staging of the tumour advances (i.e. $T_1 \rightarrow T_4$). Stage 3 bladder cancers are usually treated initially with radiotherapy though they will often bring the patient into the realm of cystectomy and either conduit-type diversion (traditional) or neobladder reconstruction (far more recent) with removal of the urethra in both cases.

Some centres advocate the use of aggressive radiotherapy prior to surgery, as some tumours may respond and thus reduce in size and/or vascularity, which makes their subsequent removal easier (so-called radiotherapy and salvage cystectomy). Overall, however, this policy may not be a good one because if the tumour fails to respond to radiotherapy, then this means that it will be more advanced by the time of surgery and also metastatic disease is correspondingly more likely.

Wound healing problems are more likely following radiotherapy, and therefore earlier surgical intervention is common, with follow-up radiotherapy later on. The combination of surgery and radiotherapy thus appears to offer a better prognosis than either in isolation. In addition, pelvic node dissection may be added to cystectomy if CT scanning reveals regional nodal disease (present in some 30 per cent of patients with T_3 disease). If there is recurrence following treatment with radiotherapy alone, or side-effects such as bleeding or bladder contracture, fistulae or incontinence, then cystectomy and some form of urinary diversion are advocated. Generally, systemic chemotherapy for advanced bladder cancer is a poor treatment option, as such bladder tumours are often unresponsive to systemic agents.

Patients may experience profound problems with body image and body image change, especially as operative procedures such as cystectomy, because of the disruption to pelvic nerves, result in a virtually 100 per cent impotence rate for males and also problems with orgasm and pelvic sensation in both sexes. Such problems may also be combined with a new urinary stoma. Therefore, helping such patients begin the process of coming to terms with such change is a key nursing responsibility.

The exact nature and nursing management of the types of surgery undertaken for such T_3-type tumours (e.g. conduit diversions or continent reservoir formation) are described in this chapter and in Chapter 7.

Prior to such surgery it is essential that the nodal and metastatic status (if any) of the patient is ascertained accurately, because such surgery is not undertaken in patients with existing metastasis. Thus, included in the preoperative work-up will be ultrasound, CT scanning (and/or NMR scanning) and pelvic X-ray studies, to try to ensure that no existing metastatic disease is present. In this way, hopefully only those patients with tumours localised to the bladder are therefore exposed to the very significant stress associated with cystectomy and diversion or neobladder formation.

Cystectomy

Cystectomy, with some form of urinary conduit formation, forms the traditional treatment for cases of T_3 bladder tumours or for extensive (normally > 60 per cent of the bladder mucosa), aggressive carcinoma in situ of the bladder. The operation is extremely extensive, taking 3–4 hours on average, and can have a very significant impact on both the patient's physical and psychological well being.

A midline incision is utilised, and the bladder than mobilised and removed, along with all of the urethra. A loop of ileum is then mobilised on its mesentery, and sutured at one end, to create the ileal 'conduit'. The ureters are then tunnelled into this, obliquely, to create an anti-reflux valve, and the open end of the loop then brought out on to the surface of the skin as a permanent, urinary stoma. The midline incision is then closed, and several drains left in situ, including a 'sump' drain, which provides drainage to the area within the abdominal cavity where the bladder was originally present.

Due to the nature of the surgery, and especially due to exploration and/or dissection deep within the abdominal cavity, pelvic nerve damage invariably occurs, resulting in an impotence rate for men of close to 100 per cent and subsequent problems with libido and/or orgasm in both sexes.

Cystectomy is therefore only normally undertaken where a 'cure' is likely, and the bladder tumour has been shown to be localised within the bladder wall (i.e. there is no obvious spread into other abdominal structures, or obvious evidence of metastases).

For patients presenting with T_4 bladder cancers, palliative urinary diversion can be undertaken. Either the ureters can be removed from the bladder, and brought out on to the surface of the abdomen as a ureterostomy, or a bilateral nephrostomy may be performed. Both of these options will allow urinary drainage and also relieve the haematuria and systemic blood loss, which can be very significant in cases of advanced bladder cancer. T_4 cancers commonly obstruct the lower ends of the ureters, and if palliative diversion is not undertaken, acute renal failure is then a common cause of death for such patients.

Patient Preparation

As cystectomy is such major surgery, patient preparation is extensive and includes:

1. Ideally, admit 2–3 days preoperatively.

2. Psychological preparation/information is vital.

3. Blood assay, this will usually include:
Full blood count, urea and plasma electrolytes, plasma glucose, hepatitis B and HIV screen, liver function tests, blood coagulation screen, blood grouping and the cross matching of at least 4 units.

4. Chest X-ray and electrocardiogram.

5. Midstream urine (for culture and antibiotic sensitivity of any isolated pathogens).

6. Urinary cytology.

7. Intravenous urogram and/or urological ultrasound.

8. CT scan or NMR scanning.

9. Bone scan, for skeletal survey.

10. Early involvement of the stoma therapist/nurse.

11. Blood transfusion, if preoperative haematuria and blood loss have resulted in significant anaemia.

12. Bowel preparation as per unit.

13. Consent.

14. Nil by mouth for 4–6 hours prior to surgery. The patient will usually be restricted to 'clear fluids' only, prior to this period.

15. Subcutaneous heparin and the fitting of thrombo-embolytic deterrent stockings, according to policy of unit.

16. Abdominal shave, as close to time of surgery as possible.

17. A mild sedative, to cover the period prior to the premedication, on the day of surgery, can be beneficial.

Also, it is important to assess the patient's peripheral veins, preoperatively, as he/she is likely to remain nil by mouth for a period of at least 5–7 days, in the postoperative period. If peripheral access is poor, then a tunnelled subclavian or jugular line (i.e. a central line) can be inserted preoperatively. The patient can then be fed preoperatively (if required), and also given all of his/her postoperative fluid replacement via this line. This then saves the patient both the pain and the discomfort caused by the repeated siting of ineffective, temporary, peripheral lines.

Specific postoperative care

The specific postoperative care of patients undergoing cystectomy centres upon:

1. A midline abdominal wound, with several drains.

2. A gastrostomy or nasogastric tube, to decompress the stomach and also allow effective aspiration of stomach contents.

A gastrostomy tube (essentially, a wide-bore Foley catheter, which is inserted into the stomach during surgery, and then brought out via the skin, in the same way as is a conventional drain) is a particularly effective option for these patients, as it eliminates the nasal and throat discomfort/pain, normally associated with a nasogastric tube.

In patients who are likely to be nil by mouth for 5–7 days (as are most cystectomy patients who have a conduit fashioned), this is a very significant advantage, in terms of patient care.

3. Two ureteric splints/stents will be sited, during surgery. It is normal for the ends of these to be visible, through the stoma bag, in the postoperative period. These remain in situ for 7–10 days, on average, and pass from the stomal loop up into the lower third of each ureter. Their function is to splint/stent the ureteric anastomosis site into the loop of ileum, whilst healing is occurring, and thus maintain the urinary flow (urine may otherwise leak, or the ureters may be obstructed by oedema, in this area, as a result of the surgery). The splints are not usually sutured in place, and either fall out spontaneously, or are gently removed by traction.

4. A peripheral or central line, for intravenous access and fluid replacement. All input and output volumes will clearly be recorded.

5. Appropriate observation of vital signs, to include urine output.

6. Stomal observations, to check blood supply of the stoma (i.e. colour, warmth, sensation, position). It is also common to see mucus in the urine of these patients, which derives from the mucus-secreting epithelium of the ileal loop.

7. Analgesics must be appropriate and given in effective doses. A subcutaneous opioid pump or epidural analgesic is ideal, during the initial postoperative period.

8. Physiotherapy, to encourage deep breathing and coughing, is obviously important, but only realistic if the patient's pain is effectively controlled.

9. Intravenous antibiotic therapy is likely.

10. Effective wound management and removal of wound drains as appropriate.

11. Gradual reintroduction to alimentation according to clinical status.

12. Early postoperative ambulation.

13. Allowing the patient time and opportunity for emotional reaction to the surgery and a new stoma. Patients should be involved in the care of their stoma as soon as this seems appropriate.

Apart from these specific measures, patients undergoing cystectomy require the routine postoperative care of any patient who has received major abdominal surgery.

In the context of bladder cancer, patients may take longer to recover from surgery, either because of preoperative malnutrition (caused by the tumour) or problems with wound healing (e.g. wound breakdown or fistulae formation) caused by radiotherapy and/or chemotherapy, in the preoperative period.

The stoma therapist/nurse fulfils a vital role in the postoperative care of patients undergoing cystectomy. This role will not only include education and advice regarding the ordering of stomal equipment (e.g. flanges, bags, etc.) but may also involve counselling or referral of the patient to other, more appropriate agencies, should problems such as impotence or loss of libido be a significant and ongoing problem in the postoperative period.

T_4 Bladder Tumours

As shown in Figure 10.2 (earlier in this chapter), T_4 tumours have invaded through the bladder wall into adjacent structures (e.g. prostate in males, uterus in females) and are thus 'fixed' and therefore cannot be surgically removed. Also, it is usual to find significant metastatic disease in such patients and, for these reasons, the treatment and nursing management of such patients with T_4 tumours therefore falls within the realm of palliative care. Common methods for managing such patients therefore include:

1. *Temporary urinary diversion* If the cancer is blocking urinary outflow at the level of the bladder neck, or is blocking the ureteric orifices, then ureterostomy or nephrostomy is likely to be undertaken. (Renal failure is often the terminal event in advanced bladder cancer due to this process of ureteric obstruction.) Temporary urinary diversion may also be undertaken if extensive haematuria is resulting from a bladder cancer, and thus causing severe anaemia in such patients (intravesical formalin and embolisation of the internal iliac artery has also been used to try to control this).

2. *Nephrostomy* if the renal pelvis is obstructed.

3. *Effective, potent analgesia* (e.g. continuous opioid infusion), as pain from both invasion of soft tissues and bony metastases is common.

4. *Radiotherapy* for palliation of bony pain (e.g. directed to pelvis or femurs) or to reduce tumour size and thus relieve compression on soft tissues or nerves, or nervous invasion by cancer cells. Radiotherapy may also be used for relief of haematuria, but clearly such X-ray treatment needs balancing against the likely side-effects, due to the bladder being low down within the pelvic cavity (and thus the intestinal tract is likely to receive radiation).

5. *Psychological care*, as for all terminally ill patients, taking account of the grieving process etc.

6. *Other care measures*, as for any patient with a terminal illness.

Thus, the effective treatment of bladder cancer at each stage of tumour development requires skilled and insightful nursing management.

Table 10.8 shows the approximate 5-year survival rates of various types of bladder carcinoma.

Table 10.8 Bladder tumour stage and likely prognosis
(Bullock et al, 1989)

Tumour stage	Prognosis*
Tis	30–40%
T_a	90–95%
T_1	40–75%
T_2	55%
T_3	25%
T_4	5–10%

*Percentage of patients likely to reach 5 years' survival.

Bullock et al (1989) suggest that lower risk bladder tumours include small, well-defined cancers (e.g. T_a, G_1), single tumours (i.e. affecting only a small part of the urothelium) and malignant disease where the rest of the bladder is essentially normal on biopsy. Conversely, high risk cancers, in terms of survival, include large, poorly differentiated tumours (e.g. T_2–T_3, G_2–G_3), large areas of mucosal dysplasia (i.e. multiple areas of premalignancy), multiple tumours and also carcinoma in situ (due to the often aggressive pattern of infiltration that characterises this type of malignant change).

RENAL CANCER

Cancers of the kidney can result either from malignant transformation of the urothelium (lining the collecting duct system) or of the renal parenchyma itself. Urothelial tumours of the kidney account for approximately 9 per cent of total urothelial cancers. In terms of malignancies of the renal substance (parenchyma), however, the two most important histological types of cancer are adenocarcinoma (accounting for some 80 per cent of renal tumours) and nephroblastoma (so-called Wilms' tumour which is usually seen in children). There are, however, a range of other types of renal tumour, both malignant and benign, and these are summarised in Table 10.9.

Of the tumours in Table 10.9, adenocarcinoma of the kidney is by far the most common. The peak incidence of adenocarcinoma is 65–75 years, and thus it is generally a cancer of older age groups. The incidence is two times higher in men and some 3 per cent of patients develop bilateral adenocarcinoma (either synchronously, i.e. at the same time, or asynchronously).

Table 10.9   Types of renal tumour

Tumours of renal parenchyma
Benign
   Adenoma
   Haemangioma
   Angiomyolipoma
Malignant
   Adenocarcinoma (formerly called hypernephroma)
   Wilms' tumour (nephroblastoma)
   Sarcoma
   Secondary tumour deposits from other primary cancers are seen, but remain rare

Tumours of renal pelvis
Benign
   Papilloma
Malignant
   Transitional cell carcinoma
   Squamous cell carcinoma
   Adenocarcinoma

Adenocarcinoma of the kidney can present as a discrete nodule or as a nodule with so-called 'satellite' nodules spreading outward around the original tumour. With higher G stage tumours (i.e. less differentiated cells) far more infiltration into normal tissue may be seen (i.e. a more diffuse pattern of spread is evident).

Spread of renal adenocarcinoma is either by invasion, into adjacent organs via the perinephric fat, or by vascular spread. Vascular spread may be either lymphatic, to the para-aortic nodes, local venous via invasion of the renal vein and thus the inferior vena cava, or more distant venous spread to sites such as the lungs, liver, bones and brain.

Renal carcinoma has a similar TNM staging pattern as for that of bladder cancer, summarised in Table 10.10.

Table 10.10   TNM staging for renal cancers

Tumour stage

T_1	Small tumour with no distortion of overall kidney structure
T_2	Large tumour distorting the kidney, but confined within the renal capsule
T_3	Spread through the renal capsule to perinephric tissues
T_4	Invasion into the abdominal wall or adjacent organs

Nodal status

N_0	No regional nodes involved
N_1	Tumour present in single regional node
N_2	Multiple regional nodal involvement
N_3	Regional nodes fixed, due to tumour invasion from nodes to adjacent structures
N_4	Lymphatic involvement beyond regional nodes

Metastases

M_0	No 'distant' metastatic illness
M_1	Distant metastatic disease present

Patients can present with a wide range of problems, not all of which may be directly suggestive of a renal malignancy. Haematuria, loin pain and a palpable mass in the area of the kidney are classical signs (the so-called 'classical triad'), but other problems may be weight loss, fatigue, anaemia, or fever, and many of these non-specific symptoms may well be the result of so-called 'toxohormones' produced by the cancer cells. Varicocele may also be seen, caused by invasion of the renal vein, which thus decreases venous drainage from the scrotal sac.

By a similar mechanism (i.e. inhibition of venous drainage) oedema of the leg may also be seen. Hormone-related problems may also be seen, due to ectopic hormone secretion by renal tumours. Thus, hypertension (due to renin secretion) or hypercalcaemia (due to ectopic parathyroid hormone secretion) are both possible.

Investigation

IVU, or, more commonly nowadays, ultrasound can be used to diagnose renal tumours, and ultrasound has the advantage of being able to distinguish a cyst from a solid mass. CT scanning can be used to stage a renal tumour (i.e. assess the degree of spread, if any) and also will allow detection of metastases within the mediastinum and lungs, if of sufficient size.

Venography and bone scanning may also be used (see Chapter 2) to help assess the degree of tumour infiltration into the vena cava or metastic spread to bone. Biopsy of possible malignant lesions via needle is not advocated, because this may disseminate cancer cells along the needle tract.

Management

If no metastatic disease is present, treatment of renal cancer centres upon radical nephrectomy (i.e. removal of the kidney, adrenal and surrounding fat, together with the upper ureter and any enlarged para-aortic nodes). The kidney is commonly removed via a thoraco-abdominal approach (i.e. the peritoneum is opened via an abdominal incision and the kidney removed anteriorly) as this allows the renal blood vessels to be ligated prior to mobilisation of the kidney, thereby preventing tumour cells from becoming dislodged and possibly spreading to other sites.

Postoperative nursing management may therefore involve caring for a patient who has undergone a modified thoracotomy, which is clearly different from the more traditional nephrectomy approach, which is a loin incision without direct penetration of the thoracic cavity. Radiotherapy may be given postoperatively if invasion into fat or para-aortic nodes is present.

The care of patients undergoing nephrectomy is described in Chapter 6.

Clearly, if a patient has only one kidney, then partial nephrectomy may be undertaken, via extracorporeal cooling. Bullock et al (1989) describe the procedure of 'bench surgery', whereby the kidney is cooled, removed, the tumour enucleated and the remnant of the kidney then autotransplanted back into the patient's iliac fossa (the normal site chosen for renal transplantation). If it is not possible to remove a malignant tumour from a solitary kidney, then dialysis will be required post-operatively, with possible transplantation later (either live donor or cadaveric) if the patient remains well.

Nephrectomy may also be undertaken in patients with metastases, but only if intractable bleeding or pain is causing particular problems. Radiotherapy may be equally effective, and radiological embolisation may also be performed, to cut off the blood supply to the kidney, thus inducing an immune response to the cancer (as the dead renal tissue then adopts the role of an antigen).

Metastatic disease, following renal adenocarcinoma, is generally poorly responsive to treatment, particularly to chemotherapy. Currently BCG and interferon (both biological response modifiers) are under trial for treatment of renal carcinoma, as these seem to be more effective. Overall, renal/adenocarcinoma results in a 5-year survival of some 30–50 per cent of patients. If penetration of the capsule or lymphatic invasion is present, then the prognosis becomes much worse. A summary of likely prognosis in terms of 5-year survival is shown in Table 10.11.

Table 10.11   Renal adenocarcinoma: prognosis (Bullock et al, 1989)

Extent of tumour growth	5-year survival (%)
Tumour confined to kidney	75
Invasion of perirenal fat	50
Invasion of regional lymph nodes and/or tumour in renal vein or vena cava	35
Metastatic illness	< 5

Nephroblastoma (Wilms' Tumour)

First described in 1899 by Wilms, this tumour accounts for approximately 10 per cent of childhood malignancies. Some 80 per cent of nephroblastomas are seen prior to the age of 5 years, with a peak at 3 years (about 5 per cent of patients have bilateral disease). However, a small number of cases are also seen in adults.

Nephroblastoma is usually a soft, pale coloured tumour and may be either cystic or contain haemorrhagic areas. The degree of differentiation ranges from well-differentiated tumours to anaplastic or spindle cell lesions with an unfavourable prognosis. As for adenocarcinoma, nephroblastoma may present with a variety of symptoms, some of which are more classically urological but others not. A palpable mass is common (approximately 80 per cent of cases) as is abdominal pain and/or haematuria. However, anorexia, weight loss, anaemia, hypertension, fever and meastatic illness, affecting either the lungs, bone and/or liver can also be seen. Nephroblastoma is investigated via IVU, ultrasound, CT scanning for staging and also bone scanning and chest X-ray (to ascertain the extent of any metastases).

The patient's urine may also be sampled for catecholamines, to help differentiate *nephro*blastoma from *neuro*blastoma (another retroperitoneal tumour).

The treatment of nephroblastoma centres upon surgery, radiotherapy and chemotherapy and, clearly, all three have implications for nursing care. Initially, nephrectomy is undertaken, again via an abdominal approach (i.e. laparotomy) which also then allows visual examination of the opposite kidney.

The most significant recent advance in the treatment of nephroblastoma has been that of chemotherapy, and agents such as Adriamycin, Vincristine and Cyclophosphamide, in combination or as single agents, can achieve good response rates, even in advanced disease. Bullock et al (1989) report an overall 5-year survival of 80 per cent, and cure in most patients who present early on in the disease. Thus, patients are likely to require both nursing management following initial surgery and also supportive care measures while they undergo chemo- or radiotherapy.

Other Renal Tumours

Other forms of renal tumour (both benign and malignant) may be hard to distinguish from adenocarcinoma, until operative removal or histology is available.

Renal sarcoma is fortunately rare (< 3 per cent of renal malignancies) as it is a highly invasive tumour (both locally and via vascular spread) and thus carries a very poor prognosis.

Tumours can also arise in the kidney which are actually metastases from other primary cancers. This may reflect the high vascularity of the kidney, though, generally, it is very rare to see such secondary tumour deposits within the kidney. The commonest primary sites for tumours which may then involve the kidney by metastic spread are carcinomas of the bronchus and breast, malignant melanoma and also lymphoreticular cancers (e.g. lymphoma). Usually such secondary renal tumours cause loin pain and haematuria, both of which may then add to the symptoms caused by the primary tumour.

Clearly the prognosis for such patients is very poor and symptoms are treated via radiotherapy or by nephrectomy.

Oncocytoma is a malignant tumour of proximal tubular cells, composed of oncocytes (well-differentiated granular eosinophilic cells). This tumour carries a good prognosis, compared to, say, adenocarcinoma, because it generally has a low rate of metastic spread.

Benign Renal Tumours

Benign renal tumours include adenomas, which tend to vary in size (typically up to approximately 3 cm) but rarely cause symptoms. However, as in the case of the ileum, such adenomas can undergo malignant change.

Angiomyolipoma

Angiomyolipoma, as the name suggests, is a tumour composed of three tissues, namely blood vessels, smooth muscle and fat cells. CT scanning may be helpful in diagnosis because fat has a characteristic tissue density. Generally, haematuria is the most common presenting symptom and angiomyolipomas can usually be removed via partial nephrectomy.

Mesoblastic Nephroma

Mesoblastic nephroma is a very rare benign tumour and is usually only seen in very young children and infants. It is composed of mesenchymal tissues and nephrectomy is usually the treatment of choice.

Cancers of the Ureter and Renal Pelvis

Cancers of the ureter and renal pelvis are rare, accounting for between 2 and 4 per cent of urothelial cancers. Again, these types of cancers are seen in the older age group, with a peak age of 65 years, and an approximate male to female ratio of two to one.

Patients with a single upper tract tumour are at risk of subsequent bladder carcinoma (some 30–50 per cent) and also upper tract tumours in the adjacent (contralateral) kidney (some 2–4 per cent). Conversely, patients with primary tumours of the bladder would appear to be at low risk of developing subsequent upper tract tumours (Oldbring et al, 1989).

Aetiology

As with bladder cancer, smoking and exposure to certain industrial dyes or solvents are associated with an increased risk of upper urinary tract transitional cell carcinomas (Shinka et al, 1988).

The majority of ureteric and renal pelvic tumours are transitional cell tumours (ureteric approximately 95 per cent, renal pelvic approximately 90 per cent).

Squamous cell cancers account for approximately 10 per cent of renal pelvic tumours, and are extremely rare within the ureter. The majority of squamous cell tumours are identified in patients with a history of chronic inflammation, from infection or calculi, and are often already invasive at the time of presentation.

Staging

The TNM staging of ureteric and renal pelvic cancers is shown below:

Stage	Pattern of spread
T_a, Tis	Confined to the mucosa
T_1	Invasion of the lamina propria
T_2	Invasion of the muscularis
T_3	Spread through the muscularis, into fat or the renal parenchyma
T_4	Spread into adjacent organs
N+	Lymph node metastases present
M+	Systemic metastases present

(From the American Joint Committee on Cancer, 1988)

Patients generally present with gross haematuria, which may also be associated with colic-type pain in the loin, due to ureteral obstruction (due to blood clots or tumour fragments).

The renal pelvis and ureter may also be obstructed, or the tumour may already have spread to involve local tissues.

Cancers of the ureter or renal pelvis have traditionally been diagnosed using IVU and retrograde ureterography. However, a ureteroscope (ureteropyeloscope) can now be used to visualise directly upper tract abnormalities, at which time biopsy of any lesion(s) can also be undertaken. Laser vaporisation of such tumours may also be possible, at the time of ureteroscopy.

Treatment

Treatment is based upon the size and staging of the tumour. Normally, nephroureterectomy is the standard treatment, owing to the possibility of spread into the collecting system on the same side as the tumour mass. When the tumour is within the proximal ureter, or in the renal pelvis, the entire ureter is removed, along with a small cuff (patch) of bladder.

Tumours of the lower ureter may be treated by partial ureterectomy, and then ureteral reimplantation. Small-volume upper tract tumours may also be treated by the instillation of BCG alone (Studer et al, 1989).

It would appear that radiotherapy has a limited role, in the treatment of such upper tract tumours, and metastatic disease is usually treated with a similar chemotherapeutic regimen as for metastatic cancer of the bladder.

Nursing care

The nursing care of these patients will therefore involve caring for a patient undergoing nephroureterectomy or reconstruction of the ureter following partial ureterectomy. Both of these procedures, and their nursing implications, are described in chapter 6.

Penile Cancer

In Europe, penile cancer accounts for approximately 2 per cent of all male tumours. Interestingly, circumcision at birth confers complete immunity against this form of neoplasm. The risk of occurence is increased where there is a high degree of penile irritation from conditions such as balanitis. This risk of malignant change is also present in some skin diseases of the penis.

Histologically, penile cancer is typically a squamous cell carcinoma, and evidence of keratinisation is usually present. Some 75 per cent of such tumours are usually well differentiated. Two types of growth are normally apparent. These are:

1. A shallow, ulcer-like tumour, typically with 'rolled' edges.

2. A fungating, papillary-like tumour.

Tumour spread

Early spread of such cancers is usually lymphatic, either from the glans and prepuce to the superficial inguinal nodes, or from deeper channels in the corpora, which may then carry the tumour to the deep inguinal, obturator and iliac nodes.

Blood-borne spread is rare, and usually arises at a late stage in the disease, involving sites such as the lung, liver and bones. Direct spread to the urethra is usually a late feature.

Treatment

Treatment of penile cancer centres around two principal options. These are:

1. Radiotherapy

2. Surgery

Penile tumours are usually radiosensitive, and the penis is readily accessible for radiotherapy.

However, tumours which are poorly responsive, or which are very advanced at the time of presentation, may then require also surgery.

Surgery, for penile cancer, utilises either:

1. Circumcision, where the lesion is contained within the prepuce only. Sadly, this is rare.

2. Penectomy, which may either be partial or total.

Partial penectomy involves:

1. The patient is placed in the lithotomy position.

2. A penile torniquet is applied.

3. Skin flaps are then marked.

4. Amputation of a portion of both corpora is then performed, with ligation of arterial branches as appropriate.

5. The urethra is anastomosed to the skin of the remaining penile 'stump'.

6. A suitable dressing is then applied.

Total penectomy involves:

1. The patient is placed in the lithotomy position.

2. A circular incision is made, around the penis, and extending into the perineum.

3. The roots of both corpora are then exposed and excised.

4. The penis is amputated, and blood vessels ligated.

5. A perineal urethrostomy is fashioned by anastomosing the bulbar urethra to the skin of the perineum.

6. An indwelling urethral catheter is then passed, and suitable wound drainage inserted.

7. The incision is then closed, and a perineal dressing applied, to help reduce post-operative oedema.

Pre-operative care

Apart from the routine care required for a patient undergoing surgery, the pre-operative preparation includes:

1. CXR and CT scan, to screen for possible metastases.

2. Bone and/or liver scan.

3. Possible lymphangiography.

4. Pre-operative shave, from umbilicus to mid thigh.

The patient will need moral support as he begins the process of trying to come to terms with such a profound change in body image.

Post-operative care

Apart from routine aspects of post-operative care, this includes:

1. Observation of the wound and drains for possible blood loss.

2. Maintaining the dressing for the first 12–24 hours, with mild compression, to help reduce oedema.

3. Observation of the wound and monitoring vital signs, for any evidence of wound infection.

4. Appropriate pain control.

5. Care of a urinary catheter, for the first 48–72 hours.

6. Intravenous fluids are likely for the first 12 hours.

7. Early ambulation.

8. Ongoing psychological care, regarding body image change (for both patient and partner, if relevant).

9. Appropriate discharge advice.

Discharge advice includes adjustment regarding voiding posture and information relating to follow up and when to seek further advice. Clearly, these patients may require ongoing support once discharged, and the use of some form of 'cancer counsellor' may be very valuable within this context.

Testicular Cancer

The incidence of testicular cancer has been increasing throughout this century. It is the most common solid tumour in men aged between 15 and 35 years and accounts for 19 per cent of total male cancer deaths within this age group (Stanford, 1988). The cause of testicular cancer is not known, but there are a number of factors which would appear related to the aetiology of such tumours.

Men with undescended or 'late' descending testes (either naturally or surgically assisted) have an approximately 11–15 per cent chance of developing a testicular malignancy. Trauma and infection (especially viral infection) have also been implicated in some patients, but neither of these would appear generalised factors at this time. Thus it is likely that some unrecognised factors are involved which could be either environmental or genetic. Four main types of testicular malignancy are recognised. These are:

1. *Teratoma* – 5–10 per cent of all tumours, and prevalent in young children and infants, though also seen in adults.

2. *Seminoma* – most common testicular tumour, and carries the best prognosis (i.e. is usually most responsive to treatment). Accounts for approximately one-third of all cancers.

3. *Embryonal cancer* – characterised by rapid growth and spread. Accounts for approximately one-quarter of all cancers.

4. *Choriocarcinoma* – 1–3 per cent of testicular tumours. Carries a poor prognosis at this time.

A patient may also present with a 'mixed' histology tumour, possessing a mixture of the above characteristics.

Treatment

Treatment of testicular cancer is dictated by the staging of the tumour. This is achieved by CT scanning, to allow assessment of the tumour and also any metastatic disease. Besides scanning, blood samples are also taken and assayed for levels of alpha-fetoprotein (AFP), human chorionic gonadotrophin (HCG) and placental alkaline phosphatase (PLAP). The plasma levels of these specific tumour markers not only help with staging but also allow monitoring of treatment response, as well as providing an indication of any subsequent tumour recurrence. (Such 'markers' are produced specifically by cancer cells.)

Tumour Staging

The staging of testicular tumours is usually performed using the so-called Royal Marsden Staging System. This is summarised in Table 10.12.

Table 10.12   Royal Marsden Staging System for testicular cancer (cited in Stanford, 1988)

Stage 1	Disease confined to testes
Stage 2	Infradiaphragmatic nodal involvement (i.e. nodes below the diaphragm level)
	(a) < 2 cm in size
	(b) 2–5 cm in size
	(c) 7 cm in size
Stage 3	Supradiaphragmatic nodal involvement
Stage 4	Extralymphatic disease
	L_1 Lung metastasis > 3 in number
	L_2 Lung metastasis > 3 in number but less than 2 cm in size
	L_3 Lung metastasis > 3 in number but greater than 2 cm in size

The care of patients undergoing orchidectomy is considered in Chapter 11. As can be seen, chemotherapy plays a crucial role in the treatment of testicular tumours, particularly when the tumour has spread outside the testicle. Currently the regimen commonly employed is a triple therapy of three drugs, abbreviated to BEP. The three drugs are Bleomycin, Etoposide and Platinum (normally cisplatin).

The side-effects of BEP therapy can be very significant, and include pulmonary fibrosis, alopecia, nausea, vomiting, nephrotoxicity, ototoxicity, peripheral neuropathy, low plasma magnesium levels and also hypersensitivity reactions. The monitoring for and prompt treatment of such side-effects are key aspects of nursing management and can do much to minimise the harmful effects of the drugs upon the patient.

In cases of recognised renal impairment, carboplatin may sometimes be substituted for cisplatin. Further, the advent of newer antiemetic drugs, such as Ondansetron (Zofran), have helped to reduce some of the more distressing side-effects to drug treatment.

The nursing management of these patients may include both supportive measures, during the administration of chemotherapy, and postoperative nursing measures, following either orchidectomy or laparotomy (for staging and removal of para-aortic metastases) or, indeed, thoracotomy (for removal of pulmonary metastases). Clearly, therefore, a partnership between nursing and medical staff, with a team approach to overall care, is essential.

Testicular cancer can also cause profound harm to the patient's concept of body image, particularly because the testes are closely identified with 'masculinity', sexual potency and the future ability to father children. Further, the combination of surgery and drug therapy can have a dramatic effect not only on the patient but also upon the family and/or significant others, particularly as some of the side-effects of treatment become apparent. The patient's status and roles within both family and society may also be threatened by the required treatment and hospitalisation periods and sexual performance may be temporarily impaired. Such patients should be offered 'sperm banking' facilities prior to treatment so that any lasting infertility (occurring as a result of treatment) will not prevent them fathering children.

Blackmore (1989) states that the nursing management of patients with testicular tumours is primarily concerned with two key areas, namely patient education and psychological support. By educating patients regarding their cancer, the required surgery and treatment, possible complications and side-effects, and also by continuing to provide both support and encouragement, patients can hopefully be assisted in working through their sense of self-loss such that they come to a more optimistic and positive outlook for their future. Early detection and treatment means that most testicular cancers now carry an excellent prognosis. Testicular self-examination should therefore be taught and encouraged, just as breast self-examination is taught within the sphere of women's health. Nurses clearly have a pivotal role to play, as health educators, and testicular self-examination should thus be an integral part of nurse education.

Guidelines for testicular self-examination are shown in Table 10.13.

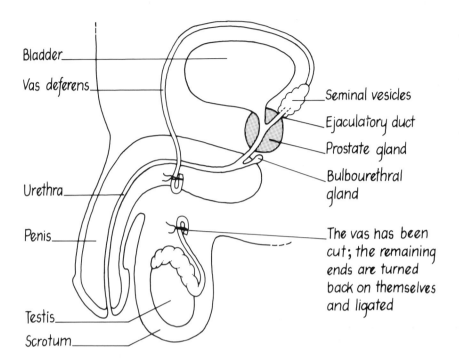

Fig 11.1 Vasectomy

VASOVASOSTOMY

This refers to the reversal of a vasectomy. The procedure may be requested due to a family tragedy where a child has been killed or perhaps a husband has remarried and wants to start a family with his new wife.

There is an approximately 80–90 per cent chance of the vas being rejoined and spermatozoa appearing in the ejaculate and a 40 per cent chance that the partner will conceive in the subsequent 2 years. However, the risk of failure is so great that vasectomy should not be undertaken unless both partners have fully decided they do not want any more children.

The procedure is most commonly performed under a general anaesthetic. A scrotal or lower abdominal incision is used. The ends of the vas are found, 'freshened' and joined together. The surgery is very delicate – whereas a vasectomy will take approximately 15 minutes to perform, this procedure usually takes 30 minutes to 1 hour.

Specifics

A full explanation of the procedure will be given. Many patients are under the misconception that the reversal of vasectomy will be as quick and straightforward as the vasectomy itself. The potential complications of wound infection, haematoma and pain will be explained as well as the fact that the success rate of the procedure is poor. To give optimum chance for healing to occur and for the surgery to be successful the patient should remain on modified bed rest both on the day of surgery and the first postoperative day, and be up for toilet purposes only. If all is well then the patient will be discharged on the second postoperative day.

Potential Complications

Moderate–Severe Pain

Because the surgery is delicate and the area vascular the patient may experience a significant degree of pain and discomfort following surgery. Pain can be controlled by the administration of adequate analgesia, as prescribed. Ensuring the scrotum is adequately supported by a well-fitting scrotal support and pad (or Netelast pants and pad) will also help relieve the pain.

Infection

The patient should not be discharged home with an untreated pyrexia. The wound should be checked for signs of infection such as oozing or inflammation. Dressings should be removed 24–48 hours postoperatively unless they require changing due to excessive oozing. Once the dressing is removed the wound can be sprayed with 'plastic skin' and left exposed. The patient should ensure that the area is kept as clean and dry as possible. Showers are recommended as opposed to baths. The patient should ensure that sutures are not soaked in the bath until at least 4 days postoperatively.

Haematoma

On occasions, large haematomas do develop and it may be necessary for the patient to return to theatre for 'evacuation of haematoma'. A regular check should be made on the wound site and scrotal area following surgery to observe for bleeding and swelling. A well-fitting scrotal support (or pad and Netelast pants) should be worn to provide both pressure to the area and also extra support and comfort.

Discharge

If all is well, patients are usually discharged home on the second or third postoperative day. Depending on the work performed by the patient, it may be necessary for him to take up to 2 weeks off work. The patient will be advised against any heavy lifting or exercise which might put strain on the area.

A scrotal support should be worn for a couple of weeks until the patient feels comfortable without it.

If the sutures are dissolvable the patient should be informed of this; if not, arrangements should be made for the sutures to be removed 7–10 days postoperatively.

Patients are advised not to have sexual intercourse for 4 weeks following surgery. An appointment should be made for the wound to be inspected 6 weeks postoperatively and for semen analysis to be performed at 3 and 4 months postoperatively.

A full explanation should be given of any analgesic or antibiotics prescribed for the patient to take home.

The patient is advised to keep the area clean and dry and to visit his general practitioner if any problems arise relating to the surgery.

LIGATION OF VARICOCELE

A varicocele is formed when the spermatic veins draining the testicle become varicose and distended. Varicoceles often feel like a 'bag of worms'.

It is believed that these veins serve as a heat exchanger mechanism, keeping the testicle cool and aiding in spermatogenesis. In one study, the surgical ligation of varicocele performed to improve fertility resulted in 80 per cent of 950 men showing improvement in semen quality and 50 per cent of their partners subsequently conceived. However, in those studies where there was a central group of patients, the conception rate was the same in the operated and control groups. Current research attempts to identify those patients who are likely to benefit from varicocele ligation.

The condition is usually asymptomatic and often only found at a routine examination. Occasionally a dragging, 'aching' feeling is experienced but it is seldom so uncomfortable that it requires supporting with a scrotal support and very rarely requires ligation.

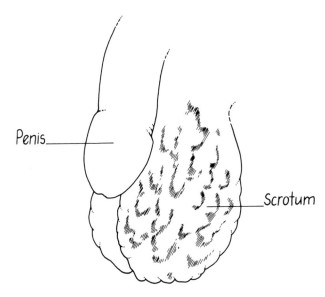

Fig 11.2   A varicocele

The surgery involves opening up the inguinal canal and all the veins except one are ligated and divided. The canal is then closed. The procedure is performed under a general anaesthetic and the patient usually discharged on the first or second postoperative day. Sexual activities can be resumed as soon as the patient feels comfortable to do so. Absence from work is usually for 1 week after discharge.

For nursing care, see Care plans A, B and C.

HYDROCELE

The outer covering of the testis is the tunica vaginalis. It has both a visceral and a parietal layer. Secretions from the tunica keep the two layers moist, allowing some mobility of the testes. The secretion is normally only a few millilitres. The testicle has a series of lymphatic capillaries which drain into the lymphatics of the spermatic cord. If these lymphatics become obstructed, fluid accumulates between the layers of the tunica vaginalis, resulting in the formation of a hydrocele.

There are three types of hydrocele:

1. *Primary hydrocele*   These are common in middle-aged men; their cause is unknown.

2. *Congenital hydrocele*   After birth the processus vaginalis may not be completely obliterated and peritoneal fluid is therefore able to enter the cavity, resulting in a

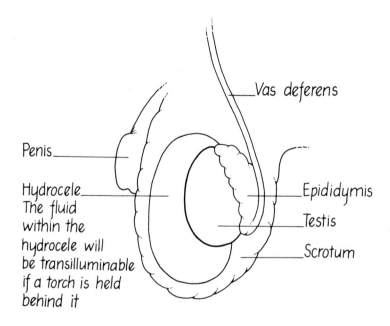

Fig 11.3   Hydrocele

hydrocele. Spontaneous closure of the processus vaginalis usually occurs, resulting in the disappearance of the hydrocele. However, if by 18 months of age spontaneous closure has not occurred the processus will have to be ligated.

3. *Secondary hydrocele* These are so called because they occur as a result of a known cause, e.g. injury to the testicle, fibrosis of the lymphatics, or secondary to heart failure.

Treatment

The treatment of hydrocele in the elderly patient is usually by aspiration of the fluid. This is performed on an out-patient basis under local anaesthetic. This method may only provide temporary relief, as the hydrocele is likely to recur.

Hydrocelectomy is performed under a general anaesthetic. It is the treatment of choice when the hydrocele persistently recurs and/or is a source of pain and discomfort to the patient. A scrotal incision is made and the sac either drained and 'bunched' with a series of sutures (thus removing the potential space for fluid accumulation) or else removed completely. The procedure often leaves the patient with a large haematoma which may take several weeks to resolve. Hence the final results of surgery are not noticeable until the haematoma has resolved.

For nursing care, see Care plans A, B and C.

Specifics

Sexual intercourse can resume 2 weeks postoperatively if the patient feels comfortable. A scrotal support should be worn until the haematoma resolves and the patient feels comfortable without it. The length of time off work following surgery is usually 2 weeks after discharge home from hospital.

SPERMATOCELE

The majority of men over the age of 40 develop tiny cysts in the sulcus between the epididymis and testis. They are thought to be diverticulae in the collecting tubules of the vasa efferentia. If these subsequently enlarge, they form multiple translucent cysts, causing the epididymis to become thin and stretched. The cysts contain clear watery fluid and also dead sperm. When many sperm are present within the cysts, they are known as spermatoceles.

Such spermatoceles can be left untreated, unless they cause pain. However, before surgery is performed to remove a spermatocele, the patient must be informed that it may result in infertility as the surgery may cause the vasa efferentia to be interrupted.

The procedure is performed under general anaesthetic and, if all is well, the patient is discharged on the first or second postoperative day.

For nursing care see Care plans A, B and C.

TESTICULAR TRAUMA

The testicles are frequently damaged as a result of sporting injuries. The injury usually causes a split in the visceral layer of the tunica vaginalis, resulting in a large painful haematocele. If left untreated over a period of weeks the haematocele will gradually subside. However, prior to this, the pressure exerted on the testicle as a result of the haematocele may squeeze it flat, resulting in permanent atrophy of the testicle and loss of spermatogenic function. If medical advice is not sought immediately by the patient, it is important that the possible loss of spermatogenic function as a direct result of the injury is explained prior to surgery.

The testicle should therefore be explored as soon as possible after such an injury. An incision is made in the scrotum, the blood clot is removed and the tear in the visceral layer of the tunica vaginalis repaired. Some of these injuries and haematoceles turn out to be tumours of the testicle – an additional reason for not delaying exploration of the testicle.

The procedure would be performed under a general anaesthetic and the patient discharged on the second postoperative day if all was well. The patient would be advised to abstain from sexual intercourse for 1–2 weeks and not to resume sporting activities for 3–4 weeks until the area is healed and comfortable.

For nursing care see Care plans A, B and C.

TESTICULAR TORSION

This can occur in both normal and undescended testicles where there is excessive mobility of the testes – allowing the testes and epididymis to rotate on its mesentery, resulting in first the venous drainage and later the arterial supply being obstructed. This leads to infarction of the testicle and requires urgent treatment. If the blood supply is compromised for longer than 6 hours it is likely that complete infarction of the testicle will result.

The patient experiences sudden acute pain in the testicle due to vascular obstruction. Occasionally referred pain is felt in the inguinal or abdominal area. The testes are tender to touch. Within 1–2 hours the testicle will appear red and become swollen, accompanied by oedema.

The torsion can be corrected by untwisting the testicle, rotating it first one way and then the other. A distinct click will be felt and the patient will experience immediate relief when the torsion is corrected.

Surgical correction of the torsion is performed under a general anaesthetic. An inguinal scrotal incision is made. The torsion is corrected and the viability of the testicle assessed. If infarction has occurred then orchidectomy is the treatment of choice. If the testicle is viable, it should be fixed to the excised edges of the tunica vaginalis and inner layer of the scrotal skin. This will lessen its mobility and guard against recurrence. If the other testicle feels equally mobile, it should be fixed at the same time. This procedure is called orchidopexy.

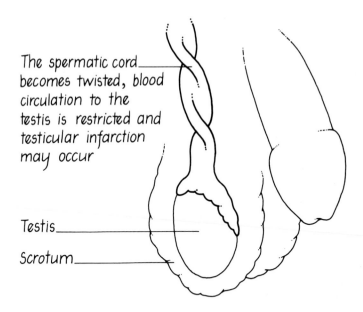

The spermatic cord becomes twisted, blood circulation to the testis is restricted and testicular infarction may occur

Testis

Scrotum

Fig 11.4   Testicular torsion

Specifics

The patient will be admitted as an emergency for urgent transfer to surgery. Prior to surgery, bed rest should be maintained and adequate analgesia administered as prescribed. The possibility of reduced fertility due to testicular infarction and/or orchidectomy being performed should be explained.

For nursing care, see Care plans A, B and C.

EPIDIDYMITIS

Acute Epididymitis

Acute epididymitis is usually the result of bacterial infection, caused by one of two principal groups of pathogens. These are:

1. *Sexually transmitted organisms* e.g. *Chlamydia trachomatis* or *Neisseria gonorrhoeae*; either alone or in combination.

2. *Non-sexually transmitted organisms*   This type of infection is often associated with urinary tract infection and prostatitis, and common causative organisms are Enterobacteriaceae and Pseudomonas.

Acute infection of the epididymis is rarely seen prior to the age of puberty, but after that occurs in all other age groups. The infection may reach the epididymis via the blood stream, or via the perivasal lymphatics. In addition, retrograde spread from the prostatic urethra and seminal vesicles can occur, a process which may be enhanced by the hydrostatic pressure associated with voiding 'forcing' infected urine into the ejaculatory ducts and through the vas deferens to the epididymis.

Genitourinary tuberculosis is also a potential cause of acute epididymitis, and remains common in areas where pulmonary tuberculosis remains a significant problem. However, in some 50 per cent of affected patients, no causative organism or underlying problem can be found.

Treatment

The condition is usually treated with a combination of:

1. Bed rest.

2. A well fitting scrotal support.

3. Appropriate analgesia, as the testicle(s) can become extremely painful.

4. Appropriate antibiotic therapy, provided a causative organism can be identified.

The nursing care of these individuals will centre upon the above priorities, as well as attempting to provide a supportive environment, where the potential embarrassment of the patient is minimised.

Unfortunately, pus and/or abscess formation within the testis can destroy the testicular substance. Further, in the longer term, atrophy of the testis is seen in 20 per cent of patients and men with bilateral disease may become infertile, due to fibrosis of the epididymal tubules.

Chronic Epididymitis

Chronic epididymitis usually results from the combination of a severe attack of acute epididymitis that has then been followed by repeated further attacks of less severity. When this happens, the vas becomes 'beaded' and shortened and the epididymis nodular and hard. The pathological changes in chronic epididymitis may cause an interruption to the vas, thus influencing the fertility of the patient. Tuberculosis remains an important cause of chronic epididymitis.

Treatment

Treatment of this condition is by appropriate antibiotic therapy, particularly if T.B. is the causative organism.

In terms of nursing management, the care is very similar to that for cases of acute epididymitis, though this will clearly vary according to the severity of the patient's discomfort.

ACUTE ORCHITIS

Viral infections account for most acute infections of the testis (e.g. rubella, infectious mononucleosis, mumps). Mumps orchitis occurs in 15–20 per cent of adult males who contract the infection, but is rarely seen prior to puberty. The diagnosis of acute orchitis can be difficult, as the symptoms are very similar to those of testicular torsion. To exclude the possibility of torsion, exploration of the testicle is required, under general anaesthesia.

Treatment

Acute orchitis is usually treated conservatively, using a combination of:

1. Bed rest

2. A well-fitting scrotal support

3. Suitable analgesic.

Some units advocate the use of steroid therapy, as an attempt to reduce the degree of subsequent testicular atrophy. There would, however, appear to be some debate over the effectiveness of this strategy.

Depending on the degree of testicular atrophy which results from the infection, patients may require counselling regarding reduced fertility or infertility. Some 50 per cent of patients subsequently develop atrophy of the affected testis, and if the condition is bilateral, sterility may clearly result.

ORCHIDECTOMY

This procedure involves removal of the testicle. It may be unilateral or bilateral, depending on the individual patient.

Bilateral Ochidectomy

This procedure is performed in patients with advanced prostatic cancer. Prostatic tumours are generally testosterone-dependent and their growth is therefore retarded when the amount of circulating testosterone is reduced. This can be achieved either by the oral or intramuscular administration of synthetic oestrogen or by the use of testosterone antagonists, such as cyproterone acetate. Surgically, testosterone production can be reduced by bilateral orchidectomy. A scrotal incision is made and the testicles removed. A dressing and scrotal support are then applied. The length of hospital stay is usually 4 days.

For general nursing care, see Care plans A, B and C.

Specifics

The specific nursing care required by the patient is for the nurse to provide comfort and support to enable the patient to come to terms with his altered body image.

The reduction of circulating testosterone is likely to reduce the patient's sexual desire and also his ability to undergo both erection and orgasm. Sterility will also occur and it is likely that such patients will also suffer a loss of perceived masculinity. The nurse should ensure he/she is there to listen and provide comfort to the patient and his family. The positive aspects of treatment can also be emphasised (e.g. the patient will probably have considerable pain reduction following surgery).

Unilateral Orchidectomy

Unilateral orchidectomy may be required following testicular torsion if the testicle is found to be infarcted. It may also be necessary following testicular trauma, where the testicle has been compressed by a haematoma causing testicular atrophy.

The most common reason for performing unilateral orchidectomy is for testicular tumours. Patients who are suspected of having testicular tumours will undergo surgical exploration of the scrotum. If malignant tissue is found then unilateral orchidectomy will be performed. The procedure is performed under general anaesthetic through an inguinal incision. Testicular biopsies are not done for suspected neoplasms, since there is risk of spreading malignant cells to healthy tissue. Most testicular tumours are prone to metastatic spread and additional treatment is therefore often required. This is dependent upon the type of tumour (see Chapter 10).

The average length of stay following unilateral orchidectomy is 5 days. However, this will depend upon the follow-up care which will be required.

For general nursing care, see Care plans A, B and C.

Specifics

The specific role of the nurse with regard to nursing care is to provide a supportive environment for the patient and to correct any inaccurate notions he may have regarding his illness. The nurse will need to provide psychological support and comfort for the patient and his partner. The patient will have to come to terms with an altered body image (e.g. he may feel less sexually attractive due to the idea of having only one testicle and therefore being different from other men). Surgical implantation of a gel-filled silicone prosthesis can be performed at a later date. It should be reinforced that although the patient will have a lower sperm count, he will still be fertile and his ability to have an erection and orgasm will not be affected.

If radiotherapy or chemotherapy are required, fertility will probably be impaired for 2 years, as the treatment has an adverse effect on spermatogenesis. If lymphadenectomy is performed the patient might suffer from ejaculatory failure, depending on the extent of surgery. One cannot overemphasize the importance of the nurse's role as a counsellor when nursing these patients. It is of vital importance that patients are allowed time and space in which to express their fears and anxieties over their diagnosis, treatment and prognosis. The patient will require frequent follow-up examinations so that any recurrence can be treated quickly.

INFERTILITY

Infertility affects some 10 per cent of all couples. In approximately one-third of these the infertility is due to a male-related problem such as a low or absent sperm count or impotence. In a further third infertility is due to a female-related problem, and in the remaining third infertility is due to problems existing in both partners.

Male Fertility

This depends on the production of viable sperm in the testes and their passage through the vas to the seminal vesicles where other components are added to manufacture seminal fluid. Fertility also depends on the ability of the male partner to both maintain an adequate erection (to enable penetration) and to undergo ejaculation. Problems may thus arise at any point in this process, resulting in subsequent infertility.

Testis

Each lobe of the testis contains seminiferous tubules and these are surrounded by Leydig cells. The Leydig cells produce testosterone. They are dormant until puberty and stimulated by the pituitary gland situated in the hypothalamus.

Spermatogenesis

Spermatogenesis begins in the seminiferous tubules under the influence of follicle-stimulating hormone (FSH) produced by the pituitary gland. The basilar membrane of the seminiferous tubules is lined with two types of cells: spermatogonium and Sertoli cells. Spermatogonium undergo growth and multiplication to become primary spermatocytes, secondary spermatocytes and finally spermatids.

The Sertoli cells provide nutrients for the spermatids. They engulf the spermatid and begin a metamorphosis which produces viable spermatozoa.

When growth is complete, sperm are released into the lumen of the seminiferous tubule and rapidly transported to the epididymis through the ductal system. As they progress through the ducts, sperm increase in vitality and vigour, undergoing further maturation. (Sperm removed from the tail rather than the head of the epididymis are more fertile.) If the sperm are not ejaculated they degenerate and are absorbed.

Spermatogenesis is continuous – the whole process takes approximately 7 days. It is sensitive to heat, occurring at temperatures a few degrees lower than body temperature. The dartos muscle within the scrotum contracts or relaxes in response to varying external temperatures, thus allowing the temperature of the testis to be regulated. (Men with uncorrected cryptorchidism remain sterile, due to the intra-abdominal temperature being incompatible with successful spermatogenesis.)

Care plan A Patient care documentation – basic preoperative care plan for a patient undergoing scrotal surgery

Patient's problem/need	Expected outcome for patient	Action
Potential anxiety due to hospitalisation and impending surgery	Patient will state he feels safe and informed about operation and will experience no excessive anxiety	1. Identify cause of anxiety by interviewing patient and providing opportunity for him to ask questions 2. Provide information about preoperative preparation using diagrams if necessary to make things clear. Inform patient where incision will be made 3. Explain about transfer to and from theatre; what to expect post-operatively, in regard to wound dressing, discomfort and provision of analgesia, length of hospital stay, etc. 4. Re-check prior to theatre whether patient still wishes to go through with surgery 5. Ensure doctor has obtained written consent before administration of premedication
Correct identification of patient	Correct patient will go to theatre with correct documentation	1. Ensure medical notes, drug chart, X-ray and results are on ward and: (a) are available at time of premedication (b) accompany patient to theatre 2. Check patient identity band with theatre request slip 3. Accompany patient to theatre
Potential injury from or loss of jewellery, dentures, contact lenses	No injury from, damage or loss of personal belongings will occur	1. Lock valuables away if patient wishes, according to hospital policy 2. Tape or remove jewellery – explain reason for doing this 3. Remove dentures, contact lenses and any prosthesis, if present 4. Ask if any teeth are loose or crowned and record
Potential postoperative infection (e.g. urine, wound)	No signs of infection will be present	1. Take patient's temperature preoperatively, report pyrexia if present 2. Observe for any skin complaint, soreness or rash around scrotal area 3. Test urine for any abnormalities, send midstream urine specimen if indicated

		4. Bath or shower patient prior to surgery 5. Provide patient with clean theatre gown to change into following bath or shower
Risk of vomiting and aspiration of stomach contents	Patient will not vomit or aspirate	1. Fast patient for 6 hours *diet*. Fast for 4 hours *fluids* prior to general anaesthetic 2. Ensure premedication given as prescribed
Risk of incontinence due to loss of voluntary muscle control whilst unconscious Potential bladder damage due to full bladder	Patient will remain continent	1. Ensure bowels have been open at least 24 hours prior to surgery (this will also reduce the chance of patient straining to have his bowels open postoperatively) 2. Give patient opportunity to void before premedication
Potential difficulty in sleeping	Patient will state that he has had a comfortable night's sleep	1. Provide environment conducive to restful sleep for individual 2. Give night sedation if prescribed and patient wishes
Ensure skin area is prepared prior to surgery	1. Infection will not occur 2. Discomfort will be reduced when dressing is removed	1. The hair will have to be removed from the area where the incision is to be made. This can be done on the ward as near as possible to the time of theatre. However, to reduce patient embarrassment and also infection risk this should be performed in theatre 2. A wide area should be shaved to reduce the chance of adhesive tape dressings being stuck on to hair – which would be painful to remove
Perform baseline recordings of pulse and blood pressure prior to general anaesthetic	Postoperative pulse and blood pressure will compare favourably	1. Perform pulse and blood pressure 2. Report any abnormalities

Care plan B Patient care documentation – general postoperative care following scrotal surgery

Patient's problem/need	Expected outcome for patient	Action
Potential problems with breathing due to anaesthetic/surgical intervention	Airway will remain clear	1. Observe and ensure clear airway 2. Stay with patient until able to maintain own airway 3. Ensure suction and oxygen available 4. Observe and record respirations after ¼, ½, 1, 2, 4 hours. Report abnormalities 5. Administer oxygen as prescribed
Potential shock	Signs of shock will not be present	1. Observe and record pulse and blood pressure after ¼, ½, 1, 2, 4 hours. Observe for falling blood pressure, rising pulse 2. Observe wound site for oozing, bleeding, haematoma, swelling of scrotum 3. Report excessive oozing. Patient to remain on bed rest for at least 2 hours immediately postoperatively 4. Be aware of signs of shock 5. Change dressing as required
Potential difficulty maintaining body temperature in immediate postoperative period	Temperature will be 35.5–37.5°C	1. Observe and record temperature after ¼, ½, 1, 2, 4 hours. Report if outside parameters 2. Ensure patient not left exposed 3. Use of 'space blanket' if temperature falls below 35.5°C
Potential pain discomfort due to surgical intervention	Pain/discomfort will be controlled to a level acceptable to patient	1. Assess degree of discomfort experienced by use of verbal and non-verbal communication 2. Position patient comfortably, ensure correct size scrotal support in situ and that it is positioned comfortably with a dressing pad to absorb any oozing from wound site 3. Give analgesia as prescribed and assess effectiveness

Potential nausea and vomiting	Patient will not feel nauseated, will not vomit	1. Observe for signs of nausea 2. Administer antiemetic as prescribed and monitor effect 3. Supply with mouthwash, vomit bowl and tissues 4. Commence on oral fluids and light diet as tolerated
Potential inability to eliminate urine and/or faeces normally	Patient will pass urine by 12–18 hours postoperatively	1. Explain to patient that he probably will not feel the urge to pass water for about 6–12 hours postoperatively, depending on amount of fluid intake. 2. Assist with adjusting and applying new dressing after passing urine 3. Ensure patient does not strain to have his bowels open 4. Administer aperient as required as prescribed if necessary and monitor its effect
Potential difficulty meeting personal hygiene needs postoperatively	Patient will state that he feels comfortable	1. Assist with postoperative wash 2. Ensure items available for regular oral care if patient not tolerating fluids 3. Assist as necessary with hygiene needs, maintaining maximum independence of patient
Care of wound site, potential infection	Infection will not develop	1. Record temperature 4-hourly, report any significant pyrexia 2. Observe wound site for oozing inflammation, large haematoma 3. Redress wound site as necessary, clean with normal saline if required and apply dry dressing and wool pad, then scrotal support 4. Daily shower from day 2 postoperatively. Ensure wound dried afterwards (hairdryer may be useful) 5. Antibiotics as prescribed (if indicated)

Care plan C Patient care documentation – discharge advice following scrotal surgery

Patient's problem/need	Expected outcome for patient	Action
To be adequately prepared for discharge home.	Patient will feel safe and secure with regard to his discharge home	1. Patient will be advised not to do anything which will cause straining around the wound site and to perform activities being aware of his own limitations
		2. In most cases sporting activities can resume 2 weeks postoperatively. In the case of vasovasostomy or orchidectomy, a 4–6-week resting period is required
		3. The patient should not do any heavy lifting
		4. Sexual intercourse can resume 1–2 weeks after discharge (except in case of vasovasostomy – 4 weeks)
		5. Patient advised to observe wound site daily for any changes, or signs of infection – oozing, inflammation, swelling, redness. If area appears infected, then patient advised to either contact GP or phone the hospital and speak to his doctor or ward staff. Antibiotics may be required.
		6. Sutures should dissolve 7–20 days postoperatively, if dissolvable. If not, then arrangements will be made prior to discharge for the sutures to be removed by the GP 7–10 days postoperatively
		7. Daily showers are recommended, as is drying the wound with a hairdryer on a cool temperature
		8. It may be necessary to take pain killers home. The nurse will explain how frequently these should be taken. If they are not sufficient to control the pain then patient is advised to contact GP or hospital. Patient advised to continue to wear the support or supporting pants for 1–2 weeks
		9. Antibiotics may also be required if the wound appears inflamed and the patient has a slight temperature prior to discharge home. The nurse will explain how frequently to take the tablets and whether they should be taken before or after food, as well as any other relevant information

4. Supplies of dressings

10. The patient should be supplied with a week's worth of pads and other dressings for discharge home. A spare scrotal support of the appropriate size, or Netelast pants should be supplied

5. Follow-up appointment

11. Prior to discharge a follow-up appointment should be made for 6 weeks postoperatively, unless further specific treatment is required

To drive a motor vehicle

1. Driving should not be undertaken for at least 2 weeks postoperatively due to the strain on the scrotal area of e.g. emergency stop

2. The patient is advised to check his driving insurance documentation as it may require him not to drive for 4 weeks postoperatively

To return to work

Once again the patient should know his own limitations. If he performs strenuous work which requires heavy lifting it may be necessary to take 2–3 weeks off work; otherwise 1–2 weeks

Viable sperm must be transported from the testis through the penis to the female reproductive tract so that fertilisation can take place. The vas widens into a broad ampulla as it ascends the pelvic cavity. The ampulla and seminal vesicles meet to form the common ejaculatory duct. The seminal vesicles produce a fluid rich in nutrients which provides for the sperm until fertilisation. At ejaculation, the seminal vesicles contract and seminal fluid is forced into the common ejaculatory duct and into the prostatic urethra, where the prostatic gland also discharges its fluid. The prostatic fluid is alkaline and believed to reduce the acidity of the seminal fluid and vaginal secretions. (The motility and viability of the sperm is greatly reduced in an acid solution.) Sperm are thus more motile in a neutral or slightly alkaline solution.

The bulbo-urethral glands add further fluid to the semen and the semen then acts as a lubricant and fluid medium for the sperm.

At ejaculation the muscle layers of the prostate gland contract rhythmically, forcing prostatic fluid into the prostatic urethra. The bladder neck muscles also contract, closing the internal urethral orifice. Powerful rhythmic contractions then result in the semen being forced along the length of the erect penis. To deposit the semen in the vagina the penis must be erect. This change is due to engorgement of the corpora cavernosa and corpus spongiosum (see Chapter 9).

Investigation of Infertility

Infertility should be regarded as a joint problem and, initially, both partners must be investigated.

The first division of patients is those who have had children before and those who have not: so-called primary and secondary infertility. Circumstances of previous pregnancies may give clues to the cause of infertility.

A sexual history is essential – it is probably not worth while investigating couples who have been having unprotected intercourse for less than 2 years. However, this must be balanced against the number of couples postponing their first attempts at pregnancy until their late twenties.

Infertility is becoming a problem later in a woman's reproductive life. Investigations may last a year or more and must not be allowed to carry the couple beyond the age at which pregnancy or possible adoption is reasonable.

Occasionally it is found that couples do not know the fertility cycle and have not been having intercourse at the appropriate time. Other sexual difficulties or even impotence may be discovered.

An important aspect of infertility clinics is to counsel the patients with regard to their prognosis. After full investigations it is possible to give the couple an estimate of their chances of conception during the subsequent year and whether treatment is likely to alter their prospects. With this information, together with the duration of infertility and the age of the woman, the couple should consider the treatment options and their likely chance of success.

Some couples will always choose to continue trying, no matter how poor the odds. Others will opt for artificial donor insemination. Some will choose to adopt children. Others will decline any further treatment and accept their infertility. These decisions are an individual matter for the couple and counselling should be based on accurate assessment of both partners.

Male Infertility

On the couple's first visit to the male infertility clinic a fertility questionnaire is normally completed by the doctor together with both partners. A full physical examination of the male partner, as well as a semen analysis, will also take place.

Fertility Investigation Questionnaire

1. *Previous marriage and pregnancies* (this will indicate whether it is primary or secondary infertility)

2. *Time attempting to conceive* – any pregnancies?

3. *Frequency of intercourse* (weekly) –
   erection
   penetration
   ejaculation

4. *Knowledge of fertility phase?* (day 14 in menstrual cycle)

5. *Previous investigation and treatment*

Past History – Male Partner

The following aspects are discussed:

- General
- Operations
- Hernia – (may cause obstruction of the vas)
- Undescended testicles – (should be corrected before age of 4)
- Varicocele – (elevated testicular temperature)
- Mumps – (if before 15 years of age, testicular damage rare)
- Epididymitis, urinary infections
- Diabetes
- Recent illnesses
- Chemotherapy   } spermatogenesis will stop for approximately 2 years following treatment
- Deep X-ray treatment (DXT)
- General health
- Frequency of shaving – (may show signs of pituitary failure)
- Emotional problems
- Smoking habits – (atheroma in arteries may cause erectile dysfunction)
- Alcohol intake – (if high may cause decreased libido)
- Current drugs

Past History – Female Partner

The following details are discussed:

- Age
- Menstrual history
- Previous pregnancies
- Previous operations
- Previous illnesses
- Family history
- Previous treatment

Investigations of Female Partner

The following are discussed or performed as appropriate:

- Biphasic temperature chart
- Endometrial biopsy
- Progesterone levels
- Tubal patency
- Cervical mucus
- Post-coital test

Examination of Male Partner

The male partner is examined for:

- Height
- Weight
- Hair distribution
- Physique
- Breasts
  (The patient may have Klinefelter's syndrome, a chromosome abnormality where there is an extra X chromosome. These patients have long limbs, small testes, gynaecomastia and female distribution of hair. They are usually infertile.)
- Abdomen may show presence of scars
- Undergarments tight/loose
- Penis:
  circumcised
  external meatus
- Testis:
  right
  left
- Varicocele
- Epididymis
- Vas
- Prostate and seminal vesicle

Investigations of Male Partner

The following tests are performed:

- Seminal analysis:
    sample 1
    sample 2
- Blood test:
    follicle-stimulating hormone
    luteinising hormone
    testosterone
    prolactin
- Vasogram
- Buccal smear
- Chromosomes
- Testicular exploration/biopsy

Testicles

The scrotal contents are examined. The size and consistency of the testis are noted. Fertility is usually supressed when both testes are 3 cm or less.

The epididymis and vas deferens are felt and any abnormality noted. Rectal examination is performed as any thickening or tenderness of the prostate or seminal vesicles may suggest infection.

The patient is examined in the standing position for the presence of any varioc&cele. These are important as they may raise the testicular temperature, causing impairment of spermatogenesis.

Penile observation

1. *Phimosis* may be present – a pinhole meatus can interfere with ejaculation and necessitate circumcision (see Chapter 9).

2. *Peyronie's disease* – development of fibrous plaques within the corpus cavernosum. This results in curvature of the erect penis, which may prevent vaginal penetration (the patient will require a Nesbit's procedure; see Chapter 9).

3. *Impotence* – this may be a cause of infertility. Psychosexual counselling may be required or surgical intervention dependent on the cause (see Chapter 9).

Seminal Fluid Analysis

This is important in the study of infertility but has its limitations. The specimen should be produced by masturbation into a clean, wide mouthed container after 3 days of abstinence. It should be examined as soon as possible (within 1–2 hours) by an experienced technician. One reading in isolation is insufficient, several samples should be examined over a period of 3 months.

The volume of ejaculate may vary. The normal range is 2–5 ml. Volumes of far less than this have been known to produce conception. If the volume of ejaculate is less than 0.5 ml, retrograde ejaculation or the absence of the seminal vesicles should be excluded.

Normal Sperm Concentration

The normal sperm concentration is 60–160 million/ml. It is only when the sperm count is less than 20 million/ml that infertility is likely to be due to a lack of spermatozoa.

Azoospermia refers to a complete absence of sperm. Oligozoospermia refers to a sperm count of less than 20 million/ml and requires further investigations.

The percentage of motile spermatozoa is important and should be more than 40 per cent at 1 hour. The quality of movement is important and the progressive movement is assessed objectively. Patients whose sperm have a persistent lack of progressive motility have a poor prognosis.

The morphology of spermatozoa is varied and even in a normal semen specimen there will be many morphological abnormalities. The prognosis is poor when most of the sperm are abnormal.

The complete evaluation of semen includes the assessment of the viscosity, pH measurement, microscopic examination for pus cells and the mixed erythrocyte agglutination reaction test for antisperm antibodies.

Additional Investigations

Endocrine assessment of the infertile male is essential in men with azoospermia or severe oligozoospermia. In these patients, plasma follicle-stimulating hormone (FSH), luteinising hormone (LH) and testosterone (T) levels are measured. The presence of any circulating antisperm antibodies is detected.

A post-coital test is valuable in the assessment of the infertile male, and also assesses factors of the partner. This test is only of value when carried out at the time of ovulation. An in vitro penetration test and crossed penetration test with donor sperm and cervical mucus may also provide useful information.

Surgical Intervention

1. *Ligation of varicocele* – this is only performed when other causes of infertility have been excluded, particularly in the wife.

2. *Undescended testicles* – the chances of improving fertility are remote but testicular biopsy may diagnose carcinoma in situ. Orchidopexy should be performed below the age of 6 years.

3. *Vasovasostomy, epididymo vasostomy.*

Azoospermia and its Treatment

This may be due to:

1. *Primary failure of the testes to produce spermatozoa.* These patients usually have small testes and a raised FSH − no treatment is possible.

2. *Obstruction* − the patient will require surgical exploration to determine the level of the block. This is only done on patients with a normal sized testis (4–5 cm) and those without a gross elevation of plasma FSH level. Under a general anaesthetic testicular exploration is carried out. The epididymis is inspected for evidence of obstruction. Vasography is performed to exclude vasal obstruction. The testes are biopsied.

If an obstruction is seen an epididymal bypass operation can be performed. (Nursing care similar to vasovasostomy). The results of the procedure vary from 'zero' where obstruction is at the head of the epididymis (associated with Young's syndrome) to 50 per cent in those with obstruction at the tail of the epididymis (e.g. due to gonorrhoea). Vasal obstruction can also occur following inexpert herniorraphy in childhood. Ten per cent of men with obstructive azoospermia have vasal or varying degrees of epididymal aplasia. Various techniques have been described for collecting spermatozoa for performing artificial insemination. Those collected from the head of the epididymis are infertile but those collected from the tail have been known to fertilize human oocytes in vitro.

The most common cause of azoospermia, at the present time, is previous vasectomy.

Treatment of Oligozoospermia

Patients with defective spermatogenesis (small testes and high FSH levels) are unlikely to respond to treatment. Any hormonal deficiencies should be identified and treated.

Other factors which depress spermatogenesis include drug treatment (e.g. Salazopyrin) and hyperthermia in a patient with viral infections. For these reasons the sperm concentration should be monitored over a 3-month period before coming to any firm conclusion. Obstructive oligozoospermia can be treated with surgery, and infection treated with antibiotics.

There is no proven treatment for idiopathic oligozoospermia.

Treatment by Drug Therapy

1. *Poor motility of sperm*   Occasionally high doses of ascorbic acid can improve motility.

2. *Infection*   Genital tract infections are a recognised cause of infertility and should be treated with appropriate antibiotics; the presence of alkaline semen and pus cells should alert the clinician. Semen, prostatic secretions and urinary cultures are necessary to confirm the diagnosis.

Hormone Therapy

A few men may benefit from hormonal treatment.

1. If the patient has a low FSH and low LH, he is treated with human chorionic gonadotrophin and human menopausal gonadotrophin or gonadotrophin releasing hormones.

2. If the patient has normal body build and normal testes, azoospermia, low FSH and testicular biopsy shows spermatogenic arrest at the spermatocyte stage, he is treated with gonadotrophin replacement therapy.

3. Men with androgen insensitivity, who have high FSH, high LH and high testosterone are treated with high doses of androgens.

4. Oligozoospermia, with low FSH and impaired spermatogenesis, is treated with tamoxifen or clomiphene citrate.

Patients with oligozoospermia should be given the following practical advice:

● Wear loose underwear
● Avoid hot baths
● Avoid regular heavy drinking
● Take exercise and try to maintain a level of health and fitness
● Do not use a lubricant with spermicidal action
● Cut down on smoking

Antibody Problems and their Treatment

Antisperm antibodies may be detected in both peripheral blood and seminal plasma. IgG antibodies are related to circulating antisperm antibodies. IgA antibodies are related to the shaking movement of spermatozoa entrapped in cervical mucus. Treatment with high doses of methylprednisolone (as much as 96 mg daily) results in a success rate of around 30 per cent.

Nursing Care

For these patients nursing care focuses on the psychological aspects of infertility. The nurse should obviously be aware that the patient with infertility has been under considerable emotional stress for a prolonged period. The main objective of the nurse is to provide a supportive environment for the patient. If the prognosis looks bleak, the nurse can explore with the couple their feelings about other options such as adoption, artificial insemination by donor (AID), or in vitro fertilization (IVF).

All of the above options have their drawbacks.

IVF

On the National Health Service, the waiting list can be in excess of 5 years. The cost of private treatment is £3000–4000 for a course of three attempts.

AID

On the National Health Service the waiting list is approximately 2 years and the success rate is 85 per cent. The cost of private treatment is £1000.

Adoptions

Couples are seldom considered over the age of 30 years.

12

Reassignment Surgery

'Sexual body image is probably more to do with what we believe we are than with the physical attributes we possess.'

Bob Price (1986)

What is Transsexualism?

A transsexual is an individual who feels an overwhelming need to function and live in the opposite sex to which he/she is born biologically. A female–male transsexual feels that she is a man trapped in a woman's body. A male–female transsexual feels that he is a woman trapped inside a man's body.

Table 12.1 Components of sexual identity

Psychological
Gender identity (sense of being male or female)
Social sex role (masculinity or femininity)
Public sex role (living or dressing as a male or female)
Sexual orientation (homosexual, heterosexual, transsexual)
Sex of rearing (brought up as a male or female)

Biological
Genetic (presence or absence of Y chromosome)
Gonadal (histological structure of ovary or testes)
Hormonal function (circulating hormones)
Interior genital morphology (presence or absence of male or female internal structures)
External genital morphology (presence or absence of exterior male or female genitalia)
Secondary sexual characteristics (body hair, breasts, fat distribution)

From Walters and Ross (1986)

Prevalence

Transsexualism is a relatively uncommon condition, but is all important to the person in whom it exists. There are approximately 25 000 transsexuals in Britain of whom 40 per cent are female to male. When considering the recorded rate of transsexualism one must be aware that many of these individuals live out their lives without ever declaring their transsexualism, and thus exact incidence and prevalence are difficult to establish (see, for example, Thomas, 1993).

Aetiology

In 1954 Harry Benjamin, a pioneer in transsexual research, coined the term 'gender role *disorientation*', which is now commonly called gender dysphoria – a disturbance of gender identity.

Transsexualism, it is argued, is a symptom of this underlying disorder. There are two main theories which attempt to explain transsexualism.

1. The gender and sexual identity of an individual are dependent on assignment by the parents (so-called sex of rearing).

2. The gender and sexual identity of an individual are biological in nature and dependent upon hormonally induced differentiation of the brain at a critical period of intrauterine development.

Onset

The onset of transsexualism may be either:

1. *Primary* – occurring during the first 10 years of life when the child begins to feel that he/she is different, identifying as a member of the opposite sex. This feeling remains constant throughout adolescence and into adulthood.

2. *Secondary* – transsexuals may always have been aware of some gender disturbance throughout life but manage to suppress it until it is brought to the fore by problems such as divorce, ageing, death or failure.

A realisation phase, when the child becomes aware of his/her identification with the opposite gender, then leads to an attempt at cross-dressing. This is usually followed by an attempt to assume the gender identity consistent with biological gender (i.e. a formal denial of his/her transsexualism). This may include taking an overtly masculine or feminine job (e.g. bricklaying in the case of a male) and the formation of heterosexual relationships which may end in a marriage, which often fails to succeed due to the suppression of transsexualism.

Medical advice may be sought for symptoms such as depression, anxiety or sexual dysfunction which are all indirectly related to the transsexualism of the individual.

Presentation

For the individual diagnosed as being transsexual there are two possible courses of action:

1. To accept his/her life as his/her biological sex *or*
2. To seek gender reassignment.

Biological sex is determined by an individual's chromosomes and therefore it is not possible to have a 'sex change' in the true meaning of the phrase (this fact has legal consequences for the transsexual, which will be discussed later in this chapter). What can be achieved are different aspects of gender reassignment – namely, social, hormonal and surgical. If successful, these represent a reasonable external attempt at 'sex change'.

Before embarking on a scheme of management, it is important to assess the individual's commitment to his/her proposed new identity. For example, is the problem really lifelong and fundamental, or may it possibly be transient? Is the individual fully aware of the extent of the readjustment he/she will have to make? Such questions have to be faced and discussed in detail.

If the ultimate goal of the transsexual is gender reassignment surgery, then referral by their general practitioner to a gender identity clinic (GIC) is desirable. The main function of the GIC is to establish that the individual is genuinely transsexual before embarking on the complicated procedure for changing gender roles.

Transsexual management begins with the encouragement of appropriate behaviour patterns for the adopted sex. GIC's require a period of 2 years' continuous 'cross-gender living' to 'prove' that the individual can function within his/her preferred gender. This first-hand experience of living, working and dressing in the chosen role is very important in proving commitment.

Cross-dressing for females is made easier by the bisexual clothing available. It has been shown that if one is given a silhouette or back view of a person to look at, the majority of people will automatically say that the silhouette is male. The male gender is applied to most people until proven otherwise. Cross-dressing for males may be more difficult due to the larger body frame, masculine voice and beard.

Hormone therapy will be prescribed by the GIC (though many transsexuals may already be taking hormones, illicitly obtained from friends).

For females, the male hormone testosterone will be prescribed. This can be given in tablet form which is taken sublingually every day. Alternatively, it can be given by monthly intramuscular injections. As a result of such hormone therapy the following changes may occur:

- Voice deepens
- Increase in body and facial hair
- Menstruation is suppressed
- Body weight increases

For males the female hormone oestrogen is given (e.g. Prenorin 2.5 mg daily). This will act to:

- Decrease facial hair (subtly)
- Promote growth of breasts (gynaecomastia)
- Cause testicular atrophy
- Promote changes in body contours, with a subsequent reduction in muscle bulk

For most male to female transsexuals, one of the biggest problems is hiding a facial beard. Oestrogens will make a subtle difference to beard growth, but cyproterone acetate (an antiandrogen) may be needed to retard growth further. Many individuals spend thousands of pounds on facial electrolysis, which is not available as an NHS treatment.

Hormone therapy cannot change the original body structure, especially in relation to hands, feet and height. Thus a small woman becomes a small man; or a large man a large woman.

Legal Issues

For successful cross-gender living, it is usually necessary for the transsexual to change his/her name either by statutory declaration or by deed poll. The services of a solicitor will be required to do this.

Having changed his/her name, an individual will be in a position to change every official record *except* the birth certificate. These include:

- National Insurance record
- Income tax
- Driving licence
- Medical card
- Passport
- Electricity, gas and phone bills
- Insurance policies
- Examination records

Birth Certificate

The Registrar General has the power to order a complete entry to be altered when he is satisfied that there has been an error of fact or substance in relation to a birth. The entry is a record of the facts at the time of birth. As long as a transsexual's sex is determined by biological criteria only, at the time of birth, the Registrar General does not have the power to make an alteration regarding gender. British courts maintain that gender is determined at birth – a view which has recently been upheld by the European Court. In the future this may change as attitudes toward transsexual identity become more sympathetic.

The inability to alter the birth certificate means that the following are affected:

1. *Marriage*   A female to male or male to female transsexual who has undergone surgery cannot marry. In English law, marriage is essentially a relationship between a man and a woman. Marriage between a female transsexual and her male partner can be prevented by the law using biological criteria. A female transsexual will regard a biological and psychological female as a member of the opposite sex but they cannot marry as the law regards them both as female.

Perversely, a male transsexual living as a woman can marry a female transsexual living as a man. Many transsexuals go abroad to marry where birth certificates are not required for marriage.

2. *Prison* Should transsexuals commit crimes in this country they could be sent to a prison determined by their original gender. A female to male transsexual could be sent to a female prison. At the discretion of the prison doctor hormone therapy may be discontinued.

3. *Pensions* A female to male transsexual should retire at 60. A male to female transsexual would not be entitled to a state pension until she is 65 years old.

4. *Life Insurance* Transsexual status must be declared on life insurance policies. Failure to do so could result in non-payment of benefit.

5. *Employment* The Sex Discrimination Act 1975 and the Equal Pay Act 1970 prohibit discrimination on the grounds of sex in places of employment. However, sex refers to the original biological sex, therefore discrimination against transsexuals is not unlawful under these Acts.

Social Issues

The transsexual must accept the possibility of permanently losing family and friends when they are informed of forthcoming changes. People will react differently, unfortunately often with anger, disbelief, guilt, shame and embarrassment. Counselling for the transsexual's family may be necessary. Of course, some transsexuals are fortunate to retain the support of family and friends. Many transsexuals find help and support from specialised organisations and make friends with other transsexuals who understand the difficulties and can thus offer advice regarding achieving a more successful cosmetic appearance.

In many cases, in order to accomplish a successful social reassignment the transsexual may be forced to move away from home in order to start afresh in his/her new identity.

The transsexual may also have difficulties in securing appropriate employment. Where their present employer is sympathetic and work is appropriate to either gender then a problem may not arise; on the other hand, it may be necessary to seek alternative employment.

SURGICAL TREATMENT

Criteria qualifying Transsexuals for Surgical Treatment

These include:

- Age 21–58 years
- Successful endocrine masculinisation/feminisation
- 1–3 years of total cross-living and working in the gender of choice
- Success in social, psychological, employment and sexual spheres.
- Freedom from psychosis or significant sociopathy (e.g. jail or drug usage).

Female to Male Gender Reassignment Surgery

Female to male gender reassignment surgery consists of:

- Bilateral reduction mammoplasty
- Hysterectomy and salpingo-oophorectomy
- Phalloplasty (construction of a penis)

Bilateral Reduction Mammoplasty

Bilateral simple mastectomy is performed, preserving the nipples.

Preoperative Management

Within the author's clinical area individuals are admitted, as a male to the male ward, or to a single room if requested (and one is available). Preoperative nursing assessment is undertaken using the model of nursing practised within the area. A full explanation is given regarding surgery and informed consent obtained.

Investigations

- Full blood count
- Group and crossmatch 2 units of blood

Postoperative Care

Postoperative care is as for an individual following a general anaesthetic and surgery.

Specific Care

A pressure dressing is strapped across the chest. This remains in position for approximately 48 hours and helps reduce swelling and bruising. A Redivac/Portovac drain is in situ. This is removed when there is minimal drainage. Sutures are usually dissolvable and therefore will not require removal.

Complications

1. *Scarring* – some degree is inevitable but this can be hidden by chest hair growth.

2. *Haematoma* – return to the theatre may be necessary for drainage.

3. *Necrosis of nipple* – the nipple blackens and sloughs.

4. *Infection* – if signs and symptoms of infection occur a wound swab should be taken and sent to microbiology and appropriate antibiotic treatment prescribed if indicated.

Hysterectomy and Salpingo-oophorectomy

Hysterectomy and salpingo-oophorectomy is the surgical removal of the uterus, fallopian tubes and ovaries.

Preoperative Management

Preoperative nursing assessment is undertaken using the model of nursing practised within the area. A full explanation is given regarding surgery, and informed consent obtained.

Investigations

- Full blood count
- Group and crossmatch 2 units of blood

Postoperative Care

This is as for an individual following a general anaesthetic and abdominal surgery.

Some transsexuals are satisfied with the above two procedures, but the majority proceed to phalloplasty.

Phalloplasty

In the past, the operation involved several stages of surgery to construct a phallus. This involved repeated admissions to hospital over a period of approximately 12 months.

Now a one-stage 'clitoral phalloplasty' can be performed. Abdominal flaps are raised from abdominal skin. The existing urethra is extended to the tip of the clitoris and clitoral skin then used to extend the urethra further.

The aim of surgery is to produce a phallus that is functional in that the 'male' can stand to void. The construction of the male urethra is a complex aspect of this surgery and there is the risk of both stricture and fistula formation. Nothing like the erectile function of the normal penis can be achieved, but at future surgery it is possible to implant Silastic penile prostheses, which will then allow for penetration during sexual intercourse.

Preoperative Management

Preoperative nursing assessment is undertaken using the model of nursing practised within the area.

A full explanation is given regarding what the patient can expect pre- and postoperatively. Informed consent is obtained. Surgery will have been discussed at length prior to admission, at an out-patient's consultation.

Investigations

● Full blood count
● Group and crossmatch 2 units of blood

Postoperative Care

This is as for an individual following a general anaesthetic and surgery.

Specific Care

Pain should be well controlled so as to promote mobility. A continuous opioid infusion is very useful for the first 48 hours.

Wound

Redivac/Portovac drain(s) remain in situ until minimal drainage. Prophylactic antibiotics are given (e.g. metronidazole 500 mg t.d.s. and cefuroxime 750 mg b.d. for 48 hours postoperatively).

Catheters

A suprapubic catheter is inserted and left on free drainage. A spigotted urethral catheter acts as a stent within the neo-urethra.
    A 'downagram' is performed at 14 days post-surgery. This is performed in X-ray. Contrast dye is inserted via the suprapubic catheter and the patient is asked to void. Any leakage from the urethra is demonstrated. If there is no leakage, then the stent and suprapubic catheter can be removed.

Complications

● Infection
● Fistula
● Necrosis of phallus
● Stricture of the neourethra
● Expectations not realised

The patient undergoing gender reassignment surgery is very vulnerable, and needs a great deal of psychological support. Just being there and having the time and interest to listen and talk with the individual is very important, for both the patient and the nurse.

Male to Female Gender Reassignment Surgery

In addition to surgical reassignment of the genitalia, many male to female transsexuals will have had other cosmetic surgery such as augmentation mammoplasty, rhinoplasty and removal of the thyroid cartilage (Adam's apple). These operations may be obtained on the NHS on the referral of the psychiatrist, though many transsexuals go private to avoid long waiting lists for non-emergency operations.

Surgical Reassignment of Genitalia

In the author's experience patients were admitted to a single room on a mixed urology ward. Preoperative nursing assessment is undertaken using the model of nursing used within the area. A full explanation is given regarding surgery to allay any worries and provide a rationale for care. Informed consent is obtained on a special consent form which specifies that the patient consents to the removal of his penis and testicles and realises that this will not change his biological sex but allow him to live more comfortably in his chosen role (a sobering thought for anyone not fully committed to this type of surgery).

Investigations/Preparations

- Full blood count – urea and electrolytes
- Group and cross-match 2 units of blood
- Shaving of hair as close to the time of surgery as possible, or in theatre itself.

Preoperative Care

The preoperative care for male to female gender reassignment surgery is directly related to the prevention of certain postoperative problems. The patient is admitted 2 days prior to surgery and commenced on fluids only. An enema is given to completely empty the bowel on the day before surgery and the patient will be given nil by mouth for 6 hours prior to surgery.

Hormone therapy must be discontinued 1 month prior to admission. Anti-embolytic stockings and/or prophylactic heparin should be given. A bath and a shave from umbilicus to mid thigh should be carried out by the patient and checked by a nurse. It must be remembered that the transsexual is usually very embarrassed about his penis and testes, so the nurse must exercise tact here. Prophylactic antibiotic therapy is commenced on the day prior to surgery.

Surgical Procedure

The operation takes 4–5 hours with the patient in the lithotomy position. The spermatic cords are transfixed and the testicles removed. The skin covering the penis and its underlying fascia is undermined and the penis is pulled out of its skin. The skin is kept intact and later pushed 'inside out' to become the lining of the 'neovagina'. The penis is pulled upwards and with a urethral catheter in situ is amputated at its roots. Dissection is carried out upwards and backwards from the root of the penis into the pelvic peritoneum, in order to create a space for the neovagina. Care must be taken not to dissect too close to the rectum as this can result in a rectovaginal fistula.

The scrotal sac is dissected, to form the labia and a clitoris. The neovagina is then sutured in place and packed with ribbon gauze. Two corrugated drains are then inserted. A second outer pack is applied to the vaginal and perineal areas and a tight T bandage applied.

Postoperative Care

This is as for any individual following a general anaesthetic and surgery, with specific care being related to the nature of the operation. Specific postoperative care, using a problem-solving approach would include:

1. *Partial prolapse of neovagina*   The neovagina is tightly packed with ribbon gauze to promote healing. Bed rest is strictly maintained for 5 days, and all food is also withheld for 5 days to prevent any bowel movement which might cause a neovaginal prolapse. Clear fluids only are allowed and nothing which will act as a bowel stimulant (e.g. cigarettes or coffee) is given. These 5 days are very difficult for the patient and the temptation to 'sneak' out of bed for some food may be too much for some patients. The nurse must provide reassurance and try to divert the patient's attention from food wherever possible.

2. *Potential shock and haemorrhage*   An intravenous infusion is usually given for the first 24 hours, after which time the patient should be taking 'clear' fluids. Routine postoperative observations are made. Special care is taken to check for bleeding from the wound site. The vagina is packed for 5 days and a pressure dressing in the form of 'meniscectomy wool' with two tight T bandages is applied. If oozing occurs the wool may be changed. The two corrugated drains are removed after 48 hours. The inner vaginal pack must not be removed.

3. *Potential infection of wound area*   The urethra is amputated during surgery and as a result may swell considerably. A urethral catheter is passed before surgery commences and remains in situ for 5 days afterwards. Chymotrypsin is given orally to reduce swelling at the urethral meatus.

When the urethral catheter is removed, a guiding suture is left in place in case the patient goes into urinary retention, necessitating the passing of a further catheter.

The patient should be warned that for some months postoperatively she may experience 'spraying' of her urine on voiding, due to the surgical refashioning of the urethral meatus.

4. *Potential closure of neovagina*   The internal pack stays in place for 5 days and is removed only by an experienced nurse or the surgeon. When the pack and the catheter have been removed the patient must be taught to dilate the vagina. It is necessary for the patient to use a Perspex dilator three times a day for the rest of her life in order to keep the neovagina patent. The dilator is 'twisted' into position gently, after lubrication with KY jelly, and retained for 10 mintues.

5. *Potential risk of DVT*   The risk of deep vein thrombosis (DVT) and pulmonary emboli is increased due to pelvic surgery, bed rest and excess of the hormone oestrogen. Active and passive exercise of the limbs and deep breathing exercises are important in the prevention of these life-threatening problems. Correctly fitted thromboembolytic deterrent stockings (TEDS) should be worn, and/or subcutaneous heparin given.

6. *Problem of anxiety*   The patient is usually very anxious to see her new vagina. It is important that she is prepared for the swelling, which may make it unsightly for the first few weeks. The stitches in the refashioned labia are removed on day 7, prior to discharge, and the patient may need reassurance that the neovagina will have a 'normal' appearance. In fact after about 6 weeks, when pubic hair has regrown, the results are usually very good. Some patients worry greatly about the depth of the vagina. This is usually between 6 and 8 inches which should be satisfactory for sexual intercourse.

There may also be some anxiety about the process of dilating, which will need a tactful and understanding approach from the nurse.

Discharge

The patient is usually discharged on the seventh postoperative day, after removal of the sutures. The patient is instructed to use a douche (or shower) daily and a Betadine pessary is used once a week for 10 weeks. She is advised to avoid constipation due to the risk of prolapse, and to carry on her dilation. (In the event of a prolapse, a colovaginal repair may be undertaken using a piece of colon to form the vagina. This surgery is more difficult, with a higher risk of complications, and so is avoided if possible.)

The patient may restart her hormones 2 weeks after surgery, which is usually a great relief as she may have started to get a regrowth of facial hair. She is advised not to do any heavy lifting for 6 weeks and to avoid sexual intercourse until after she is seen as an out-patient. Psychiatric follow-up continues at the Gender Identity Clinic.

Some patients may need to have follow-up surgery such as vaginal lengthening, refashioning of the urethra or labial reduction, but most appear happy with the results and in the author's experience seldom require further surgical treatment.

Once the site is healed and has been seen by the surgeon, the patient may, if she wishes, have sexual intercourse. The use of KY jelly is recommended as there is no natural lubrication within the neovagina. Many patients are able to reach orgasm as nerve endings are, whenever possible, left intact during surgery.

CONCLUSION

The reluctance of some surgeons to become involved in gender reassignment surgery is understandable, as it can be perceived as very mutilating to an otherwise healthy body. There is also the question of whether surgery should be performed free on the

NHS or regarded in the same light as private cosmetic surgery, which would probably render the surgery out of the reach of most transsexuals.

There remains a general lack of social awareness and tolerance of the many problems encountered by transsexuals, who are unfortunately regarded by many as social 'oddities'. Public confusion between transsexuality and homosexuality is common. Media attention tends to focus on transsexuals as 'freaks'. Female to male transsexuals were virtually unheard of in the media until relatively recently. Often, in an attempt to pass as 'normal', the transsexual may somewhat overemphasise masculine or feminine characteristics (e.g. a male to female transsexual may overapply makeup), and sadly, this may then allow them to be 'read' (exposed), leading to embarrassment. However, it may also be said that, in the author's experience, there are many transsexuals who have no difficulty in promoting an extremely credible gender image.

A high degree of nursing professionalism is the right of every individual requiring nursing care. Individuals undergoing gender reassignment clearly require a great deal of emotional and psychological support. Transsexuals are often very willing to talk about their problems, sometimes to anyone who comes to listen, and they will often do so in graphic detail. The nurse must be comfortable with his/her own sexuality in order to help transsexuals cope with theirs. Junior nurses may need the help of a more experienced nurse when dealing for the first time with individuals undergoing gender reassignment. If the nurse's feelings regarding gender reassignment interfere and are detrimental to the patient's care, then the nurse should not be put in the position of caring for such a patient. However, if the nurse is willing to be openminded he/she may well find that caring for a patient having reassignment surgery is both an enlightening and rewarding experience.

References

Price R (1986) The range of factors affecting body image. *Nursing Times* **82**(39): 30–32.
Thomas B (1993) Gender Loving Care. *Nursing Times* **89**(10): 50–51.
Walters W and Ross M (eds) (1986) *Transsexualism and Sex Reassignment*. Oxford: Oxford University Press.

13
Paediatric Urology

INTRODUCTION

The major difference in nursing care between general surgical and urological patients is probably the inevitable presence of various drainage tubes. Training nurses to care for children who are encumbered with an assortment of catheters takes time and patience but can be very rewarding. It is important that the nurse understands the different types of catheter, the reasoning behind their choice, their anatomical position, whether the catheter should or should not be draining – and why. It is vital to teach nurses the best way of securing catheters to prevent accidental removal, particularly as children are very determined and inquisitive and do not always understand the consequences of their actions.

Parents of children with congenital abnormalities require support, understanding, information and teaching to enable them to come to terms with their child's condition and help them face, with courage and hope, a future that often seems to them to be an endless round of investigations, hospitalisations, appointments and periods of despair. It is often essential to have parents resident prior to the discharge of their child to ensure that they are confident and competent to look after any appliances or long-term drainage tubes (i.e. suprapubic catheter or nephrostomy tube). Some of the conditions are so rare that the parent receives little or no assistance from the community – not because they do not want to provide it but simply because they do not know themselves. This can be a very frightening situation for parents, particularly if they live a long distance from the hospital.

The management of infants and children with genitourinary abnormalities has been revolutionised in the past 10–15 years by several factors. These include the introduction of clean intermittent self-catheterisation by Lapides in the 1970s, new surgical techniques which concentrate on creating a continent urinary diversion using bowel to augment or replace the bladder, improvements in paediatric anaesthesia which has enabled earlier surgical intervention, advances in radiological and urodynamic investigations and well-informed and motivated nursing staff.

The delicate and embarrassing nature of genitourinary problems have enormous implications in the psychological, emotional and social development of children and paediatric urological nurses have a major role to play in the pre- and postoperative management of these patients and their families.

FOETAL DEVELOPMENT OF SEXUAL ORGANS AND GENITALIA

The majority of paediatric genitourinary conditions are due to congenital abnormalities; therefore it is important to understand the normal development of the internal sexual organs and external genitalia.

The early foetus has the potential to develop both male and female internal sexual organs (see Figure 13.1a). The mullerian duct can develop into the uterus, fallopian tube and upper vagina. The wolffian duct can develop into the vas deferens, seminal vesicles and ejaculatory ducts. The mullerian duct appears to develop normally in the absence of any oestrogenic or hormonal stimulation; however, the development of the wolffian duct is stimulated by testosterone which is secreted by the foetal testis. There is a second hormone secreted by the foetal testis – a large molecular weight protein – which causes regression of the mullerian duct. The continuation of an 'androgen milieu' leads to the development of male external genitalia. Prior to this differentiation the external genitalia are the same regardless of genetic sex (see Figure 13.1b).

The testosterone from the foetal testis probably needs to be converted by 5-alpha reductase into dihydrotestosterone for the continuing normal development of male external genitalia. The testis descends from its original position in the abdomen to its final position in the scrotum by the seventh or eighth month. This descent is also dependent on the normal development of the scrotum and on other hormonal mechanisms not yet identified.

UPPER TRACT CONDITIONS

Renal Agenesis

The incidence of a child being born with no kidneys is approximately 1 in 3000, and the child is either stillborn or may only survive for a few days. As well as absent kidneys, the ureters, bladder and urethra may be affected. The child would have the typical Potter's facies of low-set ears, flattened nose and wide-set eyes as well as hypoplastic lungs due to the absence of foetal urine.

Unilateral renal agenesis is more common, affecting between 1 in 500 and 1 in 1000 of the population. The absence of one kidney may go unnoticed unless the child is being investigated for renal trauma or urinary tract infections. Treatment should only be necessary if the kidney has associated anomalies.

Fused Kidneys (Horseshoe)

Fusion of the two kidneys across the midline occurs most commonly in males, with an incidence of 1 in 600 to 1 in 1800. Usually the discovery of a horseshoe kidney in a neonate is associated with other congenital abnormalities; however, complications may occur later in life with obstruction, calculi, or reflux.

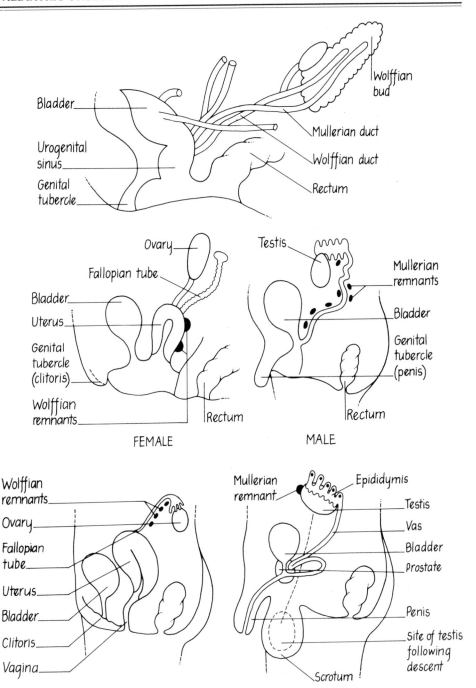

Fig 13.1   Foetal sexual development: transverse view

(a) Undifferentiated, 8–10 weeks. (b) differentiation at 12–16 weeks.
(c) Fully developed sexual organs

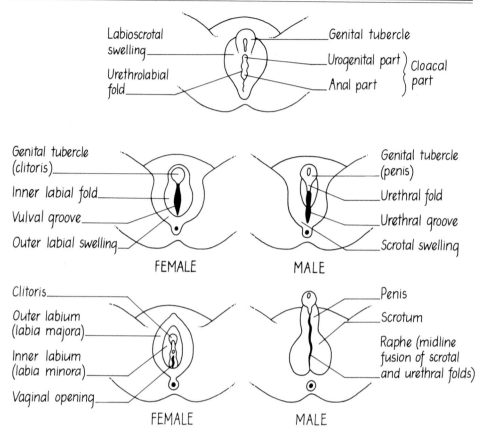

Fig 13.2   Foetal sexual development: anterior view.

(a) Undifferentiated, 8–10 weeks. (b) Differentiation at 12–16 weeks.
(c) Fully developed sexual organs

Pelviureteric Junction Obstruction

The cause of congenital pelviureteric junction obstruction or acquired pelviureteric
junction obstruction is not known but is thought to be caused in some cases by foetal
folds – invaginations of muscle and mucosa which develop into fibrous bands and
cause the obstruction. The defect results in ineffective peristalsis from the pelvis of
the kidney down the ureter. This causes dilatation of the pelvis and an increase in
intrapelvic pressure and associated hydronephrosis. Presentation can either be by
antenatal ultrasound discovering a hydronephrotic kidney or later in childhood, and
is usually associated with loin pain accompanied by a high fluid intake and
sometimes macroscopic or microscopic haematuria. In the child, investigations such
as an intravenous urogram (IVU) or diuresis renography will show the area and
degree of obstruction and associated hydronephrosis. If the differential function of
the affected kidney is less than 10 per cent with good function and there is no

obstruction on the other side, then a nephrectomy may be considered. If the function of the affected kidney is reasonable then the treatment is by way of a pyeloplasty.

Following antenatal diagnosis of unilateral or bilateral hydronephrosis, ultrasound and isotopic renography will be performed following the birth of the baby. If the function of the kidney is low, or the obstruction severe, then a percutaneous nephrostomy tube may be inserted for several weeks to see if there is any improvement in function. A decision will then be made as to whether to perform a pyeloplasty or nephrectomy, depending, of course, on the function and presence of the second kidney. Preservation of the affected kidney in infants should be attempted if at all feasible, as the kidney in this age group appears to have a greater potential for recovery than in later life.

Treatment is by pyeloplasty and some surgeons choose to inject methylene blue dye into the affected kidney above the anastomosis site at the end of surgery just before wound closure. Observations should be made postoperatively in this case for signs of blue/green urine which will indicate that the operated kidney is draining urine past the anastomosis. Depending on the severity of the obstruction, a nephrostomy tube or ureteric stent may be inserted to relieve any undue pressure on the anastomosis site, but on the whole urine drainage is by urethral catheter, with a suction wound drain. The order of the removal of these tubes and drains varies with the surgeon but usually all drains/catheters will be removed by the fifth postoperative day following a straightforward pyeloplasty.

Complications following a pyeloplasty include urine drainage via the wound drain, haemorrhage and clot retention, and stenosis at the anastomosis site, either in the immediate postoperative period or in the long term.

For this reason follow-up is by means of isotope renography and ultrasound at 3 months postoperatively and regular follow-ups for several years following surgery.

URETERIC CONDITIONS

Duplication of the Ureter

There are various forms of duplication which, depending on complexity, will depend on the severity of the child's symptoms and treatment. Duplications of the pelvis of the kidney and ureter are more common in girls and are frequently bilateral.

The simplest form of duplication is partial duplication of the pelvis of the kidney with duplication of the ureters. Problems associated with this form of duplication include a 'yo-yo' or 'see-saw' movement of urine from one pole to the other, leading to stasis of urine and associated infections. If investigations such as isotope renography show that severe renal scarring has taken place then a heminephrectomy may be considered – usually the upper pole.

Complete simple duplication is where two ureters enter the bladder separately. Where this occurs the upper pole ureter always enters the bladder below that of the lower pole. Vesicoureteric reflux is common, especially into the lower pole and if recurrent severe urine infections are a problem, a heminephrectomy may be performed.

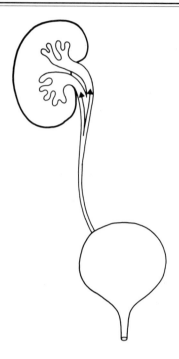

Fig 13.3   Simple, partial duplication

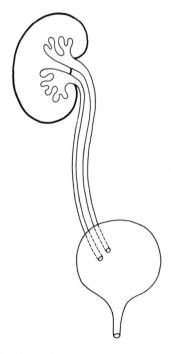

Fig 13.4   Simple, complete duplication

Symptoms of urine infections with or without outflow obstruction, especially in girls, may lead the surgeon to discover an ectopic ureter with a ureterocele. This abnormality occurs seven times more frequently in females and in 10 per cent of cases is bilateral.

A ureterocele is a bulbous submucosal dilatation at the terminal submucosal end of the ureter. It may be so large as to cause outflow obstruction. In girls, prolapse of the ureterocele may occur and the abnormality may be visible on perineal examination.

Treatment will depend on the severity and complexity of the abnormality and will vary from endoscopic incision of the ureterocele to excision of the ureterocele by open surgery with or without partial nephrectomy.

Ureteroceles may also occur without ureteric duplication and treatment is similar, with either endoscopic incision or formal excision of the ureterocele.

Another way in which a child may present with a duplex urinary system with ectopic ureters, is by persistent incontinence in females and chronic epididymitis in males. In females this is due to one of the ectopic ureters opening into the urethra below the sphincter, the vagina, or vulva. The child presents with a history of continuous wetting, despite normal voiding, and never having been 'dry'.

Rarely in boys, problems of recurrent epididymitis may be caused by an ectopic ureter draining into the posterior urethra, vas, seminal vesicle or ejaculatory duct. Treatment is by partial nephrectomy – removing the pole of the kidney which is draining into the affected ureter.

Vesicoureteric Reflux

Urinary tract infections (UTI) are the second most common infection in children. Investigations carried out on a child following a UTI may reveal a congenital abnormality which may need surgical intervention.

Vesicoureteric reflux (VUR) is the passage of urine into the ureter back from the bladder and is present in 50 per cent of children with recurrent UTI. During normal growth of a child, the base of the bladder and trigone mature and the submucosal tunnel of the ureters may lengthen and so reflux ceases. An accepted grading system for reflux was formulated by the Birmingham Reflux Study Group who classified VUR as follows:

● VUR grade I – into the lower ureter
● VUR grade II – filling but not distending the pelvicalyceal system
● VUR grade III – filling and distending the pelvicalyceal system

Diagnosis and grading is generally made following a micturating cystourethrogram.

The decision whether to operate or not is generally made by using the grading of reflux as a guide as well as the clinical presentation of the child and the social circumstances.

Usually children with VUR grades I and II will not need any surgical intervention and will cease refluxing spontaneously and are generally treated with long-term

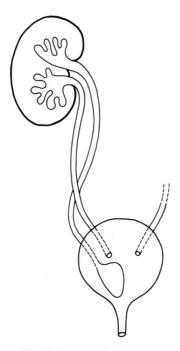

Fig 13.5   Ectopic ureterocele

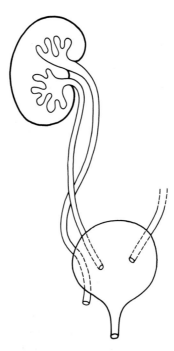

Fig 13.6   Ectopic ureter opening outside the bladder

prophylatic antibiotics. In children with grade III, reflux surgery is generally indicated to give prompt cessation of the reflux and associated renal scarring.

It has been found that there is little or no difference in the clinical outcome of treatment of children with VUR by either medical or surgical treatment (Birmingham Reflux Study Group, 1983). It is generally accepted that there is a 70 per cent chance of spontaneous cessation, compared to a 95 per cent cessation following surgery.

Careful monitoring into adulthood is necessary as there is a high risk of the development of hypertension due to reflux nephropathy. Follow-up studies indicate that approximately 10 per cent of children with renal scarring develop hypertension within 10–20 years.

Surgical treatment is usually in the form of reimplantation of the ureter in a non-refluxing manner, for instance the Politano–Leadbetter technique (Politano and Leadbetter, 1958) and the Cohen operation (Cohen, 1977).

The less invasive subureteric Teflon injection (O'Donnell and Puri, 1986) initially had some very good results but problems occurred with migration of this substance out of the bladder. Recently another product – Uroplastique – has become available and it appears so far that migration of this substance is less likely.

The postoperative management of a child undergoing ureteric reimplantation will depend on the degree of ureteric dilatation and whether ureteric plication as well as reimplantation is necessary.

If the reimplantation is straightforward the child will have a Pfannenstiel incision and usually a suprapubic catheter. Urine drainage is likely to be blood-stained for about 2–3 days and the catheter is left on drainage for 7–10 days. The catheter is then clamped and voiding re-established. Once residual volumes (checked via the suprapubic catheter) are small, the catheter is removed.

If plication has taken place, then ureteric stent catheters are inserted as well as a suprapubic catheter. Because of the long length of catheter tubing outside the body and the importance of maintenance of drainage via the ureteric stents, we tend to keep these children confined to bed to reduce the risk of accidental removal of the stents. The ureteric stents are kept in situ for 7–10 days, and 24 hours following their removal the suprapubic catheter is clamped and voiding re-established.

Frequency and urgency of voiding are not uncommon in the postoperative period.

BLADDER EXTROPHY AND EPISPADIAS

Bladder extrophy and epispadias are the most common form of a group of congenital abnormalities affecting the lower abdominal wall and urinary tract, caused by a failure of midline fusion of the ventral wall of the urogenital sinus and associated structures. The incidence is approximately 1 in 30 000–40 000 live births with a male:female ratio of 1:3–4.

All cases have a gap between the pubic bones. In epispadias (the simplest form) the bladder is formed, though often of a small capacity, but the bladder neck is incompetent and the ureters are usually incapable of preventing reflux. There are abnormalities of the genitalia. In males these include a short, broad penis with the urethral meatus opening on to the dorsal surface of the penis and upward chordee. In females there is a bifed clitoris and a short, wide urethra.

Bladder extrophy is a more severe form where the bladder lies open on the lower abdominal wall. Epispadias always accompanies extrophy and males may also have undescended testes. In females there is a cleft clitoris, separated labia or an absent vagina. There are often associated hernias – umbilical and inguinal – and skeletal abnormalities.

The most severe form is cloacal extrophy. In this condition the extrophied bladder is separated into two lateral portions, each containing a ureter, by an associated extrophy of the bowel. In this group the genital tract and development is rudimentary.

The clinical features presented by this group of patients are numerous and demand all the skill and expertise of the urological surgeon and the support and ingenuity of the multidisciplinary team. The problems include an open bladder plate with a small-capacity bladder once closed, urinary incontinence, chronic or recurrent urinary tract infections, reflux, pyelonephritis, renal failure, abnormal genitalia, an increased risk of malignant changes and a 'waddling gait' due to the skeletal abnormality. Genital development usually proceeds normally and the sexual function of girls is usually satisfactory although there is a tendency to postpartum uterine prolapse. Males are less fortunate and although some achieve normal intercourse, others are handicapped by the abnormal appearance and scarring of the penis. In theory, if the verumontanum is never damaged or infected, fertility should not be a problem, but in practice this has not been found to be the case.

The management of these children represents a major reconstructive problem and their long-term health is largely related to the efficiency of the urinary system. The 'no treatment' option is unrealistic, socially, physically and psychologically. Until the late 1970s, urinary diversion via an ileal conduit, colonic conduit or ureterosigmoidostomy was the treatment of choice. Late complications of these operations included stomal and conduit stenosis, ureterointestinal stenosis, reflux and deteriorating renal function, metabolic disturbances and malignant change. Since the late 1970s the preference has been to provide these patients with an internal, continent urinary diversion in the form of bladder substitution (e.g. Kock's pouch) or augmentation. Current management favours staged repair with the multiple aims of restoring the integrity of the abdominal wall, correcting the external appearance and the genital function, achieving urinary continence and protecting the upper tracts from reflux, and preserving renal function.

Bladder Closure

This can either be undertaken at birth or delayed until the age of 6–9 months. If surgery is delayed the skin needs careful cleansing and protection from excoriation with barrier creams. Moist sterile pads are applied to the extrophied bladder to absorb the urine; these should be changed frequently. To facilitate closure of the anterior abdominal wall, and narrow the pubic gap, it is often necessary for some kind of osteotomy to be performed. However, there is a tendency for the pubic bones to separate within a few months or years despite many different methods used to close them.

Historically, closure within 24 hours was usually done without osteotomy and these babies were nursed postoperatively with their legs bandaged together in a 'mermaid' plaster for approximately 6 weeks. More recently, closure with posterior pelvic osteotomies was undertaken after 24 hours; these babies were then nursed in 'gallows traction' for 4–6 weeks. Currently the preference is for a simple bladder closure at birth combined with salter osteotomies; these babies need to be nursed in a 'frog' plaster for 4–6 weeks postoperatively.

Most bladder extrophy babies are born at full term and like all babies are totally dependent on their parents for all their needs. Nursing neonates is a great responsibility at all times, particularly when they are sick. Changes in the infant's condition are generally extremely sudden and require immediate intervention. The skills and judgement of nursing staff must be highly developed. Inevitably the parents of a baby born with a congenital abnormality will be shocked and distressed and will need a lot of support to enable them to cope. They will have many questions and initially it should be medical and senior nursing staff who provide the consistent answers; later other members of the team will support and counsel the parents. It is important to remember that parents are unlikely to absorb more than a small fraction of all they are told and consequently they appear to ask the same questions repeatedly. Parents may need support while they go through a grieving process for the loss of their 'perfect' baby. Every effort must be made to promote 'bonding' of mother and child, and nurses require an insight and knowledge of this special relationship in order to foster it. Parents will need to be encouraged, supported and taught how to look after their baby and the nurse should remember that (s)he is an important role model in this process. The baby is likely to spend 24 hours in the intensive care unit following surgery to enable close monitoring and rapid intervention should any problems arise.

It is not the intention of the author to cover the detailed postoperative care of the neonate, merely an overview. Specific complications following surgery are wound dehiscence, stenosis of the bladder neck and reflux. While the bladder is closed, the bladder neck will still be open, incontinence will persist and the epispadias will still be present.

All male epispadiac cases will require surgical repair to some degree. In the female the external deformity is small and hardly requires any treatment. However, if this is necessary it can be delayed and done in conjunction with later surgery. It is possible to undertake the bladder neck and penile repair at the same time; however, some males do have urinary control and therefore it is preferable to delay bladder neck surgery until this can be established. The penile repair can be performed earlier to achieve a more normal appearance.

Epispadias Closure

Currently the preferred method of treatment is a simple anatomical reconstruction at either 12–15 months or 3–3.5 years. The aim is to straighten the penis, with a single stage repair, by resecting the chordee, reducing the terminal meatus, providing a urethra of uniform, satisfactory calibre and providing an adequate cosmetic result in respect of the length, direction and strength of the urinary stream, and resting position of the penis (angle of dangle!).

For 3 months prior to surgery the infant may be given a monthly injection of testosterone 50 mg to provide an adequately sized penis. Massage of the phallus with testosterone cream for several weeks prior to surgery to enlarge the penis has also been tried with limited success. The surgery and complications are similar to hypospadias repair and the nursing care is virtually the same except that the child will usually have a suprapubic as well as a urethral catheter. Suprapubic drainage continues for 10–14 days and is clamped following urethral catheter removal in order to re-establish voiding, after which it is removed. The compressive dressing is maintained for 7–10 days.

Following epispadias repair the child still has an incompetent bladder and little or no sphincter control, resulting in persistent incontinence.

Bladder Neck Reconstruction

Bladder neck reconstruction should be delayed until incontinence is proved to be present; consequently, it is usually undertaken after 4 years of age. It is generally combined with external genital repair in females and ureteric reimplantation to correct reflux, if necessary. The most common surgical procedure is the Young–Dees reconstruction.

Preoperative investigations are likely to include ultrasound scans, urodynamic studies to assess the bladder capacity, pressures and function, a urethral pressure profile designed to measure the pressure at the internal and external sphincter and assessment of renal function. Nursing care is the same as that prior to any major surgery. It is particularly important, however, to ensure that children have their bowels open prior to surgery as constipation will lead to straining in the postoperative period which may compromise the reconstruction.

Parents should be advised preoperatively that reconstruction is not an exact science and depends on many factors, including the skill and experience of the surgeon. Consequently it is possible that the child will still be incontinent or alternatively will be unable to void adequately and may need to learn self-catheterisation, postoperatively. This information is usually discussed with the parents prior to surgery at an out-patient appointment but should be reinforced at this time.

Specific postoperative care includes the following:

1. Maintaining the patency of the urinary drainage systems. The patient will always have a suprapubic catheter in situ and he or she may have a urethral catheter as well. Following implantation of the ureters there will be one or two ureteric stents (depending on whether the reimplant was unilateral or bilateral). If bilateral ureteric stents are present, nurses should be aware that there is unlikely to be any drainage from the bladder catheters, in which case gentle bladder washouts or irrigation may be necessary to remove clots from the bladder and keep the catheters patent; this does not commence for the first 24–36 hours. The ureteric stents are removed first (after 10–14 days), followed by the urethral catheter (if present) 24 hours later. The suprapubic catheter is clamped, to allow voiding, and is only removed when voiding has been re-established.

2. Females may have a vaginal pack in situ which can be removed after 24–48 hours. Vulval toiletting will help promote comfort.

3. Bed rest is recommended for 10–14 days and the child needs to be entertained and occupied.

4. A high fluid intake is necessary to maintain patency of the catheters which may necessitate intravenous fluids, but this can be discontinued as soon as the child is tolerating oral fluids.

5. Intravenous antibiotics are usually prescribed for the first 24–72 hours. These are sometimes followed by a course of oral antibiotics although these may not commence until after the removal of the catheters.

6. Constipation must be avoided (as mentioned previously). It can be difficult to persuade children to eat enough roughage, although most like grapes and other fruit, and it may be necessary to give a laxative or suppository if there has been no bowel movement by day 3.

Following this operation 20–30 per cent of patients achieve continence. For those who do not there are several options and these should be fully discussed with the family. The choices include:

1. Further surgery to tighten the bladder neck, which will almost definitely mean the child will need to be prepared to learn, and do, intermittent catheterisation. (This is often the best option for females.)

2. Bladder augmentation, which may also require the child to self-catheterise.

3. The placement of an artificial urinary sphincter; this option may be negated by the prohibitive cost (approximately £3000 at present).

There is a further choice for males which is to wait until puberty and prostatic development, which may increase the outflow resistance sufficiently to achieve continence.

Apart from continuing incontinence (usually secondary to a small capacity bladder and inadequate outflow resistance), other complications include bladder neck obstruction leading to urinary retention and, potentially, hydronephrosis.

Bladder Augmentation

Following bladder neck surgery many children remain incontinent with a debilitatingly small bladder capacity. The bladder can be augmented using any part of the bowel – colon, ileum or ileocaecal segment. If the bowel is unsuitable it is possible to do a gastrocystoplasty.

Specific preoperative preparation includes:

1. The physical and psychological preparation of the child and family, which entails giving detailed information regarding the need for careful and effective bowel clearance, the number and function of catheters/tubes/drains, etc, following surgery and how long they are likely to be required, and providing the family with an opportunity to discuss their own fears and worries.

2. Different surgeons prefer different methods of bowel preparation, but it usually includes aperients, enemata and washouts. The use of intestinal antibiotics to sterilise the bowel is not recommended today but they are still used by some surgeons. A fluid diet is often recommended for 2 or 3 days but it is important to remember that children do not have the same reserves as adults and prolonged starvation is not recommended. During this period of preparation the induced diarrhoea adds to the child's discomfort.

3. The presence of mucus in the urine should be explained, as parents find it worrying if they are not prepared for it.

Specific postoperative care includes:

1. *Parenteral fluid administration*

2. *Nasogastric decompression* until bowel sounds return or the child passes flatus.

3. *Wound drainage.* The quantity and type of drainage should be measured, assessed and recorded. This can be removed when there has been no further drainage for 24 hours.

4. *Control of postoperative pain.* The most effective and comfortable method of achieving this in the initial postoperative phase is by continuous infusion of opioids. These can be administered just as effectively – and more safely – by the subcutaneous route, as opposed to the intravenous route. Nursing staff need to be vigilant in observing and monitoring the child for signs of excessive sedation and respiratory depression and should know exactly what to do should this occur (slow or stop the infusion and notify the doctor) as per local policy. Other analgesics such as co-proxamol and Voltarol are effective as the child's condition improves.

5. *Maintaining the patency of urinary catheters* (usually both suprapubic and urethral). Due to the presence of mucus these catheters are liable to become blocked. Gentle milking, intermittent washouts or continuous irrigation with small volumes of fluid can be utilised. Encouraging a high oral intake also helps. Parents may need to be taught to do bladder washouts at home if the child is discharged with a catheter.

Complications of bladder augmentation include high residual urines which may necessitate clean intermittent self-catheterisation, continuing incontinence, mucus retention leading to infections, and stone formation and perforation. This type of surgery has not been performed for long enough to assess the possibility of long-term malignant changes.

The Artificial Urinary Sphincter

The artificial urinary sphincter (AUS) made its debut in 1972 and has proved to be of immense benefit in the management of urinary incontinence in patients with neuropathic bladder. It has not been approved for general use but preliminary trials with other groups of patients have shown it has some value.

Prior to implantation it is essential to establish that the incontinence is due to an incompetent bladder neck and not detrusor instability. If the latter is present it must be demonstrated that the instability can be controlled – either pharmacologically or by other methods. Outflow must be unobstructed and the patient able to void efficiently. The bladder should be of a good capacity and normal compliance. Urodynamic studies can provide this information. Renal function should be assessed and any significant vesicoureteric reflux must be corrected before the device is implanted. The tissues at the proposed site of implantation must be well vascularised as there is a risk of erosion and/or incomplete urethral occlusion in the presence of poor-quality tissue.

Careful assessment of the patient's physical, psychological and educational abilities is necessary. The child needs to have sufficient intelligence, motivation and manual dexterity to operate the device. It is important to explain the risks and limitations, as well as the advantages, of the device. Ideally the surgery should be carried out after puberty so children do not need to have the device revised as they grow (and whatever increased resistance provided by the prostate in males will have occurred), but this may not be acceptable socially and developmentally.

The most important factor governing success or failure is infection. There should be no instrumentation of the lower urinary tract for 48 hours preoperatively. A midstream urine specimen should be sterile – surgery may be deferred in the presence of an infection. Skin (including the hair) preparation with a bactericidal solution (such as Hibiscrub) is recommended for 36–48 hours prior to surgery and the rectum should be empty. These patients should be first on the theatre list.

The sphincter is composed of three parts: the cuff, which comes in 11 sizes; the pressure-regulating balloon, in four sizes; and the pump. The components are joined by tubing.

Postoperatively, the child is unlikely to have any drainage tubes in situ, but is likely to require antibiotics. The care is similar to that described for simple orchidopexy (see page 339).

There is a period of persistent incontinence postoperatively as the tissues must be allowed to heal completely before the device is activated. This period ranges from 4 to 12 weeks.

The AUS (Figure 13.7) is a mechanical device with the potential for malfunction of any component. Blockage of the tubing may be caused by kinking, air bubbles, fluid leakage and incorrect 'tailoring' of the tubing at insertion. Erosion may occur due to improper cuff sizing, incorrect balloon selection or infection. Meticulous preoperative preparation reduces the risk of infection but nurses should be alert to the potential. Patients should also be advised to seek early treatment at all times if they suspect an infection. Incontinence may persist after the device has been activated. This is usually due to incorrect cuff or balloon choice, leakage of fluid from any component or tubing, or uncorrected detrusor instability.

Patients should always have an X-ray after activation of the device.

URETHRAL/PENILE CONDITIONS

Posterior Urethral Valves

The most common form of outflow obstruction in boys is posterior urethral valves, and the child may present at birth, or later on in childhood, depending on the severity of the obstruction. The valves are sail-shaped membranes that arise from the verumontanum, extend distally and are attached to the anterior lateral walls of the urethra. The prostatic urethra dilates, and the detrusor muscle of the bladder hypertrophies. The renal changes range from mild hydronephrosis to severe dysplasia, depending on the severity of outflow obstruction in foetal development and the promptness of diagnosis.

The diagnosis of posterior urethral valves may be suspected antenatally with the discovery of severe oligohydramnios on maternal ultrasound. Advances have been made towards antenatal catheterisation of the foetus while in utero to prevent further renal damage.

At birth the baby may have a palpable, distended bladder, poor or absent urinary stream and signs of renal failure.

Treatment begins with catheterisation and correction and stabilisation of any electrolyte imbalance. Dialysis may be necessary in severe cases. Diagnosis is confirmed by a micturating cystourethrogram and once the baby is stabilised medically, the valves may be ablated using a diathermy hook.

The condition may go unnoticed if obstruction is not severe. Babies may present later with a history of poor urinary stream, vomiting, failure to thrive and urinary tract infections. In older children presenting symptoms may be poor stream, haematuria, infections or incontinence.

Careful monitoring is necessary throughout childhood after the 'disruption' of the valves due to the resulting problems of bladder instability because of the thick-walled trabeculated bladder and varying degrees of renal dysplasia.

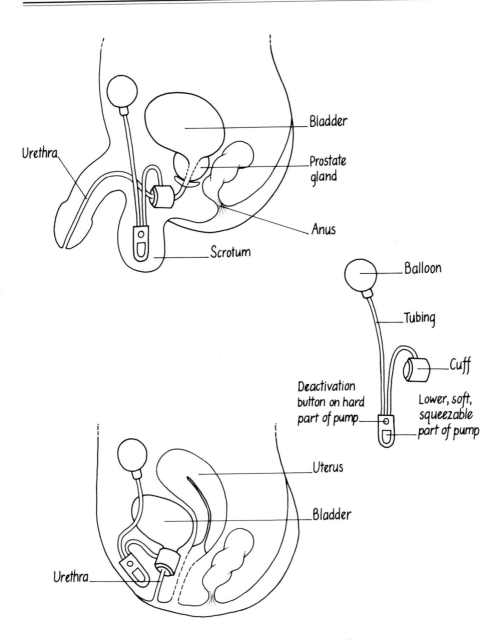

Fig 13.7 Positioning of the artificial sphincter

(a) Position in the male. (b) Components of the pump. (c) Position in the female. The sphincter is activated as follows. The pump is first located and the tubing above it grasped, thereby immobilising it. Using the other hand, the lower, soft part of the pump is squeezed several times until it is flat. The cuff is now deflated (open) and micturition can occur. The cuff reinflates, automatically, within several minutes

Hypospadias

This is one of the most common congenital abnormalities, occurring in approximately 1 in 300 live male births. At around 10 weeks of foetal development a urethral groove develops in the genital tubercle. This deepens and closes over to form the urethra. Hypospadias results from incomplete closure of the groove with the urethral meatus terminating on the ventral surface (underside) of the penis. Chordee (longitudinal bands of fibrous tissue in the corpus spongiosum tethering the penis in a downward, flexed curve) is often present and can be mild, moderate or severe. Other associated conditions include cryptorchidism and intersex; upper tract anomalies appear to be no greater than in the general population. Hypospadias represents a spectrum of deficiency (approximately 65 per cent are of the anterior variety), consequently there is no single repair suitable for all forms. Table 13.1 shows a classification according to the position of the urethral meatus prior to surgery and common repairs in use today.

Table 13.1   Classification of hypospadias repair

Classification	Surgical Repair
Glanular	MAGPI (meatal advancement and glanuloplasty incorporated); IPGAM (reverse MAGPI); Mathieu (meatal-based) flap
Distal shaft	Mathieu flap; pedicle preputial patch and tube; onlay island patch
Midshaft	Duckett's repair; transverse preputial island graft
Penoscrotal and perineal	Bladder or buccal mucosal graft (this involves obtaining a strip of mucosa from either the bladder or the cheek or inner lip, tubularising it and placing it in the penis). The use of buccal mucosa is a very recent variant and more time is needed to assess its viability

Hypospadias is usually detected at birth during routine inspection and symptoms vary according to the degree of severity. These may include:

● Difficulty with micturition
● Retention of urine (if meatal stenosis is severe)
● A thin stream
● An altered position for voiding – sitting (penoscrotal/perineal) or holding the penis upwards (midshaft), which can cause embarrassment and psychological distress
● Potential difficulties with sexual intercourse when severe chordee is present.

The aim of hypospadiac surgery is to straighten the penis by releasing the chordee, reduce the terminal meatus, construct a hairless urethra of uniform, satisfactory calibre and provide a cosmetically acceptable penis by creating a symmetrical glans and shaft with normalization of voiding and erections.

The timing of the surgery is very important. The optimal psychological window for hypospadias repair is between 6 and 18 months, as this will minimize the emotional effects of surgery. In the USA they aim to complete surgery within this time frame although in Britain the goal is for surgery to be completed by the time the child starts school (5 years). Some of the psychological factors that need consideration are:

- The bonding of parents and child, which may be impaired by the baby not being 'perfect'
- Genital awareness and sexual orientation
- The child's own body image

Multistaged repairs were standard in the 1960s and 1970s and are still used today for the more difficult repairs, but contemporary preference is for the single-stage repair which offers patients the benefits of simplification of treatment and one general anaesthetic, and surgeons the opportunity to utilize virgin tissue, devoid of scars and disruption of the normal blood supply. Difficulties experienced in operating on young children include the risks of anaesthesia and the size of the penis; advantages include the fact that the younger child is more easily managed and appears to have less memory of the operation through subsequent development.

The successful management is contingent upon adequate preoperative parental teaching and meticulous attention to detail in postoperative care. Hence nursing staff have a vital role to play. In some centres in the USA hypospadias surgery is routinely done on a 'day case' basis, with no reported adverse affects. However, in Britain the preference is still for hospitalization until removal of the compressive dressing (usually 5–7 days) except in the simplest of repairs.

Nursing consideration in the preoperative period should include:

1. *Psychological preparation* It is important to warn parents and the child that the penis may look bruised and swollen following removal of the dressing and that the appearance will resemble that of a circumcised penis.

2. *Obtaining and sending a midstream urine specimen* (as well as routine ward urinalysis) as any infection will jeopardize healing.

3. *Obtaining a flow rate recording* for objective comparison postoperatively.

4. *Ensuring that appropriate blood samples have been obtained* (haemoglobin estimation and group and cross match; the penis has a very good blood supply, therefore there is a potential for haemorrhage).

The specific postoperative care includes the following:

1. Ensuring all urinary catheters/stents are patent and draining. Virtually all patients will have some form of urinary diversion as premature voiding is undesirable and may lead to wound dehiscence and fistula formation. One of two types of drainage are generally used: (a) the self-retaining balloon catheter draining into a bag and (b) a 'dripping stent' (a thin silastic tube placed through the neourethra and into the bladder) which is secured by one stitch to the glans penis and drains continuously into a nappy. A recent variation of this is the 'voiding stent', where the end of the tubing lies outside the external urinary sphincter, allowing intermittent voiding.

These latter methods appear to decrease bladder spasms (an impression with which the author concurs). Urinary diversion continues for an average of 7–14 days, depending on the extensiveness of the repair and the assessment of healing by the appearance of the penis following removal of the dressing. Patients who have had a bladder mucosal graft (BMG) will usually have a suprapubic as well as a urethral catheter in situ. At the appropriate time the urethral catheter will be removed first and voiding re-established, with the suprapubic catheter clamped, prior to its removal. Catheters should be adequately secured to the child's skin and should not be taped to the leg or the bed linen. Gentle 'milking' of the catheter may be necessary, especially if the drainage is heavily blood-stained, to maintain patency, but this can increase bladder spasms so should be avoided if possible. Following a BMG it may be necessary to perform a bladder washout using small (10–30 ml) volumes of sterile saline or water and a meticulous aseptic technique. The drainage bag must always be situated lower than the bladder and tubing must be observed at regular intervals to prevent 'kinking' and obstruction. The child often complains of the urge to pass urine even though the catheters are draining adequately and the nurse will have to provide much reassurance.

Great care must be taken when removing catheters to prevent damage to the neourethra. If a balloon catheter is used it is essential that the balloon is completely deflated prior to removal and equally obvious that any retaining sutures are cut. If there is any resistance encountered on withdrawing the catheter the procedure should be halted and the doctor notified. Following the removal of catheters, observation of urinary output is essential, leakage or dribbling from the meatus or suture line, the angle and the strength and fluidity of the stream should be noted and reported to the medical staff. A flow rate recording should be obtained for objective comparison during follow-up (the first void following catheter removal does not usually reflect an accurate assessment). Reassurance is necessary as the child is often frightened or reluctant to pass urine.

2. *Observing for signs of bleeding* It is important to monitor and record vital signs postoperatively with particular reference to signs of shock. Most patients will have some form of compressive dressing in place which provides three functions: assisting with haemostasis and containment of oedema; immobilization of the penis and drainage tube; and protection of the suture line. This dressing usually takes one of two forms: in the simpler repairs an occlusive, self-adherent dressing such as Tegaderm or Opsite. Parents are often distressed and frightened by the visualisation of the penis beneath the dressing and need much reassurance. Surgeons claim this dressing is easily removed but nursing staff would not necessarily agree. In the author's experience it can be very difficult to remove even after bathing. This type is usually removed after a few days (2–5).

The second form of dressing is silastic foam – this is provided in a quick-setting, liquid form which is poured into a mould surrounding the penis. After setting, the mould is removed and the dressing secured to the skin with Elastoplast or a similar adhesive tape. This is easier to remove after the child soaks in a bath for about 30 minutes. There is usually a retaining suture in the tip of the glans which is secured to the outside of the dressing and it is very important to remove this suture prior to removing the dressing. The dressing is generally removed at 7 days postoperatively although the range is from 5 to 10 days.

The child and parents should be warned that the penis may look very swollen and bruised initially but that this will resolve spontaneously and the final appearance may not manifest itself for several weeks.

3. *Postoperative pain control*   Children undergoing penile surgery are usually given a caudal anaesthetic (see section on Circumcision). Most children obtain adequate analgesia from Panadol, older children may require something stronger initially such as co-proxamol or Voltarol.

4. *Adequate fluid intake* is essential to ensure the catheters drain freely and do not block; this can tax the patience and ingenuity of even the best of paediatric nurses. The child may require an intravenous infusion initially but this should be discontinued as soon as oral intake is established. The nurse should ensure that fluids are balanced so the child will still eat and not fill him/herself up with inappropriate drinks.

5. *A well-balanced diet* is necessary to promote healing. Children in hospital often lose interest in eating; the food may not be visually appealing and is prepared differently; they may be eating more sweets and crisps than usual as a form of compensation.

6. *Prevention of constipation* is important to prevent straining, excessive tension on the sutures, increased incidence of bladder spasms and compromised urinary drainage. Systemic measures such as a mild laxative (e.g. lactulose) or local measures such as suppositories should be given if the child has not had a bowel movement by day 3. Explanations and reassurance are again necessary as the child is often frightened that passing a stool will be painful.

7. *Preventing bladder spasms*   These are due to irritation from the catheter and can lead to forcible expulsion of urine via the neourethra with serious adverse effects. Spasms are difficult to control and cause much distress to both child and parents. Anticholinergics (e.g. Probanthine), muscle relaxants (e.g. diazepam) and opiates (used more commonly in the USA) may be helpful.

8. *The routine use of antibiotics* is controversial, with some surgeons denying their value, some restricting their use to those patients with open urinary drainage (dripping stents) and others who prescribe them routinely, particularly after catheter removal. It is important to anticipate the potential problem of infection following instrumentation of the urinary tract and to monitor the child's temperature regularly, notifying medical staff if it is elevated above 37°C.

9. *Restricting mobility* by confining the child to bed promotes healing and helps prevent accidental removal of drainage tubes; it is recommended for all but the simplest repairs, and should continue until the dressing is removed (5–10 days).

Attention to general hygiene must be maintained appropriately during this period and parents are usually anxious to assist after being taught what to do. Boredom is a potential problem and should be prevented by age-appropriate games, toys and supervised play.

10. *The genital area* should be kept clean and dry; daily or twice daily baths are encouraged following removal of the dressing, depending on the state of the wound. It is particularly important to keep the urethral meatus free of any scabs which could obstruct the flow of urine and cause wound breakdown and fistula formation. The child may find the use of a hair dryer, instead of a towel, more comfortable to dry the genital area.

11. *Prior to discharge*, parents should be given a date and time to attend the out-patient clinic (usually after approximately 6 weeks). They should be warned about any potential problems and advised who to contact should they occur (the ward or the GP). It is essential that children are prevented from playing with 'ride astride' toys (bicycles and rocking horses) for a few weeks after surgery and they will probably find loose clothing (boxer shorts and track suits) more comfortable than tight trousers.

Complications following hypospadiac surgery include the following:

1. *Fistula formation* – as high as 30 per cent. 'Pinhole' fistulas may close spontaneously and this may be encouraged by teaching the child to occlude the fistula with his finger whilst voiding. The authors have seen and been surprised by the spontaneous healing of some comparatively large fistulas. Surgical repair may be necessary but this should not occur for at least 3 months to ensure complete healing.

2. *Persistent chordee* – will need further surgery.

3. *Meatal stenosis and retraction* – this is seen infrequently in the single-stage repair.

4. *Urethral diverticulae and strictures* – usually due to postoperative infection or stenosis of the neourethra/meatus, sometimes due to poor surgical technique.

5. *Poor cosmetic results and potential sexual problems in later life* Some studies and reports suggest that with hypospadias there is a sense of inferiority, poor body image and poor or late onset of sexual activity. Other reports refute this. The potential problems should be recognised so early intervention can be provided if necessary.

Female Hypospadias

In this condition the vulva appears superficially normal, but on closer inspection the urethral meatus is abnormally positioned on the anterior vaginal wall, a short distance within the vaginal introitus. Minor degrees of this abnormality are relatively common and require no treatment. Severe deformities are rare and usually complicated by urinary obstruction, a trabeculated bladder and urinary reflux; other cases may include bifurcation of the vagina and a degree of vaginal outlet obstruction. These cases will require surgical repair.

Circumcision

The foreskin (prepuce) probably serves a useful purpose in protecting the glans and meatus from ammoniacal irritation from urine-soaked nappies during infancy. It is normal not to be able to retract the foreskin behind the glans penis before the age of 2 or 3 years; in fact any attempt to do this should be actively discouraged. However, should the condition (phimosis) persist beyond the age of 3 years or recurrent balanitis (irritation and infection under the foreskin) occur with ballooning of the prepuce and/or pain during voiding, circumcision should be considered. There is some evidence to suggest that circumcision is beneficial in reducing the incidence of penile cancer in later life and a decreased incidence of carcinoma of the cervix. Circumcision is also performed to comply with some religious beliefs.

The operation is ideally suited to day case surgery (as described under Orchidopexy). Other care specific to penile surgery includes the following:

1. *Caudal anaesthesia* This has a dual purpose in that it provides effective pain control in the initial postoperative phase without recourse to strong analgesia (such as pethidine) and the vasoconstriction provides a relatively blood free field for the surgeon in an area that has an excellent blood supply. The child (if he is old enough to understand) and parents should be advised that he may get a headache and feel dizzy if he gets up too quickly after surgery; he should be encouraged to lie flat for about 6 hours. He is likely to complain of loss of function and/or sensation of the lower limbs and may experience some discomfort and 'pins and needles' as the caudal anaesthetic wears off; gentle massage may promote comfort. The nurse should observe the lower limbs for colour, sensation, warmth and movement in the immediate postoperative period. The first time the child gets up he should be accompanied by a parent or the nurse as a safety precaution.

2. *Risk of haemorrhage* Primary or reactionary haemorrhage (due to vasodilation or a slipped suture) could occur immediately and up to 48 hours after surgery; parents should be advised of how and where to apply direct pressure, the use of a cold compress and to call the GP immediately, day or night. (They may be advised to call the ward, depending on local policy).

Secondary haemorrhage can occur as a result of infection; parents should be advised to look out for signs of infection: fever, local discharge, increased pain or discoloration and to call their GP if they are worried. The use of cold packs should be carefully monitored and supervised to prevent more damage occurring. The nurse should inspect the penis for bleeding prior to discharge.

3. *Difficulty with micturition* The child should pass urine before being discharged. The child should be observed for signs of discomfort; the nurse can palpate the

abdomen to assess the degree of retention and should notify the doctor appropriately. Several steps can be taken to encourage the child to void: change of position and mobilization; the application of warm packs to the abdomen; analgesia; the sound of running water; a warm bath, although this may be contraindicated immediately postoperatively; and increased oral fluids. Parents should be advised to contact their GP (or the hospital) if pain and difficulty persist longer than 12 hours.

4. *Swelling* The best treatment for this is to reduce activity, advise the careful and supervised use of ice/cold packs and ensure the child wears loose clothing (boxer shorts and track suits).

Postoperative complications include haemorrhage, damage to the glans penis, amputation of the glans penis and urethral fistula.

CONGENITAL ABNORMALITIES OF THE TESTES

Undescended Testes – Cryptorchidism

The testis begins in the gonadal ridge of the foetus, high in the abdominal and behind the peritoneal cavity, and by the time of birth it should have descended into the scrotal sac via the inguinal canal which forms the channel between the abdomen and the scrotum. By 3 months of foetal life the testes should lie close to the inguinal region and by 7 months they should have passed down through the inguinal canal into the genital swelling which then fuses to form the scrotum. On completion of testicular descent the inguinal canal is closed off by fusion of the processus vaginalis; if this fusion does not occur there is a risk of fluid from the abdominal cavity collecting in the scrotum, creating a hydrocele.

The absence of one or both testes from the scrotum requires careful examination by palpation in order to differentiate between true cryptorchidism (failure of or arrested descent of the testis), the ectopic testis (where the testis has emerged from the external inguinal ring but has not entered the scrotum) and the retractile testis (where the testis can be found in the groin at the external inguinal ring but can be gently manoeuvred into the scrotum).

The complications of undescended testes include:

● Inguinal hernia
● Torsion
● Infertility
● Psychological effects
● Malignancy

The aim of treatment is to secure the testes sufficiently early to allow maximum functional potential.

Orchidopexy

The optimum age for a child to undergo orchidopexy (the operation to bring the testis down and secure it in the scrotum) is 2–3 years. Unfortunately the diagnosis is often not made until the child is much older; these children should have surgery as soon as practical and prior to puberty.

There is very little required in the way of specific preoperative preparation prior to a simple orchidopexy; however, if there is a possibility of a laparatomy being performed, serum should be obtained and sent to the laboratory for routine haemoglobin estimation and group, and saved; the nursing staff should check that this has been done.

A child with no other health problems undergoing a simple orchidopexy may be a suitable candidate for 'day case' surgery and this should be encouraged, provided that the social circumstances are appropriate. It is vital to ensure that the child and parents are adequately prepared prior to the admission, either during the initial out-patient appointment or on a preoperative ward visit. Written information should be provided for reference as it may be some months before the child is called for surgery. The benefits of a preoperative ward visit, particularly for those patients having 'day surgery', cannot be overemphasised. For the child and family it helps to reduce anxiety through familiarisation with the ward environment, providing the opportunity to express their fears and worries regarding the diagnosis, the surgery and the postoperative care. These fears may include the possibility of delayed development, a lifetime of hormone therapy, the fear of malignancy and reduced fertility. Nursing staff should be prepared to provide information about causes, available treatments and the ultimate effect on reproduction. They should therefore familiarise themselves with the facts regarding the individual's condition and reinforce what they have already been told by medical staff. Nursing staff are better able to assess the family's ability to cope with the postoperative care following a meeting of this type and can mobilise community support as necessary.

The specific pre- and postoperative teaching should include the following:

1. *Fasting prior to surgery*   Parents should be advised of the exact time to stop their child eating and drinking (no solids or milk for 6 hours and no clear fluids for 4 hours prior to surgery).

2. *Arrival time on the ward* and whether or not the child should have a bath at home.

3. *Control of postoperative pain*   Panadol is usually sufficient to keep a child comfortable following orchidopexy. Parents should be advised of the appropriate dose and frequency of administration.

4. *The risk of haemorrhage*   Reactionary haemorrhage can occur up to 3 hours postoperatively; this is caused by vasodilation of the small veins in the scrotal skin. Rarely, patients may need to return to theatre for cautery to these veins but the bleeding will usually stop spontaneously. The scrotum should be inspected prior to discharge and parents advised to contact their own GP or the hospital (as per local policy) if they notice any bleeding or discoloration of the scrotum. They should be reassured that the bruising will disappear although it may take a week or two.

5. *Scrotal oedema* Swelling is not uncommon following surgery and restricting mobility for several days postoperatively is helpful in reducing swelling and pain. Parents should be advised to put away 'ride astride' toys such as bicycles and rocking horses and prevent their child from playing with these for about 2 weeks postoperatively. Play with siblings and others will need to be supervised for a week or two, but this should not prevent the toddler or preschool child returning to playgroup after a week or so provided the staff are aware of the recent surgery and are happy to provide the extra vigilance necessary. The child may find snug-fitting underpants more comfortable than boxer shorts as these provide more support.

6. *Stitches* There will be a small groin incision usually secured with dissolvable sutures subcutaneously and two or three Steri-Strips to the skin, and a couple of stitches on the underside of the scrotum; these do not require removal. The incisions are usually left uncovered and the Steri-Strips can be removed after about 5 days, by the child or parents.

7. *General hygiene* The groin and scrotal incisions should be observed and kept clean and dry for a couple of days after which the child can start bathing again. If there is any swelling, increased local tenderness or discharge from the incisions the GP should be notified, as it may indicate an infection which requires antibiotic therapy.

Ward staff should liaise with the GP and/or the health visitor prior to the child's discharge and the parents should be aware of whom to contact should any problems arise – day or night.

The child who has undergone a laparotomy and orchidopexy will need to stay in hospital for a longer period – generally 5–7 days – if there has been significant handling of the bowel whilst locating the testis. The general principles surrounding any patient following abdominal surgery will apply.

1. *Parenteral fluid administration to maintain adequate hydration* A burette type administration set with safety valve and Luer lock should be utilised routinely for all paediatric patients to ensure accurate administration of small volumes of fluid, prevent accidental 'overloading', and reduce the risk of accidental disconnection.

2. *Wound drainage* (vacuum type) will be present, to prevent haematoma formation. This is removed, according to the surgeon's instructions, when there has been no drainage for 12–24 hours – generally by day 3.

3. *Nasogastric decompression* may be utilised, although the routine use of nasogastric tubes following abdominal surgery is being questioned and reassessed. In the author's experience children tend to find the nasogastric tube the most uncomfortable 'accessory' and are always more cheerful following its removal; however, inserting a nasogastric tube in an alert, postoperative child is an unpleasant procedure requiring all the skills of persuasion, patience and dexterity which the paediatric nurse possesses and the advantages/disadvantages must be assessed very carefully.

All cannulae and tubing should be firmly secured to the patient's skin. If the child is old enough to understand, the need for each item should be explained, using appropriate language and diagrams, as this helps the child to tolerate them. The use of restraints to prevent 'fiddling' and dislodgement (either accidental or intentional) is discouraged; divertional therapy is recommended.

Early mobilization is encouraged to reduce the risk of complications.

Prior to discharge, the child should be given a date and time to attend the outpatient clinic 6–12 weeks after the operation.

Testicular Torsion

Torsion of the testis is caused by twisting of the spermatic cord and blood vessels. It is not an uncommon condition and may occur in childhood at any age, most often around puberty (Blandy and Moors, 1989). The testis will only be viable for 6–8 hours if its blood supply is impaired, therefore this is considered a surgical emergency. The surgeon may attempt to untwist the torsion manually after prescribing a strong analgesic (such as pethidine). The nurse should stay with the child following administration of the injection and help to calm, distract and reassure him. Surgical exploration is essential even if the attempt is successful and the initial pain is relieved. If the diagnosis is confirmed the opposite testicle must be explored as the same underlying condition which allowed the torsion to occur initially is often present.

Nursing care follows that described for the child undergoing orchidopexy.

Hydrocele

The normal space around the testicle contains a trace of fluid which allows it to move within the scrotum and helps protect it against minor injury. This fluid increases in certain conditions: lack of fusion of the processus vaginalis, obstructed testicular lymphatic drainage, testicular disease and malignancy. Most hydroceles are idiopathic.

Treatment initially consists of 'tapping' the hydrocele – aspirating the fluid using a small plastic cannula. This is a minor procedure and can be done on an out-patient basis with the child sedated. If the fluid collection recurs quickly, the child will need a small operation to close the processus vaginalis or treatment of the underlying cause.

Testicular Tumours

Malignant testicular tumours account for not more than 1 per cent of all solid tumours in infancy and childhood. Table 13.2 is a simplified classification of

Table 13.2 Classification of testicular tumours

Classification	Incidence	Treatment
Tumours of germ cell origin		
Embryonal carcinoma	Most common testicular tumour in infancy and childhood (approximately 50%) and usually confined to the age group up to 4 years. Metastases develop readily (approximately 30%)	Orchidopexy and bilateral retroperitoneal lymph node dissection; prophylactic chemotherapy is controversial though generally recommended only in patients with metastases. Three out of ten children die from metastases, usually within 2 years of surgery
Seminoma	Found only in older boys and comprises less than 5% of the testicular neoplasms in this age group; up to 10% of this group have metastases when diagnosed	Orchidectomy followed by irradiation of the para-aortic and iliac area; chemotherapy recommended only when metastases are present; mortality about 10%
Teratoma	Accounts for approximately 30% of testicular tumours in children. Majority of patients are under 4 years old. The tumour may be congenital and metastases are rare	Orchidectomy; retroperitoneal lymph node dissection and postoperative chemotherapy are less indicated in the paediatric as opposed to the older age group
Mixed germ cell tumours		
Tumours derived from specialised gonadal stroma	Relatively frequent (20% of all testicular tumours). Metastases are extremely rare	Orchidectomy
Rare or unclassified testicular tumours		
Metastatic (secondary) testicular tumours	There is a higher incidence of secondary tumours in children than in adults	Orchidectomy and bilateral retroperitoneal lymph node dissection, irradiation and chemotherapy

testicular tumours found in children based on Mostofi's (WHO) classification, the incidence and recommended treatment. There is no way to distinguish benign testicular tumours from malignant ones by clinical investigation. Biopsy is contraindicated because of the danger of tumour spillage and consequently these patients should be prepared for orchidectomy – the excision of the testis, vas and vascular pedicle. If there is any evidence of lymphatic spread of the tumour a radical retroperitoneal lymphadenectomy will also be performed. The preoperative investigations may include ultrasound and CT scanning, urography, lymphography, chest X-ray and the collection of serum for measurement of tumour markers and hormonal status.

The focus of nursing care revolves around providing psychological and emotional support during this very difficult period as well as physical preparation and care of the child. The nurse should explain the investigations, in language the child understands, and be available to assist as necessary. Some of the investigations are unpleasant and time consuming, so the child might require sedation. The dye used in some of the radiological investigations may stain the skin and the urine. This resolves spontaneously after a few days but the child and family should be forewarned.

Chemotherapy is unpleasant and the preferred regimen of drugs is subject to frequent change and consequently should always be used under the direct supervision of a well-trained, specialist team. The side-effects include bone marrow suppression, loss of hair and severe vomiting, though the last can be controlled by drugs.

Testicular cancer today can nearly always be cured and knowing this can be of enormous help to children and families in providing the encouragement they need in the months of treatment that may be necessary.

References

Birmingham Reflux Study Group (1983) Prospective trial of operative versus non-operative treatment of severe vesicoureteric reflux: two years observation in 96 children. *British Medical Journal* **287**: 171–174.

Blandy JP and Moors J (1989) *Urology for Nurses*. London: Blackwell Scientific Publications.

Cohen SJ (1977) The Cohen reimplantation technique. *Birth Defects* **13**: 391–395.

O'Donnell B and Puri P (1986) Endoscopic correction of primary vesicoureteric reflux: results in 94 ureters. British Medical Journal **293**: 1404–1406.

Mostofi FK and Price EB (1983) *Tumors of the Male Genital System*. Washington, DC: Armed Forces Institute of Pathology.

Politano VA and Leadbetter WF (1958) An operative technique for the correction of vesicoureteric reflux. *Journal of Urology*. **79**: 932–941.

Bibliography

Abernathy E (1987) Biological response modifiers. *American Journal of Nursing* **87**: 458–459.

Armstrong CN and Walton T (1990) Transsexuals and the Law. *New Law Journal* **140**: 1384–1390.

Association of Continence Advisors (1988) *Directory of Continence and Toiletting Aids.* London: Association of Continence Advisors.

Badenoch D (1987) *Aids to Urology.* Edinburgh: Churchill Livingstone.

Birch BRP and Miller RA (1989) Percutaneous nephrolithotomy. *Surgery* **70**: 1680–1683.

Blandy J (1984) *Lecture Notes on Urology,* 3rd edn. London: Blackwell Scientific Publications.

Blandy JP (1986) *Operative Urology* 2nd edn. Oxford: Blackwell Scientific Publications.

Blandy JP (1991) *Lecture Notes on Urology,* 4th edn. London: Blackwell Scientific Publications.

Blandy JP and Moors J (1989) *Urology for Nurses,* 3rd edn. London: Blackwell Scientific Publications.

Boyd SD, Feinberg SM and Skinner DG (1987) Quality of life survey of urinary diversion patients. *Journal of Urology* **138**: 1386–1389.

Brundage D (1991) *Renal Disorders,* St Louis: CV Mosby and Co.

Bullock N, Sibley G and Whitaker R (1989) *Essential Urology.* London: Churchill Livingstone.

Canning DA, Perman JA and Jeffs RD (1989) Nutritional consequences of bowel segments in the lower urinary tract. *Journal of Urology* **142**: 509–511.

Chaple C and Christmas T (1990) *Urodynamics Made Easy.* Edinburgh: Churchill Livingstone.

Charig CR, Webb DR, Payne SR et al (1987) Comparison of treatment of renal calculi by open surgery, percutaneous nephrolithotomy and extra-corporeal lithotripsy. *British Medical Journal* **292**: 879–883.

Coe FL et al (1988) Pathophysiology of kidney stones and strategies for management. *Hospital Practice* **23**(3): 185–189; 193–195.

Cumming J, Worth PHL and Woodhouse CRJ (1989) The choice of suprapubic continent catheterisable urinary stoma. *British Journal of Urology* **60**: 227–230.

Das G, Dick J, Bailey MJ et al (1987) Extracorporeal shock-wave lithotripsy: The first 1000 cases at the London Stone Clinic. *British Medical Journal* **295**: 891–893.

Dowdell P (1983) Nursing care study: Sex change operation. *Nursing Mirror* **156**(27): 46–51.

Ducket JW and Snyder H (1985) Use of the Mitrofanoff principle in urinary reconstruction. *World Journal of Urology* **3**: 191–193.

Ducket JW and Snyder MC (1986) Continent urinary diversion: variations on the Mitrofanoff principle *Journal of Urology* **136**: 58–62.

Edwards Hood L (1987) Interferon: getting in the way of viruses and tumours. *American Journal of Nursing* **87**(4): 459–463.

Franks LM and Teich NM (eds) (1990) *Introduction to the Cellular and Molecular Biology of Cancer,* 2nd edn. New York: Oxford Medical Publications.

Gabriel R (1985) *Postgraduate Nephrology,* 3rd edn. London: Butterworth Heinemann.

Hinchliff SM and Montague SE (1988) *Physiology for Nursing Practice.* London: Baillière Tindall.

James J (1984) *Handbook of Urology.* London: Harper and Row.

James J (1984) *Handbook of Urology.* London: Lippincott Nursing Series.

Jeter K, Fallo N and Norton C (1990) *Nursing for Continence.* Philadelphia: WB Saunders.

Kaisary AV (1991) BCG Treatment for superficial bladder tumours. In: *Recent Advances in Urology/Andrology*, Hendry WF (ed). Edinburgh: Churchill Livingstone.

Kellett MJ, Wickham JEA and Russell RCG (1988) Percutaneous cholecystectomy. *British Medical Journal* **296**: 454–455.

Lasater S (1990) Testicular cancer – a peri-operative challenge. *AORN Journal* **51**: 513–519.

Lavin M (1987) Mutilation, deception and sex changes. *Journal of Medical Ethics* **13**: 86–91.

Lerner J and Khan Z (1982) *Mosby's Manual of Urological Nursing*. St Louis: CV Mosby and Co.

Lothstein LM (1983) *Female-to-male Transsexualism: Historical, Clinical and Theoretical Issues*. London: Routledge and Kegan Paul.

McCabe SV (1988) Male-to-female transsexualism: a case for holistic nursing. *Archives of Psychiatric Nursing* **2**(1): 48–53.

Milroy E (1991) Urethral stenting for stricture. In: *Recent Advances in Urology/Andrology*, Hendry WF (ed). Edinburgh: Churchill Livingstone.

Mundy AR (ed) (1988) *Current Operative Surgery: Urology*. London: Baillière Tindall.

Price B (1986) The range of factors affecting body image. *Nursing Times* **82**(39): 30–32.

Rees M (1993) He, she or it? *Nursing Times* **89**(10): 48–49.

Ross JRW and Wilson KTW (1990) *Anatomy and Physiology*, 7th edn. London: Churchill Livingstone.

Scott R (1982) *Urology Illustrated*. Edinburgh: Churchill Livingstone.

Scott R and Russell L (1983) *Urology Illustrated*, 2nd edn. London: Churchill Livingstone.

Snell RS (1988) *Clinical Anatomy for Medical Students*, 3rd edn. London: Churchill Livingstone.

Stanford JR (1987) Testicular self-examination: Teaching and practice by nurses. *Journal of Advanced Nursing* **12**: 13.

Stevens M (1989) Screening urines for bacteriuria. *Journal of Medical Laboratory Sciences* **46**: 194–206.

Sturdy DE (1986) *An Outline of Urology*. Bristol: J. Wright.

Tanagho EA and McAninch JW (eds) (1992) *Smith's General Urology*, 12th edn. London: Prentice Hall International.

Thompson FD and Woodhouse CRJ (1986) *Disorders of the Kidney and Urinary Tract*. Edinburgh: Churchill Livingstone.

Thompson FD and Woodhouse CRJ (1987) *Physiological Principles in Medical Science. Disorders of the Kidney and Urinary Tract*. London: Edward Arnold.

Uldall R (1977) *Renal Nursing*. London: Blackwell Scientific Publications.

Walters W and Ross M (eds) (1986) *Transsexualism and Sex Reassignment*. Oxford: Oxford University Press.

Watson JE (1990) *Medical–Surgical Nursing and Related Physiology*, 3rd edn. Philadelphia: WB Saunders.

Watson GM and Wickham JEA (1989) The development of a laser and a miniaturised ureteroscope system for ureteric stone management. *World Journal of Urology* **7**: 147–150.

Wickham JEA (1982) *Recent Advances in Surgery: The Management of Renal Calculus Disease*. Edinburgh: Churchill Livingstone.

Wickham JEA and Buck AC (1990) *Renal Tract Stones: Metabolic Basis and Clinical Practice*, 633–639. Edinburgh: Churchill Livingstone.

Wickham JEA and Miller RA (1983) *Percutaneous Renal Surgery*. Edinburgh: Churchill Livingstone.

Woodcock J, Watkinson C, Taber S and Dick J (1988) Smashing the stones. *Nursing Times* **84**(33): 40–43.

Woodhouse CRJ (1991) The Mitrofanoff principle for continent diversions. *WCET Journal* **11**: 12–15.

Yates A (1987) Sexual healing. *Nursing Times* **83**(32): 29–30.

Index